INTRODUCTION TO OCCUPATIONAL HEALTH IN PUBLIC HEALTH PRACTICE

INTRODUCTION TO OCCUPATIONAL HEALTH IN PUBLIC HEALTH PRACTICE

BERNARD J. HEALEY
KENNETH T. WALKER

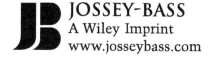

JOSSEY-BASS
A Wiley Imprint
www.josseybass.com

Published by Jossey-Bass
A Wiley Imprint
989 Market Street, San Francisco, CA 94103-1741—www.josseybass.com

Readers should be aware that Internet Web sites offered as citations and/or sources for further information may have changed or disappeared between the time this was written and when it is read.

Jossey-Bass books and products are available through most bookstores. To contact Jossey-Bass directly call our Customer Care Department within the U.S. at 800-956-7739, outside the U.S. at 317-572-3986, or fax 317-572-4002.

Jossey-Bass also publishes its books in a variety of electronic formats. Some content that appears in print may not be available in electronic books.

Library of Congress Cataloging-in-Publication Data

Healey, Bernard J., date.
  Introduction to occupational health in public health practice/Bernard J. Healey, Kenneth T. Walker.—1st ed.
    p.cm.
Includes bibliographical references and index.
ISBN 978–0–470–44768–0 (pbk.)
1. Industrial hygiene. 2. Public health. I. Walker, Kenneth T., date. II. Title.
RC967.H414 2009
363.110973—dc22
                                                        2009021651

FIRST EDITION
PB Printing   10 9 8 7 6 5 4 3 2

CONTENTS

PART THREE
PUBLIC HEALTH ISSUES IN OCCUPATIONAL SAFETY AND HEALTH

PART FOUR
EVALUATION AND LEADERSHIP ISSUES IN PREVENTION

FIGURES, TABLES, AND EXHIBITS

FIGURES

TABLES

EXHIBITS

INTRODUCTION

In the United States the workplace can be hazardous to one's health through injuries and disease. Although the average worker spends more than forty hours every week in the workplace, many workers are unaware of the potential dangers present in their home away from home.

When young men or women begin their first job, usually at a young age, they are not aware that they have entered a world of potential health problems. This can be a very dangerous period in their lives because they are now exposed both to the possibility of workplace injuries and to the possibility of developing chronic diseases later in life from health behaviors developed or supported in the workplace environment.

According to the Bureau of Labor Statistics (2007), a worker is injured every five seconds and every ten seconds a worker is temporarily or permanently disabled. Individuals usually spend a majority of their lives in the places where they work, and these years in the workplace are the same years when they may be incubating chronic diseases or experiencing serious injuries that often cause disabilities and poor health later in life.

HEALTH IN AMERICA

Length of life has definitely improved in the United States since the early 1900s, and most people can expect to live well into their eighth decade of life. The majority of this increase in life expectancy can be directly attributed to the many public health accomplishments made possible by dedicated workers in the field of public health in this country. The reduction in tobacco use, better nutrition, more physical activity, proper immunizations, and effective health education programs are just a few of the initiatives developed and implemented by public health departments during the past hundred years. Unfortunately, too many Americans still experience premature death, disability, or poor quality of life.

The *healthy people* concept, which was introduced by the U.S. Surgeon General's Office a few decades ago, has helped us continue our progress in helping Americans to achieve good health for themselves and their family members. The most recent report, *Healthy People 2010* (U.S. Department of Health and Human Services, 2000), has established even more aggressive but achievable goals and objectives to improve the health of all Americans.

It is now time to expand this public health success story to the workplace. There is a captive audience in the workplace who want to be healthier and an employer who wants to keep employees healthy and productive. All that is required is leadership to make the workplace a healthy place to earn a living and experience healthy aging.

WORKPLACE HEALTH

Twenty years ago injury was a leading cause of death in the United States, with 143,000 fatalities in 1983. Today over four hundred deaths a day result from injuries, including injuries happening in the workplace. Injuries are the second leading cause of death in this country before the age of seventy-five. The large numbers of injuries that occur on a daily basis lend themselves very well to a public health model of prevention. According to Finkelstein, Corso, and Miller (2006), an injured worker misses an average of 11.1 days of work and the productivity losses associated with the injury are the value of the goods never produced because of the injury.

Chronic diseases—such as heart disease, cancer, and diabetes—are the leading causes of death and disability in the United States. As the burden of chronic diseases in the United States increases, greater efforts will be made to identify and implement interventions that successfully reduce disease risk, especially in the workplace. These diseases account for seven of every ten deaths and affect the quality of life of ninety million Americans. Although chronic diseases are among the most common and costly health problems, they are also among the most preventable. McGinnis and Foege (1993) point out that daily habits such as smoking, inactivity, eating a poor diet, and using alcohol and their consequences contribute to the development of virtually all morbidity and mortality in industrial nations. Adopting healthy behaviors such as eating nutritious foods, being physically active, and avoiding tobacco use can prevent or control the devastating effects of these diseases.

Employers are becoming more interested in dealing with the economic losses suffered each year as a result of injuries and illness suffered in the workplace. These losses include higher health insurance costs for the employer and loss of employee productivity. Employers are faced with a real need to reduce costs associated with producing a product and the need to have healthy employees who come to work rather than using sick leave to tend to illness and injuries that may have been acquired in the workplace.

GOVERNMENT INVOLVEMENT

The federal government became deeply involved in occupational safety and health after the passage of the Occupational Safety and Health Act in 1970. This act created the Occupational Safety and Health Administration (OSHA) and the National Institute for Occupational Safety and Health (NIOSH) to protect American workers from dangers to their health in the workplace.

OSHA is housed in the Department of Labor; it is responsible for creating standards and using those standards to protect the American worker from injury, illness, and death in the workplace. NIOSH is headquartered at the Centers for Disease Control and Prevention, because of its investigative role. It is the research component of the Occupational Safety and Health Act and through the use of the science of epidemiology has helped to discover the causes of injury and disease in the workplace. Through the use of public health expertise, researchers are then able to develop programs to reduce or eliminate workplace injuries and disease.

Despite the success of OSHA and NIOSH over the last few decades, there are still those who dislike any form of business regulation. The conservative governance of the last several years in this country has cut OSHA and NIOSH budgets, experimented with reorganizations and taken away some of these agencies' power, and even tried to abolish these agencies.

There could be a leadership role for OSHA and NIOSH in bringing together partnerships between the businesses they regulate and public health agencies. Such collaborations will be necessary if we are to improve the overall health status of the American worker. In order to make a difference in workers' health we have to go beyond the talent and resources found in any one agency. Because there is a very large difference between what is known about injury and illness prevention in the workplace and what is actually being done to prevent these important health problems, we can accomplish a great deal through collaboration among multiple stakeholders.

PUBLIC HEALTH OPPORTUNITIES

Public health efforts in this country are carried out by numerous agencies with a mandate to improve the health of the population. These agencies have produced remarkable success stories on very limited budgets. In addition they are receiving more new challenges to deal with, including bioterrorism preparedness, emerging infections, the AIDS pandemic, and now avian and swine influenza.

Moreover, in recent years public health agencies have shifted their focus from communicable diseases to the behaviorally caused chronic diseases. These diseases have a very long incubation period and cannot be cured, only treated or prevented from ever starting. Even though chronic diseases and injury prevention programs have high costs at the start, they do very well when cost-benefit analysis is applied to the outcomes associated with them.

The public health success with identifying the causes of chronic diseases needs to be expanded into an effort of preventing the occurrence of these diseases or at the very least postponing their complications until later in life. This knowledge should be of great value to corporate America in reducing chronic and noncommunicable disease costs. Public health has a tremendous opportunity to help businesses reduce the costs of health insurance and keep their employees healthy and productive. The return to the public health field could be the availability of resources from businesses and a captive audience of employees who are practicing prevention techniques and whose results can be documented.

ROLE OF PREVENTION

The Institute of Medicine report titled *The Future of the Public's Health in the 21st Century* (2003) recommends that the corporate community and public health agencies work together to strengthen health promotion and disease prevention programs for employees and their communities. The results of the Framingham study (discussed in Chapter One) have given us guidance for reducing the incidence and damage caused by chronic diseases such as cancer, diabetes, heart disease, and arthritis among all members of society. The answers produced in the Framingham study need to be given to employers to help them develop programs to prevent chronic disease occurrences in the workplace.

This book was written to discuss the many health problems facing the American worker as he or she ages in the workplace. The authors' premise is that a number of these health problems can be prevented if public health skills are applied in the workplace. The opportunity to eliminate or reduce injuries and many illnesses in the workplace is within reach of employers, employees, and public health officials. Now is the time to learn about this wonderful opportunity that has presented itself and to do the right things to make the workplace safe and healthy.

This book begins with a discussion of the history of public health in the United States, paying particular attention to the many successes of public health programs in the last century. This leads to a discussion concerning the need for public health expertise to understand and reduce occupational illness and injury occurrences. The reader is also introduced to the many uses of epidemiology in developing injury and illness surveillance systems that can help all concerned to better define occupational health problems.

A discussion of occupational safety and health history and the importance in protecting workers from morbidity and mortality follows, and a discussion of OSHA and NIOSH helps the reader understand the various problems faced by workers as they earn a living. Special attention is given to the types of injuries and illnesses that occur in the workplace and the role of legislation in reducing these occurrences.

The text then moves to a discussion of specific public health problems and their potential solutions, paying particular attention to public health prevention strategies for the workplace. The topics in this section of the book include workplace stress, drug and alcohol abuse, worker exposure to toxins, workplace wellness programs, and emergency planning and bioterrorism in the workplace. This book also looks at ergonomics, communicable diseases, vision and hearing problems, and health disparities as they affect the employer and employee. Additional topics include the economics of public health prevention activities in the workplace, the need for program evaluation, and a discussion of leadership and partnerships in keeping the American worker safe, healthy, and productive.

ACKNOWLEDGMENTS

We would like to begin by acknowledging the dedicated people who work in public health and who, despite limited resources, have accomplished so much in making the United States a better place to lead a healthy life. This is really a book about their success stories and their attempt to bring the healthy people concept to the places where people work to earn a living. Once you are bitten by the bug of serving others by making the world a safer place to live, you can never stop being a public health person.

During the process of writing this book we met many dedicated people who demanded professionalism in everything they tried to accomplish. One such person was John P. Sestito, surveillance program coordinator in the Division of Surveillance, Hazard Evaluations and Field Studies, National Institute for Occupational Safety and Health. He was there to help Bernard Healey with the chapter on injuries in the workplace. He shared his work and went out of his way to make this chapter the best that it could be.

Four more individuals to whom we are truly indebted helped us with the writing of particular chapters. They are Bridget McKenney Costello, Alison Healey, Kristin Joseph, and Jason R. Smith. Their biographies appear in the next section.

During the entire research and writing of this book we were surrounded by intelligent, caring individuals who cared only about making our ideas better. We are very fortunate individuals to have the opportunity to write a book for a national publisher but equally fortunate to have been able to work with such talent.

THE AUTHORS

Bernard J. Healey is professor of health care administration and director of the graduate program in health care administration at King's College in Wilkes-Barre, Pennsylvania. He began his career in 1971, as an epidemiologist for the Pennsylvania Department of Health, retiring from that position in 1995. He has been teaching undergraduate and graduate courses in business, public health, and health care administration at several colleges for more than thirty years. During his tenure with government, he completed advanced degrees in business administration and public administration. In 1990, he earned a PhD degree at the University of Pennsylvania.

Kenneth T. Walker is a certified safety professional operating his own safety consulting company in Tunkhannock, Pennsylvania. He is retired from the position of industrial hygiene and safety and emergency response manager for Procter & Gamble Paper Products Company in Mehoopany, Pennsylvania. He has received advanced training in ergonomics, electrical safety for general industry, and construction safety and has completed numerous courses at National Safety Council Congress and Exposition sessions and American Society of Safety Engineers Professional Development Conferences. He is also a retired U.S. Army captain. He holds an MS degree from the University of Scranton.

THE CONTRIBUTORS

Bridget McKenney Costello is assistant professor of sociology at King's College, where she teaches courses in social problems, gender, and culture. She earned her PhD degree in sociology from the University of Pennsylvania, concentrating in social inequality and cultural consumption. Her scholarly works have investigated trends in school redistricting since Brown *v.* Board of Education, the changing occupational health profile of women, trends and correlates of pseudoscientific belief, the gendered reception of mainstream and alternative scientific information, and the educational trajectories of disadvantaged students, including the aspirations and outcomes for low-income mothers. Currently, she is launching a study of cultural influences on individual health practices.

Alison Healey has managed the New York City bureau of an international financial magazine for Thomson Financial, has written and edited copy for a biweekly magazine and daily electronic news updates, and has also written and edited news stories and feature articles for this publication and its supplements, as well as comprehensive sector-specific management reports. She covered North American project finance activity, including but not limited to energy and infrastructure sectors. She is currently employed by Northeast Counseling conducting crisis assessments of children and adolescents in Northeast Counseling offices and emergency rooms. She determines the lethality of crisis patients and consults with on-call psychiatrists. She also conducts psychosocial assessments and links new patients to outpatient medication and therapy services. In addition, she teaches abnormal psychology, general psychology, and stress and coping at Marywood University, in Dunmore, Pennsylvania. She earned her MA degree in clinical/counseling psychology from Fairleigh Dickinson University and her MA degree in journalism from Temple University.

Kristin Joseph is a registered and licensed dietitian with more than ten years of experience in the field of nutrition. She has counseled individuals and groups on improving their eating and lifestyle habits and has conducted more than three hundred print, TV, and radio interviews on topics such as weight management, child and adolescent nutrition, school nutrition, and nutrition for disease prevention. She has also worked as a newspaper correspondent covering health and nutrition topics. She earned her BS degree at Indiana University of Pennsylvania and completed a postgraduate internship at Texas Woman's University in Houston, where she also earned an MS degree in nutrition. Experienced in the areas of clinical practice, community nutrition, and nutrition education, she acts as a resource to health professionals, consumer leaders, the media, and employee wellness programs.

Jason R. Smith is an optometrist in private practice at Forty Fort Eye Associates in Forty Fort, Pennsylvania, and the founder of Home Eye Care, which provides eye care to homebound and nursing home patients. He is currently the staff optometrist at fifteen nursing homes in Luzerne County. He is a 1993 graduate of the New England College of Optometry in Boston, and in 1999 he received an MS degree in health care administration from King's College in Wilkes-Barre, Pennsylvania. He is the first and only optometrist to receive this degree from King's College.

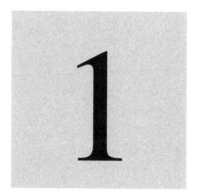

1

PUBLIC HEALTH PREVENTION FOCUS

CHAPTER

1

HISTORY AND IMPORTANCE OF PUBLIC HEALTH

After reading this chapter, you should be able to

- Understand the use of the skills of public health in the prevention of workplace illness and injuries.

- Understand what public health departments do and how they accomplish their goals.

- Discuss the advantages of partnerships between workplaces and public health departments.

- Explain the evolution of public health responsibilities in the United States.

It is difficult for most people to understand what public health does because they very rarely if ever have to deal with a public health department. Public health agencies become visible only when a health problem receives extensive media coverage. Yet the work that has been completed by public health over the last century is one of the main reasons for the long life expectancy of most Americans.

One way to understand public health is to compare a physician and a public health professional. The physician is most concerned with the health of his or her individual patient whereas the public health professional is concerned with the health of the community. More broadly, the medical care system in our country focuses attention and resources on the individual and the cure of disease whereas the public health system is concerned with the population and the prevention of disease.

Shi and Singh (2008) point out that many people believe that public health is nothing more than a massive welfare system. The agency responsible for the good health of Americans is not a welfare program but a separate agency of government that is supplemented by many nonprofit public health agencies. Every organization should have an interest in the important programs that protect and promote the health of all citizens. It is unfortunate that most people do not come to really understand public health until there is an emergency and that they forget about public health after the emergency ends.

Schneider (2006) believes that public health is concerned with the prevention of disease and the promotion of health. This definition places public health in the area of primary care. McKenzie, Pinger, and Kotecki (2005) argue that public health involves governmental actions to promote, protect, and preserve the health of a population. However, public health activities are also performed by nongovernmental agencies. The perception of public health agencies as responders to health emergencies prevents even health policy experts from understanding the contribution that could be made by public health departments in solving the current health care problems in this country. These departments do many things that prevent disease but that are never publicized and therefore are not known by the average person.

The public health system is always working at making good health available for all individuals. It is usually seen as a silent component of health services, one that demands few resources and still produces immense value for all of our citizens in terms of better health for all. This system employs some of the most dedicated health professionals to be found in any part of this country's health care system. These individuals have special skills that could be extremely useful in helping employers keep their workforces healthy and free from disease and injury.

A BRIEF HISTORY OF U.S. PUBLIC HEALTH

As just described, the valuable contribution made by public health professionals year after year is largely taken for granted. People think of public health and public health departments only when an emergency threatens their health and they need guidance and answers from public health officials and the various governmental agencies that they represent. Problems like E. coli in our food supply, anthrax in the mail, contaminated water, or drug-resistant tuberculosis bring public health to the forefront until the crisis subsides, and then public health departments seem to disappear until we need their help again.

Many definitions of public health point to a science dedicated to the improvement of the health of everyone. In 1926, Winston defined public health as "the science and art of preventing disease, prolonging life and promoting health through the organized efforts and informed choices of society, organizations, public and private, communities and individuals." McKenzie et al. (2005) define public health as the health status of the population, including governmental action to promote, protect, and preserve people's health. Novick, Morrow, and Mays (2008) define public health as "organized efforts to improve the health of communities." Vetter and Matthews (1999) argue that public health is "the process of promoting health, preventing disease, prolonging life and improving the quality of life through the organized efforts of society." And Turnock (2009) points out that public health represents a collective effort to deal with unacceptable realities that usually result in poor life outcomes that could have been prevented.

These various definitions of public health also offer a vision of **population-based medicine** rather than medical care centered around a specific individual. They emphasize prevention of health problems rather than a cure for health problems. If fully employed, the principles of public health could provide an answer to many of the problems that plague our current medical care delivery system. There also seems to be a major role for public health involvement in workplace health and safety issues.

Awofeso (2004) identifies six major approaches to public health that have been taken over the centuries:

- Public health as health protection (antiquity to 1830s)

- Public health as sanitary movement (miasma control) (1840s to 1870s)

- Public health as contagion control (1880s to 1930s)

- Public health as preventive medicine (1940s to 1960s)

- Public health as primary health care (1970s to 1980s)

- The "new public health"—health promotion (1990s to present)

These approaches offer a number of insights into the history of public health in the United States. There has been an emphasis on control of disease, regulation of some parts of the health care system, and more recently a stronger role in the development and implementation of prevention programs. The word *control* is frequently heard when describing the historical development of public health: control of disease, control of the free movement of people (quarantine), and control of certain high-risk behaviors.

Public health departments in the late 1800s and early 1900s became very successful at controlling the spread of diseases but were not so good at preventing these diseases from occurring in the first place. This changed with the development of vaccines that virtually eliminated childhood illnesses. In addition, the discovery of penicillin allowed public health departments to cure many sexually transmitted diseases in special clinics that concentrated on the control of venereal diseases. Public health professionals were trained to interview those infected with venereal diseases, find their sexual contacts, and bring them to treatment. This strategy resulted in a reduction in these diseases until public health resources were reduced through budget cuts.

It has taken a long time for the emphasis to begin to shift from the word *control* to a new word, *prevention.* Public health departments are now assuming greater roles in prevention that entail keeping people healthy and free from disease. Unfortunately, up to this time, limited budgets never allowed these departments to truly prevent anything except through the use of vaccines.

Nevertheless, from these earlier approaches came a number of very effective public health programs that saved lives, reduced morbidity, and added several years to the average life span of most Americans. In antiquity, in the very early years of the development of public health, people believed that disease was somehow caused by supernatural forces and therefore that epidemics were a punishment by god or other spiritual forces. When epidemics of plague, leprosy, cholera, and the like occurred, it was thought very little could be done about these outbreaks, some of which had mortality rates greater than 30 percent of the population.

Miasma control, an approach beginning in the 1830s, was usually the result of industrialism and urbanization that allowed public health conditions to worsen. The United States and other countries moved from farming to manufacturing, and people moved from farms to cities. People working and living closer together provided an environment for disease to develop and spread rapidly from person to person. According to McKenzie et al. (2005), the major theory of disease at this time was that vapors or miasmas were the cause of many diseases and that these diseases, resulting from a filthy environment, could be eliminated only by cleaning and other environmental precautions. A famous report by Edwin Chadwick, titled *Report on an Inquiry into the Sanitary Condition of the Labouring Population of Great Britain*, documented the influence of filthy conditions on the occurrence of disease.

Lemuel Shattuck's 1850 *Report of the Sanitary Commission of Massachusetts* was one starting point for the development of public health in the United States. This report called for the development of public health departments that would have the responsibility for handling the public health concerns of the population of a locality or state. This report was a response to the need to have the authority to deal with infectious diseases and environmental problems, and it focused on state and local responsibility to deal with these issues.

The next era of public health involved the germ theory of disease, first proposed by Louis Pasteur in 1862. Discoveries in this era revealed the identity of such bacterial diseases as typhoid fever, leprosy, tuberculosis, cholera, diphtheria, and tetanus. This era also saw the founding of the American Public Health Association, the start of local public health departments, and the pasteurization of milk. It was now known that many diseases were caused by microbes and that the spread of disease could be controlled through public health activities. As the public health departments were established, they were given the goal of protecting the health of the community. In order to accomplish this goal these departments were granted powers to enforce public health laws and regulations. These powers included quarantine, isolation, immunization, and investigative powers.

Public health was now ready to move to the next stage of development, which involved the effort to prevent communicable diseases and to focus that prevention on high-risk groups. The discovery of penicillin gave physicians a weapon that could be used to cure many communicable diseases. The development of vaccines allowed the virtual elimination of many childhood diseases. Public health departments became very good at organizing and implementing mass immunization campaigns, which were credited with preventing enormous morbidity and mortality from communicable diseases.

The science of epidemiology was also developing. In 1849, John Snow, a London physician, had used epidemiological techniques to discover the cause of the spread of cholera in a particular city district. Having previously studied the transmission of cholera through contaminated water, Snow surveyed households of cholera victims and traced their water supply to the Broad Street well, one of three wells being used in that area. Once the suspect well was closed at his urging, the outbreak ended.

A study conducted by Doll and Hill in the 1950s implicated the use of tobacco in causing a form of cancer rarer at that time than now, lung cancer. This study paved the way for additional chronic disease studies that linked secondhand smoke to the same deadly form of cancer. Tobacco became identified as the leading cause of death for 430,000 Americans every year. Secondhand smoke was identified as a cause of over 80,000 additional deaths from lung cancer. After Doll and Hill's study, it seemed a natural follow-up to start using epidemiology to evaluate high-risk health behaviors as a potential cause of other chronic diseases. Epidemiology was now ready to deal with diseases involving very long incubation periods that had no visible starting point.

Epidemiology has been called the basic science of public health by people who work in the field of public health, and in fact most of the major accomplishments of public health are a direct result of exhaustive studies conducted by epidemiologists. Epidemiology focuses on human populations and has been used in the determination of the causes of many chronic diseases. This science relies heavily on the use of descriptive and analytical statistics to determine the major risk factors of disease (Schneider, 2006).

One of the most important studies ever conducted involved an epidemiological evaluation of chronic noninfectious diseases in Framingham, Massachusetts. This cohort study, begun in 1947, evaluated the relation of heart disease to factors that included high blood pressure, serum cholesterol, and cigarette smoking. Oppenheimer (2005) argues that this successful epidemiological study, which coined the term *risk factor*, was also able to uncover the causes of many other chronic diseases.

The **Framingham Heart Study** was instrumental in proving the value of involving a community in a collaborative effort designed to improve the health of that community. This was an important first step in the expansion of population-based medicine, which allowed a differentiation between the medical care system and public health departments. It also demonstrated that even when goals are different, there is real value in collaboration with others.

The next phase of public health development involved an interest in providing health care that was geared toward the community. This focus on primary care involved greater consideration of socioeconomic concepts and an evaluation of all of the determinants of good health. Public health started to move closer to the community through federal and state grants that encouraged the formation of **local health departments** with city or county health responsibilities. Public health at this time involved an increased focus on the prevention of diseases that were long term or chronic in their etiology. The country was gaining in its war against communicable diseases, and public health departments began to move resources to the control of the epidemic of noncommunicable chronic diseases. This effort began with a concentration on heart disease, stroke, and cancer. In recent years public health has also moved toward dealing with physical inactivity, diet, tobacco use, and obesity.

Public health entered the current **health promotion** era in 1979. Public health officials became convinced that population-based medicine would have a much better chance than individually focused medical care of solving the major problems found in the U.S. medical care delivery system. It also seemed obvious to some public health leaders that if we could keep individuals free of chronic diseases, we could reduce the costs of health care delivery and at the same time reduce the numbers of individuals who require access to health services. At this time prevention should have become the main focus of public health efforts, leaving the medical care delivery system to focus on cure. However, many public health professionals continued to support programs that focused on control of disease rather than on preventing disease. This failure to put the primary emphasis on prevention was a result of budget reductions and a bureaucratic structure that was unable to move beyond disease counseling and testing. A good example of this failure is found in the public health response to HIV in the early years of that disease. Public health agencies seemed to believe that counseling and testing of individuals could somehow prevent the HIV epidemic from growing. They were wrong.

HEALTHY PEOPLE 2010

Many people in the United States have long had an interest in the prevention of health problems. This interest is evident when we look at the strong support for the elimination of childhood diseases through the funding of vaccine development and distribution by public health departments. At the same time, there was also a long-term reluctance to move past the care of children and young adults with well-developed prevention programs.

Then, in 1979, the *healthy people* concept came into being, documented in a report titled *The Surgeon General's Report on Health Promotion and Disease Prevention*. This report was responsible for the start of a national discussion on the relationship of personal health behaviors to the development of many serious diseases and injuries, and the Healthy People program represents a change from the physician and hospital emphasis on the individual to the public health focus on the population. Healthy People program objectives were then outlined in a 1990 report. The latest report, *Healthy People 2010* (U.S. Department of Health and Human Services, 2000), establishes twenty-eight broad *focus areas* for the Healthy People program (see Table 1.1). These focus areas contain 467 target objectives for communities to use in the effort to improve the health status of their residents.

TABLE 1.1.   **Healthy People 2010 focus areas**

Access	Injury/Violence Prevention
Arthritis, Osteoporosis, Chronic Back Conditions	Maternal, Infant, Child Health
Cancer	Medical Product Safety
Chronic Kidney Disease	Mental Health and Mental Disorders
Diabetes	Nutrition and Overweight
Disability and Secondary Conditions	Occupational Safety and Health
Environmental Health	Oral Health
Educational and Community-Based Programs	Physical Activity and Fitness
Family Planning	Respiratory Diseases
Food Safety	Public Health Infrastructure
Health Communication	Sexually Transmitted Diseases
Heart Disease and Stroke	Substance Abuse (including alcohol)
HIV/AIDS	Tobacco Use
Immunization and Infectious Diseases	Vision and Hearing

Source: U.S. Department of Health and Human Services, 2000.

In giving concrete goals and objectives to communities, the Healthy People initiative helps these communities to increase collaboration and to build community agreement with and support of constant improvement toward a healthier community. The objectives are tracked and reported as moving in the right direction, moving in the wrong direction, showing no change, or being untrackable. This ongoing evaluation process allows public health agencies to measure results and attempt to change community-supported programs that are not working. It is not a perfect process, but for those interested in the health of the community it represents a step in the right direction.

One of the focus areas for improvement in *Healthy People 2010*, as shown in Table 1.1, is occupational safety and health. This section has very specific, measurable objectives that employers can apply to their place of employment and motivate employees to achieve (Table 1.2 shows the areas that these objectives address).

TABLE 1.2.   **Healthy People 2010: short titles of occupational safety and health objectives**

No.	Objective Short Title
20-1	Work-related injury deaths
20-2	Work-related injuries
20-3	Overexertion or repetitive motion
20-4	Pneumoconiosis deaths
20-5	Work-related homicides
20-6	Work-related assaults
20-7	Elevated blood lead levels from work exposure
20-8	Occupational skin diseases or disorders
20-9	Worksite stress-reduction programs
20-10	Needle stick injuries
20-11	Work-related, noise-induced hearing loss

Source: U.S. Department of Health and Human Services, 2000.

One issue that has long inhibited the accomplishment of workplace health and safety objectives has been uniting the players in the process and offering appropriate incentives to make collaboration happen. The interest is now present for the development of strong partnerships between employers and public health agencies for the improvement of the health of workers, which benefits everyone.

RESPONSIBILITIES OF PUBLIC HEALTH

The general consensus of those who work in public health is that the **core responsibilities of public health** include

- Assessing and monitoring of the health of the community in order to identify health problems and health priorities

- Developing public policies to solve identified local, state, and national health problems and health priorities

- Ensuring that all populations have access to appropriate and cost-effective care, including health promotion and disease prevention services, and evaluating the effectiveness of that care.

These responsibilities all entail prevention of disease and protection of the health of the population. They are carried out by a cadre of dedicated public health professionals working for federal, state, and local public health departments. Public health professionals' duties are usually defined in terms of minimum program requirements, and involve communicable disease control, laboratory services, health education, environmental health, epidemiology, maternal and child health services, public health nursing, and chronic disease control. (As we have noted, the word *control* does not support the development of public health efforts in prevention and indicates that there is still much to do in shifting the public health focus.)

PUBLIC HEALTH ACCOMPLISHMENTS

Public health departments have been key players in many of the great achievements of medical care over the last century. They had very little support in terms of staffing and financial resources, and they also had to be innovative within a very restrictive bureaucratic structure. Their success is a direct result of dedicated employees, a strong culture, and a desire to improve the health of the community. In addition, one of our public health departments' greatest strengths has always been the ability to partner with others in the reduction of diseases in the community. Exhibit 1.1 lists their major accomplishments.

These accomplishments that resulted from public health programs are very impressive, and they were made possible by the formation of partnerships involving community leaders, including leaders from the business community. It must also be revealed,

EXHIBIT 1.1.   **Ten great public health achievements—United States, 1900–1999**

Vaccination

Programs of population-wide vaccinations resulted in the eradication of smallpox; elimination of polio in the Americas; and control of measles, rubella, tetanus, diphtheria, Haemophilus influenza type b, and other infectious diseases in the United States and other parts of the world.

Motor-Vehicle Safety

Improvements in motor-vehicle safety have contributed to large reductions in motor vehicle–related deaths. These improvements include engineering efforts to make both vehicles and highways safer and successful efforts to change personal behavior (for example, increased use of safety belts, child safety seats, and motorcycle helmets and decreased drinking and driving).

Safer Workplaces

Work-related health problems, such as coal workers' pneumoconiosis (black lung), and silicosis—common at the beginning of the century—have been significantly reduced. Severe injuries and deaths related to mining, manufacturing, construction, and transportation also have decreased; since 1980, safer workplaces have resulted in a reduction of approximately 40% in the rate of fatal occupational injuries.

Control of Infectious Diseases

Control of infectious diseases has resulted from clean water and better sanitation. Infections such as typhoid and cholera, major causes of illness and death early in the 20th century, have been reduced dramatically by improved sanitation. In addition, the discovery of antimicrobial therapy has been critical to successful public health efforts to control infections such as tuberculosis and sexually transmitted diseases (STDs).

Decline in Deaths from Coronary Heart Disease and Stroke

Decline in deaths from coronary heart disease and stroke have resulted from risk-factor modification, such as smoking cessation and blood pressure control coupled with improved access to early detection and better treatment. Since 1972, death rates for coronary heart disease have decreased 51%.

Safer and Healthier Foods

Since 1900, safer and healthier foods have resulted from decreases in microbial contamination and increases in nutritional content. Identifying essential micronutrients and establishing food-fortification programs have almost eliminated major nutritional deficiency diseases such as rickets, goiter, and pellagra in the United States.

Healhier Mothers and Babies

Healthier mothers and babies are a result of better hygiene and nutrition, availability of anti-biotics, greater access to health care, and technological advances in maternal and neonatal medicine. Since 1900, infant mortality has decreased 90%, and maternal mortality has decreased 99%.

Family Planning

Access to family planning and contraceptive services has altered social and economic roles of women. Family planning has provided health benefits such as smaller family size and longer interval between the birth of children; increased opportunities for preconception counseling and screening; fewer infant, child, and maternal deaths; and the use of barrier contraceptives to prevent pregnancy and transmission of human immunodeficiency virus and other STDs.

Fluoridation of Drinking Water

Fluoridation of drinking water began in 1945 and in 1999 reached an estimated 144 million persons in the United States. Fluoridation safely and inexpensively benefits both children and adults by effectively preventing tooth decay, regardless of socioeconomic status or access to care. Fluoridation has played an important role in the reductions in tooth decay (40%–70% in children) and of tooth loss in adults (40%–60%).

Recognition of Tobacco Use as a Health Hazard

Recognition of tobacco use as a health hazard in 1964 has resulted in changes in the pro-motion of cessation of use and reduction of exposure to environmental tobacco smoke. Since the initial surgeon general's report on the health risks of smoking, the prevalence of smoking among adults has decreased, and millions of smoking-related deaths have been prevented.

Source: Adapted from *Ten Great Public Health Achievements—United States, 1900–1999,* 1999.

however, that public health has had its share of failed programs. One of the most notable occurred in 1976 when the government's response to the reporting of one case of swine flu at Fort Dix, New Jersey, was perceived as a complete failure. A mass immunization program was instituted to protect the public from a potential epidemic, but the outbreak never materialized and the vaccinations resulted in several cases of Guillain-Barré syndrome that caused paralysis. Failures like this went a long way toward making people fear large public health interventions.

The third accomplishment listed has to do with the improvement of workplace safety, which can go a long way toward the improvement of community health.

Turnock (2009) points out that workplaces are safer today but more needs to be done to protect workers from disease and injuries. Public health departments are capable of using epidemiology and sophisticated surveillance systems to reduce injuries and develop disease screening and intervention programs. This can be accomplished only if businesses and public health work together in the reduction of illness and injuries in the workplace.

EMPHASIS ON PREVENTION NOT CONTROL

Public health is facing enormous challenges in this new century that range from communicable diseases and chronic diseases to bioterrorism. Public health departments are confronting the challenges of HIV, tuberculosis, influenza, diabetes, tobacco use, physical inactivity, and obesity. All these diseases and high-risk health behaviors have become epidemic and require the attention of public health agencies and the expansion of prevention programs. Control of disease has long been key to the function of public health programs. An example of this philosophy is found in the way public health departments approach their responsibilities concerning communicable diseases. Public health professionals assigned to work in communicable disease programs are trained in investigation techniques along with counseling skills. Their job is to find individuals infected with communicable diseases, bring them to treatment, and find their contacts, who will also be treated. In years past infected individuals could also be quarantined in order to protect the general public from infection. The problem with this strategy is that nothing has been prevented, only controlled. That is why many diseases are increasing in incidence until a serious effort is again made to control their spread among the population. This strategy never worked with communicable diseases and certainly will not work with our current epidemic of chronic diseases.

If you were alive in 1900 you could expect to live until age forty-nine. Today most of us have a life expectancy of seventy-nine years of age. This increase in life expectancy has been facilitated by successful prevention activities that were developed and implemented by public health agencies. There has been a remarkable reduction in deaths from heart disease, strokes, and many forms of cancer. Most childhood diseases have been virtually eliminated because of the expansion of immunizations. These public health initiatives have not only extended our life expectancy but in many instances have also improved our quality of life.

Great progress has also been made in the understanding of injuries and, more important, how to prevent them. In the years since the establishment of the Occupational Safety and Health Administration in 1970, progress has similarly been made in assuring safe and healthy workplaces. Nevertheless, according to the Institute of Medicine (2003), an average of 137 individuals die each day from work-related diseases and an additional 16 die from workplace injuries. The National Institute for Occupational Safety and Health (NIOSH, 2005) reports the direct and indirect costs of workplace injuries and illnesses to be $171 billion a year for all employers.

The Institute of Medicine reports that many of these costs could be avoided with greater attention being paid to worksite safety and health training and a long-term commitment to the workplace goals established by *Healthy People 2010.* Public health departments need to spend a great deal of time and effort helping small employers who do not have trained staff available to develop the required prevention programs. Smaller employers experience higher levels of workplace hazards than larger employers do. It is at this level that the development of surveillance systems and wellness programs will reap large benefits.

More effort must be made by employers and public health departments to partner with each other. Better and more frequent communication needs to occur between employers and public health agencies housed in the community. **Evidence-based prevention programs** that promote workplace health and safety and that are cost effective and produce the desired results need to be developed. Such collaboration efforts can go a long way toward improving workers' health and making employers more productive. Employers and public health agencies make up a winning partnership, and the time for implementation is now.

This country and its medical care system have never placed a great emphasis on the value of prevention programs. In fact a large number of individuals have argued that prevention programs are not worth what they cost. They also point out that it is virtually impossible to prove the value of programs that prevent because one cannot prove that without the intervention something bad would have happened. Cohen, Neumann, and Weinstein (2008), for example, argue that the use of preventive measures can cost more than they save. But whether or not a preventive measure is a good investment is dependent on the type of intervention and the population using the intervention. This is why it is so important to fund research to determine whether an intervention is highly effective at avoiding higher costs at a later time or whether our resources should be devoted to finding a cure. This is essentially the rationale for public health to develop best practices for preventive care procedures. Fleming (2008) argues that we need to do much to gather the best data we can about the best clinical practices. He believes that such data have not become available because of a financing mechanism that does not reward evidence-based practice.

The Trust for America's Health (2008) reports that the evidence is now pointing to the value of prevention in saving and improving lives and also in reducing the escalating costs associated with health care delivery in this country. The Trust for America's Health believes that investing $10 per person each year on proven prevention efforts, such as increased physical activity, improved nutrition, and smoking cessation programs, could result in a savings of $16 billion annually within five years. This represents a $5.60 return for every $1.00 invested.

Turnock (2009) argues that the use of certain policies and programs can also reduce health risk and ultimately improve the health of the 141 million full-time and part-time workers in this country. The Task Force on Community Preventive Services has begun a systematic review of the programs that work best in promoting healthy behavior and ultimately improve the health of employees.

PUBLIC HEALTH AND OCCUPATIONAL HEALTH

Workplace accidents and violence can be reduced through the use of epidemiology so that causes can be determined and prevention strategies can be developed and implemented. Chronic diseases that are developing in a large number of workers as they age and many of the high-risk health behaviors that are developed and continued during the working years can be slowed or prevented through workplace health education and health promotion programs.

The value of public health in such efforts is that these agencies have the expertise and incentive to work with OSHA and NIOSH to keep the workplace healthy and free of disease and injuries. In the past there has been very little interest by public health departments in forming partnerships with employers in developing workplace wellness programs. That attitude is changing as employers seek health promotion from public health agencies and public health agencies actively pursue the goals put forth by *Healthy People 2010.*

The workplace offers the ideal opportunity to keep people healthy. Workers usually spend forty hours a week or more in their place of employment, and they are a captive audience for many health promotion activities. This captive audience could receive health promotion information at the workplace, screening programs to detect disease at an early stage, and employer-provided incentives for employees and their families to stay healthy.

Awofeso (2004) argues that health promotion has three components: education, prevention, and protection. These are the components that can ensure a safe and healthy workforce. Satcher (2006) points out that the current epidemic of overweight and obesity is causing Americans to reverse all the life-span increases achieved in the past one hundred years.

The increasing cost of health care is threatening the very survival of many businesses in the United States. As governor of Arkansas, Mike Huckabee (2006) argued that wellness programs provided in the workplaces of America would result in a more cost-efficient workforce that would improve this country's productivity and its ability to become competitive with other countries. Huckabee wanted state governments to encourage wellness programs for their employees and serve as a role model for other employers.

Benjamin (2006) calls for the business community to develop a relationship with public health departments to improve the business climate and build a more productive workforce. Employers and public health departments have to work together as wellness partners. If this can be achieved, the result will be a reduction in health care costs and an improved economic climate. These opportunities must be exploited by employers and public health and the time is now.

Schulte et al. (2007) point out that obesity and workplace risks may be related. Research is needed to explore the relationship of the work environment to the development of obesity and the extent to which obesity may increase the risk of occupational disease and injury.

Table 1.3 shows the leading causes of death in the United States in 2001. According to the Centers for Disease Control and Prevention (CDC), chronic diseases (italicized in Table 1.3) claimed the lives of more than 1.7 million Americans and were responsible for seven out of ten deaths in 2001. These diseases account for 70 percent of the $2 trillion bill for medical care in this country. These diseases are also preventable if high-risk health behaviors are eliminated or never begun. The use of tobacco is one of the high-risk health behaviors instrumental in causing many of these chronic diseases.

Tobacco use by workers is clearly one of the most important triggers of worker illness, disability, and death in this country. It is also linked with a tremendous loss of productivity and loss of wages in the workforce. There is no doubt that this dangerous product is responsible for a dramatic reduction in the profits of many companies in

TABLE 1.3. **Most common causes of death, United States, 2001**

Condition	Rate
Diseases of the heart	246.8
All cancers	195.6
Stroke	57.7
Chronic lower respiratory diseases	43.6
Unintentional injuries	35.5
Diabetes mellitus	25.2
Influenza and pneumonia	21.8
Alzheimer's disease	19.0
Nephritis and nephrosis	13.9
All other causes	192.4

Note: Rates are age adjusted to the 2000 total U.S. population. Italics indicate chronic disease or condition.
Source: Centers for Disease Control and Prevention, 2005.

America, and many companies are not even aware of the loss. The CDC reports ("Annual Smoking-Attributable Mortality . . . ," 2005) that smoking cost the nation about $92 billion in the form of lost productivity in the years 1997 to 2001, up from $10 billion from the annual mortality-related productivity losses for the years 1995 to 1999. The new lost productivity estimate combined with smoking-related health care costs (reported at $75.5 billion in 1998) exceeds $167 billion per year. This represents an enormous loss in profits for American businesses.

There are only two ways to reduce consumption of this deadly and costly product in the workplace: regulation of the use of tobacco in the workplace and development of workplace smoking cessation programs that include education and therapy. Employers are not doing a good job currently of providing recommended preventive care. In fact, less than 10 percent of employers offer optimal coverage for smoking cessation programs. However, Harris, Cross, Hannon, Mahoney, and Ross-Viles (2008) point out that employers are potential partners with public health in preventing chronic disease for a number of reasons. These reasons for partnering include

- Employers' power over workplace environments

- Increases in health care costs and decreases in worker productivity because of illness

- Employers' control over whether health insurance covers preventive care aimed at avoiding chronic diseases and their potential complications

Tables 1.4, 1.5, and 1.6 display information about a study conducted by Harris et al. (2008) that made use of Workplace Solutions, a program developed by the American Cancer Society. This program attempts to increase employers' use of fifteen evidence-based practices (divided into five categories) to prevent or control chronic diseases among employees. The study involved eight employers in the Pacific Northwest, and it found that Working Solutions resulted in a large increase in the employers' use of evidence-based best practices aimed at the prevention of cancer and other chronic diseases in their places of employment. The largest change involved the increased use of tobacco cessation treatment in the workplace, which can result in a significant reduction in cancer and other chronic diseases. The use of cancer-screening programs also improved significantly.

Tobacco cessation programs provided in the workplace can result in a tremendous reduction in the rate of smoking by employees and offer employers the opportunity to have a considerable positive impact on the health of their employees. Help from public health professionals can represent the difference between success and failure in such workplace wellness initiatives. Harris et al.'s study offers a good example of how collaboration between public health professionals and employers can have a significant impact on the implementation of evidence-based prevention programs in the workplace.

TABLE 1.4. Employer chronic disease prevention best practices, by practice type, eight Pacific Northwest employers, American Cancer Society Workplace Solutions Pilot Study, 2005–2006

Practice Type	Best Practice	Relevant Community Guide Recommendation(s)	Relevant USPSTF Recommendation(s) and Prevention Priorities [CPB/CE/Total Score]
Insurance benefits	1. Provide full coverage for tobacco cessation treatments, including prescription medications, over-the-counter nicotine replacement therapy, and counseling.	Reduce out-of-pocket costs for tobacco cessation.	Tobacco-use screening and cessation intervention [5/5/10]
	2. Provide full coverage for breast, cervical, and colon cancer screenings.	Reduce out-of-pocket costs for breast cancer screening.	Breast: mammography [4/2/6]; cervical: Pap smear [4/3/7]; colorectal: any of 4 tests [4/4/8]
	3. Provide full coverage for influenza vaccination.	Reduce out-of-pocket costs for vaccinations.	Annual vaccination for adults age 50 and older [4/4/8]
	4. Require health plans to send reminders to members and network providers about preventive health services.	Provide client and provider reminders for breast, cervical, and colon cancer screening and influenza vaccination.	
	5. Require health plans to track delivery of preventive health services and send performance feedback to network providers.	Assess providers' delivery of recommended cancer screenings and influenza vaccination and give feedback.	

(continued)

TABLE 1.4. Employer chronic disease prevention best practices, by practice type, eight Pacific Northwest employers, American Cancer Society Workplace Solutions Pilot Study, 2005–2006 (*continued*)

Practice Type	Best Practice	Relevant Community Guide Recommendation(s)	Relevant USPSTF Recommendation(s) and Prevention Priorities [CPB/CE/Total Score]
Workplace policies	6. Ban tobacco use at worksites.	Use smoking bans and restrictions (to reduce environmental smoke).	
	7. Post "Use the Stairs" reminder signs near elevators.	Use point-of-decision prompts to increase physical activity.	
	8. Provide facilities for physical activity.	Enhance access to physical activity facilities, in combination with informational outreach.	
	9. Make healthy food choices available and affordable.	Offer multicomponent interventions aimed at diet, physical activity, and cognitive change.	
	10. Require and provide sun protection for employees who work outdoors.	(Insufficient evidence for required use in occupational settings, but recommended for adults in recreational settings.)	Currently under review by USPSTF

Workplace programs	11. Sponsor a tobacco cessation quit-line, including nicotine replacement therapy.	Offer multicomponent interventions that include client telephone support to increase tobacco cessation.	Tobacco-use screening and cessation intervention [5/5/10]
	12. Provide annual influenza vaccination on site.	Enhance access to vaccinations, in combination with intervention to increase community demand.	Annual vaccination for adults age 50 and older [4/4/8]
	13. Offer a workplace physical activity program.	Encourage individually adapted health behavior change to increase physical activity.	
Tracking	14. Survey employees' health behaviors to track effectiveness of health promotion efforts.	NA	
Communication	15. Conduct targeted health promotion campaigns, focusing on key health behaviors and use of preventive health care.	Offer multicomponent interventions to increase breast and cervical cancer screening and vaccination; provide small media and one-to-one education to increase breast cancer screening.	

Notes: USPSTF, United States Preventive Services Task Force; CPB, clinically preventable burden; CE, cost effectiveness; NA, not applicable. Recommendations are summaries from the USPSTF and the *Community Guide* (a CDC publication containing USPSTF evidence-based public health recommendations and findings), as well as health impact and cost-effectiveness scores from the USPSTF's prevention priorities. Possible scores for both CPB and CE range from 1 to 5, with 5 indicating greatest value. Some practices do not have Advisory Committee on Immunization Practices (ACIP) or USPSTF recommendations, as indicated by blank cells.

Source: Slightly adapted from Harris et al., 2008.

TABLE 1.5. Employer characteristics and chronic disease prevention best practice scores at baseline and follow-up, eight Pacific Northwest employers, American Cancer Society Workplace Solutions Pilot Study, 2005–2006

Employer	Industry	Number of Employees	Best Practice Implementation Score at Baseline, %	Best Practice Implementation Score at Follow-Up, %	Change in Implementation Score, Percentage Points
1	Financial	51,000	43	85	42
2	Retail trade	11,712	58	58	0
3	Government	13,000	42	59	17
4	Agriculture	7,500	33	56	23
5	Manufacturing	8,710	27	75	48
6	Government	115,522	37	52	15
7	Retail trade	45,000	23	37	14
8	Manufacturing	12,390	39	71	32

Note: Best practice scores calculated by adding the scores for all best practices and then dividing by the total number of best practices (14 was the denominator for employers without outdoor workers, because best practice 10 [promote sun protection] was not applicable to them; 15 was the denominator for employers with outdoor workers).

Source: Harris et al., 2008.

TABLE 1.6. Implementation rates of chronic disease prevention best practices at baseline and follow-up, eight Pacific Northwest employers, American Cancer Society Workplace Solutions Pilot Study, 2005–2006

Best Practice	Mean Implementation Score at Baseline, % (95% CI)	Mean Implementation Score at Follow-up, % (95% CI)	Mean Change in Implementation Score, Percentage Points (Range)	p Value
1. Cover tobacco cessation treatment	35 (14–56)	66 (35–97)	31 (0–75)	.03
2. Cover recommended cancer screenings	78 (71–86)	96 (88–100)	18 (0–25)	.03
3. Cover influenza vaccination	69 (44–93)	88 (76–99)	19 (0–100)	.25
4. Send preventive services reminders	0	38 (0–81)	38 (0–100)	.25
5. Track delivery of preventive services	0	50 (0–95)	50 (0–100)	.13
6. Have a tobacco ban	72 (46–98)	72 (46–98)	0	1.00
7. Have "Use the Stairs" signs	13 (0–42)	25 (0–64)	12 (0–100)	1.00
8. Provide physical activity facilities	63 (28–97)	71 (39–100)	8 (0–33)	.50
9. Provide healthy food choices	31 (0–62)	50 (11–89)	19 (0–100)	.63

(continued)

TABLE 1.6. Implementation rates of chronic disease prevention best practices at baseline and follow-up, eight Pacific Northwest employers, American Cancer Society Workplace Solutions Pilot Study, 2005–2006 (*continued*)

Best Practice	Mean Implementation Score at Baseline, % (95% CI)	Mean Implementation Score at Follow-up, % (95% CI)	Mean Change in Implementation Score, Percentage Points (Range)	*p* Value
10. Promote sun protection	0	0	0	NA
11. Have a tobacco cessation quit-line	25 (0–64)	63 (19–100)	38 (0–100)	.25
12. Provide on-site influenza vaccination	63 (29–96)	81 (52–100)	18 (0–100)	.25
13. Have physical activity programs	25 (0–64)	63 (19–100)	38 (0–100)	.25
14. Track employee health behaviors	25 (0–64)	50 (5–95)	25 (0–100)	.50
15. Use health promotion campaigns	30 (5–55)	50 (23–77)	20 (0–100)	.22
Total best practice score*	38 (29–47)	61 (49–74)	23 (0–48)	.02

Notes: NA, not applicable. Best practices scored from 0 to 1.00. Means rather than medians presented for ease of interpretation of change in scores from baseline to follow-up. *p* values derived from two-tailed nonparametric sign tests.

*Calculated by adding the scores for all best practices and then dividing by the total number of best practices (14 was the denominator for employers without outdoor workers, because best practice 10 was not applicable to them; 15 was the denominator for employers with outdoor workers).

Source: Harris et al., 2008.

SUMMARY

Public health departments have a long history of developing and implementing programs that are successful in reducing morbidity and mortality from disease. In recent years, public health has proven its value in responding to the epidemic of chronic diseases in our country. Our cost crisis in health services and our need to reorganize medical care delivery are providing a unique opportunity for public health to assume a leadership role in the new system of health care. Expertise in the development of prevention programs is necessary if we are to succeed in delivering good health to all Americans at a cost we can afford. Nowhere is the need for prevention greater than in the workplaces throughout the United States.

There is a need for programs with a proven record of success in the prevention or postponement of the development of chronic diseases. The workplace is an ideal location for the development, implementation, and evaluation of evidence-based prevention programs. It has large numbers of people who are in the right age group to benefit greatly from successful prevention programs. And the employer has an incentive to keep employees healthy and free from diseases and injuries—increased productivity and profits.

Public health needs to form partnerships with employers in order to keep workers healthy. Public health has the prevention expertise, and employers have the captive audience along with additional resources needed to make health promotion efforts a success. The opportunities can be seen in highly successful smoking cessation programs. Elimination of tobacco use by workers will go a long way toward the reduction of many of the costly chronic diseases that are now epidemic in the United States.

KEY TERMS

core responsibilities of public health
evidence-based prevention programs
Framingham Heart Study

health promotion
local health departments
population-based medicine

QUESTIONS FOR DISCUSSION

1. Why do public health agencies and employers have an interest in forming partnerships to deal with the epidemic of chronic diseases in the United States? Name and explain the reasons.

2. What are some of the greatest success stories of public health departments?

3. How can epidemiology, along with the development of disease and injury surveillance systems, keep workers healthier and more productive?

4. What is an example of a public health function that would help employers improve the health and safety of their employees?

CHAPTER

2

EPIDEMIOLOGY OF OCCUPATIONAL SAFETY AND HEALTH

After reading this chapter, you should be able to

■ Understand why epidemiology is important in the field of occupational safety and health.

■ Explain the value of workplace surveillance systems in understanding the causes of occupational illnesses and diseases.

■ Understand the chain of infection in disease causation.

■ Discuss the use of rates in defining workplace health problems.

■ Explain how the case definition used by epidemiologists can help to define workplace health problems.

Since their creation in 1970, the Occupational Safety and Health Administration (OSHA) and the National Institute for Occupational Safety and Health (NIOSH) have attempted to use public health concepts in the protection of workers and their workplace environment. This is an awesome task for any governmental agency, especially given that workplace improvement will almost always take away from a business's bottom line, or profit. These federal agencies are effectively demanding that employers invest in something with returns that cannot be immediately seen, despite the fact that employers may not consider long-term improvement to workers' quality of life and potential reductions in future liability costs a worthwhile investment. There are currently very few studies that have applied cost-benefit analyses to disease and injury prevention programs in the workplace in order to see the real value of such efforts.

Since OSHA and NIOSH came into being four decades ago, employers have been forced into taking a public health approach to their workplaces. This is a new role, one that employers were not properly prepared for and were very reluctant to begin. Nevertheless, they have had to assume new responsibilities to protect employees from injury and disease in order to avoid paying hefty fines for violating the 1970 law. This law also forced change on existing federal and state agencies that dealt with health and safety.

INTRODUCTION TO EPIDEMIOLOGY

Prior to the passage of the Occupational Safety and Health Act, public health departments had developed a tool kit of ways to deal with injuries and diseases. The most important of these tools is **epidemiology,** which in various forms has been part of medicine as well as public health since antiquity. Epidemiology examines the health of the population rather than the health of the individual. This tool has served us well over the years by solving many of the mysteries surrounding the causation of many illnesses and diseases. This public health science has now expanded into the analysis of workplace injuries, illnesses, and chronic diseases.

There is substantial evidence that Hippocrates used an epidemiological approach when recording outbreaks of communicable diseases such as plague, cholera, and dysentery. But as the science and art of epidemiology grew in stature and understanding, its many applications also expanded. According to Friis and Sellers (2009), epidemiology is a sound method of investigation that employs statistical techniques to evaluate a hypothesis about causation of a disease. If you gather enough accurate data about an event and use sound statistical analysis, you can usually understand why it happened and possibly how to prevent it. As a result, chronic diseases, injuries, environmental and occupational exposures, and personal behaviors are now frequently studied with epidemiological methods.

Epidemiology studies the determinants, distribution, and frequency of disease. The epidemiologist applies a concept called the **chain of infection** to explain how disease is transmitted from an infected individual to someone who is not infected. It is a time-tested method for solving medical problems of unknown etiology. Like a detective methodically solving a crime by determining cause, the epidemiologist attempts to understand a disease by determining the causative factors. Detectives work with motives, circumstances, and profiles of the victim and the criminal. Epidemiologists analyze the disease, injury, or illness; profile the patients; and look at circumstances or environments, habits, and motivations for healthy or unhealthy lifestyles. Epidemiologists may evaluate both ill and well individuals in an attempt to find the reasons some people get ill and others do not. The usual starting point for this type of investigation is gathering data from ill and well individuals through surveys. Then an attempt is made to uncover the determinants of the disease and document locations and numbers of old and new cases. The data gathered from ill and well individuals who may have been exposed to the possible determinants allows the development of a rough hypothesis to explain causation. The epidemiologists now begin building a *case definition*. This case definition includes clinical and personal qualities of the people experiencing the health event under investigation.

Figure 2.1 illustrates the process through which injury, disease, and many other health events occur. The pathogen in this chain of infection can be anything that causes harm and makes our bodies ill. Therefore this epidemiological process can also be used to understand multiple health hazards in the workplace.

Epidemiology can be the starting point of the planning process for the control and prevention of occupational injuries and disease. The first thing needed by the epidemiologist is a well-defined case definition for each of the possible health hazards found in the various businesses throughout the United States. This allows the labeling of health events according to location, time, and person.

In Chapter One we discussed some famous instances of identifying health hazards through epidemiological techniques: the process of interviewing used by John Snow in the mid-nineteenth century to identify the well that was the source of a cholera outbreak in London; the study by Doll and Hill that linked lung cancer with tobacco use in the 1950s; and the continuing analytical study of heart disease in Framingham, Massachusetts, begun in 1947. Over the years the **Framingham Heart Study** has revealed that by changing a few health behaviors (stopping smoking, eating a better diet, controlling weight, and engaging in physical activity), individuals can reduce their chances of developing heart disease. The initial successes of this study signaled that epidemiology was moving rapidly into the important area of chronic disease causation, even though chronic diseases are usually caused by multiple factors. Epidemiology was now ready to deal with diseases involving complex etiologies, long incubation periods, and no clear-cut starting point.

One of the most feared words in any epidemiologist's dictionary is *epidemic*. This much-abused term simply means more cases of a disease or other event than one would normally expect. The word *epidemic* can be used to describe excess cases of

FIGURE 2.1.   *The chain of infection.*

Pathogen — Reservoir — Mode of Transmission — Host

communicable diseases, chronic diseases, injuries, or environmental and occupational health problems. Rowitz (2006) argues that the definition of *epidemic* includes "the level of contagiousness, small facts or events that have large and long-lasting consequences, and how to prevent additional cases which can occur suddenly or at a dramatic moment." Examples of epidemics are all around us every day. The City of New York is experiencing an epidemic of diabetes, the nation is preparing for a pandemic of avian and swine influenza, women are experiencing an epidemic of heart disease, and some occupations are experiencing an epidemic of homicides. It is interesting to note that all four of these epidemics can be prevented with the help of public health expertise, which can lead to a better understanding of the behaviors that predispose individuals to the problem being studied.

One of the most important tools used by the epidemiologist in an investigation is a *rate*. In fact, it is noted by those in public health that what separates an epidemiologist from other scientists is the development and comparison of rates in order to form a hypothesis. A rate is a measure of some event, condition, disease, injury, or illness in relation to a unit of population during some specific time period (Figure 2.2). It is much easier to compare health events when the population exposed and infected is taken into consideration. A rate of illness, disease, or injury makes more sense when evaluated in terms of morbidity rates for other illnesses, diseases, or injuries. A rate of cause of death makes more sense when it is evaluated in terms of mortality rates for a number of diseases, illnesses, or injuries.

Many types of health event rates used in epidemiology are also useful for making comparisons in the workplace. The most important rates for an epidemiologist in this

FIGURE 2.2. *Determination of a rate.*

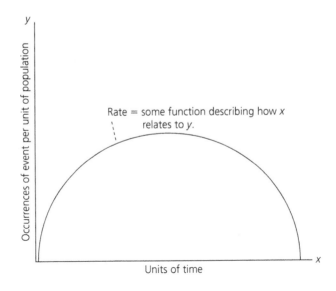

setting are the incidence rate, prevalence rate, and the attack rate. The **incidence rate** is useful in a short-term evaluation of a developing epidemic of some type of workplace hazard or illness. It looks at new cases of a specific health problem over a short period of time. The denominator is the population at risk; the numerator is the number of new cases occurring during a given period of time.

The **prevalence rate** looks at things like disease and workplace hazards over a longer period of time, such as a year. It is defined as the proportion of persons in a population who have a particular disease or attribute at a specified point in time or over a specified period of time. It is very useful for looking at long-term exposure to workplace hazards and changes in the reporting of chronic diseases in workers over the long run. The **attack rate** is a variant of the incidence rate and is derived from evaluation of a narrowly defined population observed for a short period of time. One other useful rate is the *severity rate*, which looks at productivity loss associated with an occupational injury or illness.

In order to have reliable rates, one must be using good data gathered from an established **surveillance system.** In order for a surveillance system to be reliable at gathering data, it must be mandated by some type of internal or external formal authority, such as the government or a company's top management.

SURVEILLANCE SYSTEMS

According to the Centers for Disease Control and Prevention (2009c), public health surveillance encompasses data collection for infectious and chronic diseases, injuries, environmental and occupational exposures, and personal behaviors that promote health and prevent disease. The techniques used in public health surveillance are not disease specific; they can be applied to gather data about a variety of health conditions, exposures, and behaviors of concern to public health agencies. Public health surveillance is based on a simple premise: understanding a problem is essential to solving it. The CDC (2009c) defines surveillance as the "ongoing, systematic collection, analysis, and interpretation of health data essential to the planning, implementation, and evaluation of public health practice, closely integrated with the timely feedback of these data to those who need to know."

Analysis of surveillance data often begins by summarizing it according to event or problem, person, place, and time—that is, looking for patterns of disease or health outcomes among different populations, in different places, at different times. Identifying who got sick, where they went prior to becoming sick and while sick, and when and for what duration they were sick, yields valuable information about the types of disease control and prevention efforts that are needed and the people who need to be targeted in order to most efficiently limit or prevent the spread of disease.

Examining surveillance data focused on health promotion and disease prevention behaviors for trends is as important as focusing on the disease and injury occurrences themselves. For example, knowing the patterns of vaccination coverage helps us understand why cases of vaccine-preventable diseases are declining, and knowing

FIGURE 2.3.   *The triad of disease.*

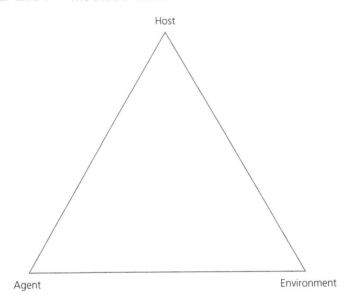

patterns of caloric intake and physical inactivity helps us explain changing trends in the incidence of obesity and the increase of type 2 diabetes cases.

The epidemiological concept of the *triad of disease*—agent, host, and environment—is extremely useful in explaining how diseases and injuries happen (Figure 2.3). It was developed by public health epidemiologists and is now being used by NIOSH researchers. It is a starting point for viewing any health problem or issue. It is especially useful when attempting to understand workplace illness and injury. For example, researchers investigating a workplace might identify a workplace chemical as an agent, a storage container as an environment, and a set of workers as the host. The researchers are then able to consider how a health problem might occur and move to a prevention rather than a cure strategy. In other words, you can determine a prevention plan before you experience a workplace hazard.

The process of surveillance starts with a problem statement. The problem can be disease, injury, a syndrome, environmental contamination, or anything else that requires better data for its understanding. This process has even been used successfully in solving marketing and management problems. It is important to define the real problem and not symptoms of a larger problem.

The second step in surveillance involves risk factor identification, or finding the cause of the problem. The risk factor can be a bacterium, virus, secondhand cigarette smoke, obesity, or faulty machinery in the workplace, and so forth. Epidemiology has allowed our country significant success in determining the cause or causes of many health problems. These successes have been shared with the workplace, but we still have a long way to go in making our workplaces even safer.

The third step in the surveillance process is to find out what works to solve the problem under consideration. The best way to do this is to look at a number of potential solutions and apply cost-benefit analysis to find the one with the greatest chance of success at the lowest cost in resources. This is an important step in that you are forced to make value judgments about the various options that could solve the problem while also considering the costs associated with your decision.

A consideration in all these steps is whether the surveillance system used to gather data should be active or passive. A *passive system* requires alerting the sources of the needed data that you are interested in receiving their data, and requesting their cooperation in the process. When you do this, you are assuming that if they see the data you requested, they will call you. An *active system* requires alerting the data source that you plan on contacting it at a prescribed time each week to ensure a timely reporting process. The active system works best when you are faced with the possibility of an epidemic.

Consider that in 1900 in the United States, the leading killer was a communicable disease (tuberculosis), whereas in 2010, the leading killer will be a disease usually caused by health behaviors that can be prevented (heart disease). McGinnis and Foege (1993) took these data one step further and determined that the real causes of most heart disease are tobacco use, poor diet, excess weight, and physical inactivity. With this revelation, the country was ready to use epidemiology to develop health promotion programs to educate people to prevent chronic diseases.

Furthermore, life expectancy in 1900 was only forty-nine years of age; that figure has now increased by almost thirty years. This increase in life expectancy is due in large part not to better medical care but to a better understanding of how disease occurs and how to prevent it. As a result of learning the real causes of disease, medicine has started to shift its emphasis from curing individuals to preventing illness and disease.

Dever (2006) argues that of the methods of epidemiology being made available through surveillance data, one of the most important is the concept of risk analysis. Using the parameters of high-risk health behaviors, we are better able to understand the major diseases of today and predict the major diseases of the future. We can also better understand and learn how to prevent workplace injuries and illnesses. Levy, Wagner, Rest, and Weeks (2005) found that information from good surveillance systems can be used to detect trends, clusters, associations, and causes of disease and injuries and is one of the answers to reducing morbidity and mortality in the workplace.

EPIDEMIOLOGY STUDIES

Several types of experimental studies can be used in research generally and by epidemiologists particularly to prove causation. These studies are usually used at the end of a sequence of less demanding and less costly studies that have led researchers to a hypothesis about causation. Now this hypothesis must be tested. Experimental studies to prove causation are complex and expensive to develop, implement, and evaluate.

Many of the studies used in the beginning of an investigation are quite simple and proceed to a more complicated form as time permits and resources become available.

The simplest study in epidemiology is a *descriptive study*, which simply gathers data and describes what is happening. There is no attempt to determine the cause of the event being observed. An *analytical study* takes the same data and attempts to prove causation. A *case control study* usually looks at retrospective data in an attempt to determine causation of the event. A *cohort study* is prospective in that it follows individuals and selected traits into the future and watches, for example, whether cohort members remain well or become ill as they grow older. Christoffel and Gallagher (2006) note that successful epidemiological studies require good data in order to get meaningful results. Among the good sources for health data are health records, vital statistics data, and the National Electronic Injury Surveillance System.

In the case control study, all types of data may be gathered on both the cases and the controls to attempt to determine causation. According to Christoffel and Gallagher (2006), the case control study allows researchers to calculate an odds ratio, which is nothing more than a representation of the likelihood of incurring a disease or injury when an associated factor is present. Christoffel and Gallagher also point out that the odds ratio can be used with cohort and cross-sectional study designs as well. Figure 2.4 is an example of a two-by-two matrix (a conventional format used by epidemiologists) displaying data needed for calculating an odds ratio.

The major objective of epidemiological studies is to prove causation. Rothman and Greenland (2005) argue that causal inferences are self-taught and early learning experiences. We learn about causation at a very early age through our experiences with life. Rothman (2002) defines the differences between the sufficient and the component causes of an occurrence. A *cause* is a condition that was necessary for occurrence of a specific outcome. A *sufficient cause* is an event that by itself can cause a specific outcome. A *component cause* is one of several events that must occur in some order to cause a specific outcome.

FIGURE 2.4. *Example of matrix displaying study outcomes.*

	Cases	Controls
Exposed	A (90)	B (40)
Unexposed	C (10)	D (60)

A = Number of persons with disease and exposure of interest.
B = Number of persons without disease but with exposure of interest.
C = Number of persons with disease but without exposure of interest.
D = Number of persons without disease and without exposure of interest.

Many workplace injuries, illnesses, and chronic diseases have a number of component causes. For example, when type 2 diabetes manifests, it is usually a result of more than one high-risk health behavior. A strong relationship between cause and outcome usually offers an incentive for more researchers to study that cause. A result that is repeated in several well-run studies offers stronger support to the hypothesis that a particular factor is in fact a cause of the injury or illness at issue.

HEALTH HAZARD EVALUATIONS

A *health hazard* is something that can produce a negative effect on people's health, either immediately or over time. The World Health Organization (1999) has identified the major steps in an assessment of health hazards: hazard identification, risk characterization, exposure assessment, and risk estimation. Completing a successful hazard assessment requires the help of well-trained individuals in public health who are dedicated to preventing health problems in the workplace.

When NIOSH conducts a *health hazard evaluation* (HHE), it is a study of a workplace. This study framework, according to Levy et al. (2005), includes the monitoring of both hazardous exposures and the health outcomes from those exposures. Staff from NIOSH visit the workplace and meet with the employer to discuss health hazards and review records about exposure and health. They may survey employees and conduct a battery of medical tests. When the evaluation of the workplace is complete, a written report is provided. This process is very similar to an epidemiological investigation by health officials.

For example, NIOSH staff carrying out a health hazard survey might ask employees the question displayed in Exhibit 2.1.

EXHIBIT 2.1. Sample NIOSH survey question

Do you think a health hazard exists in your workplace? Do any of the following stories resemble situations at your workplace?

A factory worker was feeling numbness and tingling in her fingers. She learned that three coworkers had the same problem, and two had headaches while at work but not over the weekend. Some workers said the air at work smelled bad. Their supervisor noticed the smell but didn't think it was anything to worry about.

A manager noticed that employees in one work area had more skin rashes in the past year than the year before. He wanted to know why, but didn't know what to do.

A work crew was putting cement tiles on a roof. They were working outside, but the air seemed dusty. The saws used to cut the tiles were noisy. Someone told them that this work was dangerous and they should have it checked out.

TABLE 2.1.   **Examples of NIOSH surveillance activities in the workplace**

NIOSH Division:	Analyzes and Collects Data On:
The Surveillance Branch in the Division of Respiratory Disease Studies (DRDS)	Occupational respiratory disease
Surveillance and Field Investigations Branch in the Division of Safety Research (DSR)	Occupational injuries
Division of Surveillance, Hazard Evaluations, and Field Studies (DSHEFS)	Nonrespiratory diseases and illnesses, such as dermatitis, lead and pesticide poisoning, and cancer
Pittsburgh and Spokane Research Laboratories	The mining industry

Source: NIOSH, 2006.

Generally, NIOSH responsibilities are to

- Analyze and interpret existing data

- Undertake data collection efforts to fill gaps in surveillance data

- Provide support to state agencies to conduct occupational surveillance and associated prevention efforts

- Fund and conduct research on surveillance methods

- Work with federal, state, and private sector partners to improve occupational health surveillance

The NIOSH surveillance program involves both intramural and extramural activities. Several NIOSH divisions and laboratories include units focused on surveillance to discover workplace problem areas (see Table 2.1).

Fatalities are of particular concern to NIOSH and OSHA. Fatal occupational injury rates in 2002 were highest in mining (23.5 per 100,000 workers); agriculture, forestry, and fishing (22.7); construction (12.2); and transportation and public utilities (11.3). The rate for all private industry was 4.2 per 100,000 workers (Bureau of Labor Statistics, 2009). Figure 2.5 shows the ten leading industries for fatalities in the United States. Now a plan must be developed by OSHA and NIOSH to deal with these locations of highest fatalities.

FIGURE 2.5.   *Fatal occupational injury rates by industry division, 2002.*

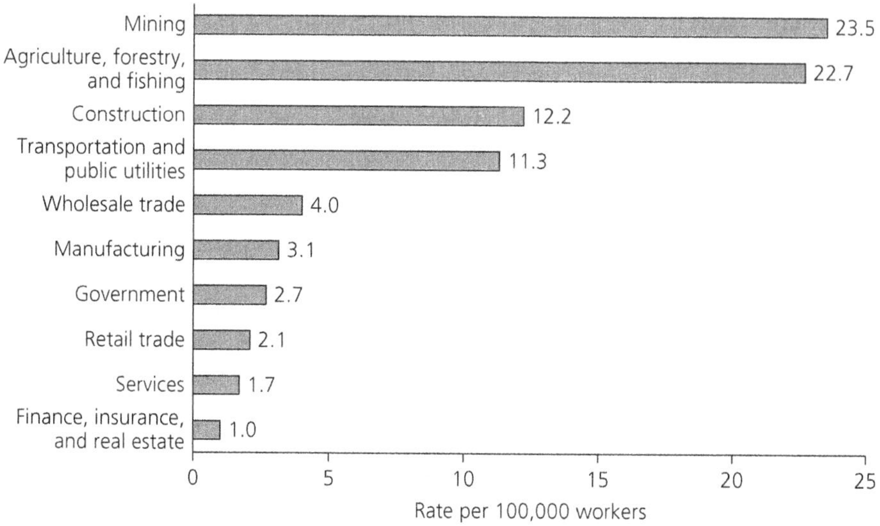

Source: Bureau of Labor Statistics, 2009.

PUBLIC HEALTH SYSTEMS IN THE WORKPLACE

Public health is concerned with protection of the entire community from illness and the prevention of disease. This mandate would certainly include the millions of people who go to work in small and large businesses. As we have discussed, protection of workers in the workplace presents a unique set of problems for public health agencies because of some employer resistance and the costs associated with the development of workplace prevention programs.

Public health agencies do, however, have the requisite skills to offer to the workplace. They can offer educational solutions to the problems causing morbidity and mortality in the workplace as well as in the community by providing programs and services that enable employers to discourage workers from practicing high-risk health behaviors such as tobacco use, poor diet, eating that leads to obesity, and physical inactivity. Workers that practice these behaviors are likely to do so both at work and at home. Reducing these high-risk health behaviors at home will require strategies similar to the ones used to reduce workplace injuries and environmental illness.

People require the expertise of public health agencies in order to live a healthier life both in the community and in the workplace. In fact, there is an important role for public health in the shaping of a vision of better health for everyone by eliminating the causes of poor health. In other words, establish obtainable goals for preventing illness and injury in the community and the workplace. According to Rowitz (2003), one of the major functions of public health is to ensure that services required to achieve agreed-upon goals are in fact provided. Public health leadership is required to develop plans for improving health by establishing and implementing the needed programs and then evaluating the success or failure of these programs.

CHRONIC DISEASE EPIDEMIOLOGY IN THE WORKPLACE

According to the CDC, chronic diseases such as heart disease, cancer, and diabetes are the leading causes of mortality in the United States. Chronic diseases account for seven of every ten deaths and affect the quality of later life for over ninety million Americans. Chronic diseases are noncommunicable and degenerative. It seems ironic that they are incurable once they occur but prior to occurrence are almost totally preventable. This is the reason why it makes sense to concentrate scarce resources on prevention rather than cure. Prevention of diseases that are very costly once their complications develop makes good economic sense. It also seems to be a sensible plan to seek out individuals in the workplace who are already experiencing the symptoms of one or more chronic diseases in order to prevent the complications that can occur from these diseases. In other words, while OSHA and NIOSH are fulfilling their mandate of protecting the safety and health of the worker in the workplace, they could also deal with the growing chronic disease epidemic found in the same workplace. Epidemiological tools should be used to gather information about chronic disease in the workplace and create a prevention plan.

McGinnis and Foege (1993) argue that the major contributors to mortality in this country are health behaviors. "In 1990 they were tobacco (an estimated 400,000 deaths), diet and activity patterns (300,000), alcohol (100,000), microbial agents (90,000), toxic agents (60,000), firearms (35,000), sexual behavior (30,000), motor vehicles (25,000) and illicit use of drugs (20,000)." If these behaviors are the causes of chronic diseases later in life, we need to develop specific health promotion programs to prevent these behaviors long before they begin. This is an enormous task for any one agency, but it can be made easier if it is shared with several agencies working for the same goal through workplace regulation and educational programs.

Employers can better understand the potential problem with chronic diseases in the workplace by conducting a health survey to discover the major high-risk health behaviors being practiced by their workers at home and at work. Many of these behaviors, such as tobacco use, physical inactivity, and poor diet, will in time produce chronic diseases in many of the workers, eventually resulting in increased sick days, reduced productivity, and increased disability among employees. There will also be a substantial increase in health insurance premiums and an eventual increase in the percentage of the insurance cost paid by the employee. Because these economic and human costs associated with chronic diseases developing in employees will have a negative effect on the profit level of the company, the health survey is a helpful tool with which to start developing a workplace chronic disease prevention program.

SUMMARY

The tools of epidemiology, following a long history of success in public health, have been brought into the workplace to deal with occupational safety and health. The starting point for applying epidemiological methods to solve the problem of disease causation is using a questionnaire and implementing effective surveillance systems in order to apply the chain of infection concept to uncovering the causes of illness and chronic disease in the workplace. Employers can then use the data collected in these ways, in combination with issues and guidelines already established by OSHA and NIOSH, to analyze and improve health and safety conditions for employees.

Chronic disease epidemiology has had many successes with diseases that have long incubation periods and no cure.

We have described the changes in the leading causes of morbidity and mortality in the United States over the last one hundred years from communicable diseases to chronic diseases. In the workplace unintentional injuries have become the leading cause of years of potential life lost (YPLL) for those under the age of sixty-five. That is why epidemiology has been added to the tool kit used by NIOSH investigators. Both the mission of OSHA and the surveillance and investigative pursuits of NIOSH could complement the many activities already being undertaken to deal with chronic disease. Because NIOSH is already a part of the CDC it seems a logical step to include OSHA too in beginning to track and attempt to prevent the high-risk health behaviors that cause chronic diseases both in the community and in the workplace.

KEY TERMS

attack rate
chain of infection
epidemiology
Framingham Heart Study

incidence rate
prevalence rate
surveillance system

QUESTIONS FOR DISCUSSION

1. What is the value of establishing active and passive surveillance systems in the workplace?

2. What is the role of epidemiology in uncovering workplace health and safety issues?

3. Should public health departments and employers form partnerships to reduce injuries and illnesses in the workplace? Explain the reasons for your answer.

PART

2

OCCUPATIONAL SAFETY AND HEALTH

CHAPTER

3

HISTORY AND IMPORTANCE OF OCCUPATIONAL SAFETY AND HEALTH

After reading this chapter, you should be able to

- Understand the major health and safety problems found in U.S. workplaces.

- Describe the long-term effects of the epidemic of work-related chronic diseases in this country.

- Discuss the role that public health needs to play in U.S. occupational safety and health.

- Discuss the need for health care delivery reform.

- Explain how levels of personal health and health care costs and access are interrelated.

In 1900, workers in this country were faced with a high probability of suffering disease and injury in the workplace (McKenzie, Pinger, & Kotecki, 2005). Because both occupational injury and disease were increasing frequently in the United States, there were numerous attempts over the years to develop legislation at the federal level to protect people's health while they were at work. However, the political will to take on big businesses and make them comply with protective measures for their employees was not present at first. There were no clear incentives for employers to protect workers, and people had to work to live. Eventually, however, as Bayer (2000) states, increasing dangers to health in the workplace leading to greater morbidity and mortality among workers eventually led to the establishment of the Occupational Safety and Health Administration (**OSHA**) in 1970.

OSHA was given the regulatory authority to protect workers against hazards in their work environment. This new federal agency became part of the Department of Labor and began fulfilling its mandate in 1971. Its mission was complex: to prevent work-related injuries, illnesses, and deaths by issuing standards that could be enforced to protect the worker in the workplace. In its early days of operation, however, OSHA was poorly regarded, as it implemented many regulations that businesses considered burdensome, unnecessary, and confusing.

The same legislation that created OSHA established the National Institute for Occupational Safety and Health (NIOSH). This agency charged with investigating worker safety and health and considered OSHA's research body is headquartered at the Centers for Disease Control and Prevention (CDC) in the Department of Health and Human Services. In addition to conducting research, NIOSH makes recommendations relating to the dangers of exposure to hazardous substances and other dangerous conditions in the workplace.

OSHA is responsible for the safety and health of over 110 million workers at 7 million worksites and has a total staff of about 2,200 employees (McKenzie et al., 2005). This agency has done a remarkable job over the years of reducing workplace morbidity and mortality rates. The Institute of Medicine (2003) points out that even with this success, 16 workers still die on the job every day from injuries and more than 14,000 a day experience an injury or illness. According to the BLS (2009) the nonfatal workplace injuries and illnesses among private sector employers declined from 4.4 cases per 100 full-time workers to 4.2 cases per 100 in 2007. This is good news but more work needs to be done.

McKenzie et al. (2005) argue that OSHA must ensure that workers in the private sector are not being exposed to recognized hazards at their place of work that may cause morbidity and mortality. This is a massive undertaking, which includes developing an understanding of the nature of the many occupational diseases, establishing active surveillance systems in the workplace, and creating primary prevention systems designed to reduce the development of work-related diseases. Many of OSHA's goals and objectives for the workplace are the same as the occupational safety and health goals put forth in the **Healthy People 2010** program and followed by **public health** departments across the United States. As we discussed in Chapter One, Focus Area 20 of Healthy People

2010 addresses occupational safety and health. The goal for this area is to "promote the health and safety of people at work through prevention and early intervention." As outlined in Table 1.2 in Chapter One, the Healthy People 2010 objectives for occupational safety and health (U.S. Department of Health and Human Services, 2000) address

Work-related injury deaths

Work-related injuries

Overexertion or repetitive motion

Pneumoconiosis deaths

Work-related homicides

Work-related assaults

Elevated blood lead levels from work exposure

Occupational skin diseases or disorders

Worksite stress-reduction programs

Needle stick injuries

Work-related noise-induced hearing loss

In the 1990s, NIOSH and other agencies collaborated in developing a set of priority research areas to study the economic impact of the workplace injury and disease burden and to support a research plan for the twenty-first century (see Table 3.1). The resulting National Occupational Research Agenda (**NORA**) depends heavily on good surveillance procedures in order to accurately forecast workplace health issues and develop comprehensive solutions to these problems. NORA surveillance results in collecting, analyzing, and interpreting large amounts of workplace data in the areas shown in Table 3.1. After being examined and interpreted by epidemiologists, these data are disseminated to OSHA and to employers to help them improve workplace health. NORA offers the possibility of developing measurable objectives for research activities and the ability to evaluate performance of the agencies responsible.

Despite such efforts, there needs to be, as Bayer (2000) points out, a major change in the attitude of the government toward workers' exposure to injury and disease if this country is ever going to achieve the mission established for OSHA almost forty years ago. This agency's performance does not receive high marks under the scrutiny of cost-benefit analysis. When workplace hazards are discovered, maximum penalties need to be levied in order to give incentives to all businesses to comply with OSHA regulations. Greater collaboration with other federal agencies such as the Environmental Protection Agency (EPA) will make enforcement of laws and regulations more effective. In addition, as we discussed in Chapter Two, close relationships between public health departments and businesses need to be established in order to deal more effectively with worker exposure to the determinants of communicable and chronic diseases.

TABLE 3.1.   **NORA research categories**

Category	NORA Priority Research Areas
Disease and Injury	Allergic and Irritant Dermatitis Asthma and Chronic Obstructive Pulmonary Disease Fertility and Pregnancy Abnormalities Hearing Loss Infectious Diseases Low Back Disorders Musculoskeletal Disorders of the Upper Extremities Traumatic Injuries
Work Environment and Workforce	Emerging Technologies Indoor Environment Mixed Exposures Organization of Work Special Populations at Risk
Research Tools and Approaches	Cancer Research Methods Control Technology and Personal Protective Equipment Exposure Assessment Methods Health Services Research Intervention Effectiveness Research Risk Assessment Methods Social and Economic Consequences of Workplace Illness and Injury Surveillance Research Methods

Source: NIOSH, 1996.

According to the CDC (Workers' Memorial Day. . . . ," 2009) workplace injuries and illnesses are still an important problem in this country. In fact April 28 is set aside each year by the CDC to remember workers who have died or been injured in the workplace. Even though current rates of workplace injury and acute disease are much lower than they were before OSHA began establishing regulations, these rates can still be improved. Moreover, most workplace health statistics do not even consider the large number of these workers who are incubating **chronic diseases** caused by high-risk personal behaviors, diseases that will most likely adversely affect their quality of life as they grow older in the workplace. The Bureau of Labor Statistics reports that the cost for workplace injury and disease is an estimated $89 billion a year. These costs include the costs associated with the injury or illness that will be reflected in higher costs for health insurance for the employer. Other costs that need to be included are lost productivity along with disability pay for the injured or ill worker. According to the CDC (2009c), more than half of Americans are living with one or more chronic diseases as they grow older. And many of these individuals are becoming disabled, developing chronic diseases, and reducing their quality of life in later years as a direct result of their work environment. Many of these diseases were developing during their working years and could have been prevented. If the cost of chronic diseases acquired during the years in the workplace is included, the cost of workplace injury and illness rises to well over a trillion dollars. Moreover, now that epidemiologists are shedding more light on the development of chronic diseases, it has been proven that many of the high-risk health behaviors that foster chronic disease are connected with the workplace. For example, Schulte et al. (2007) point out that there is strong evidence that obesity and overweight may be related to adverse work conditions.

Simon & Fielding (2006) argue that public health and businesses share a strong interest in a healthy population. As we argued in Chapter Two, many of the public health strategies that have been used so successfully in the public health achievements of the past seem appropriate for helping workers to remain healthy and productive as they age. Public health agencies work for everybody, including the workplace population. Public health should, therefore, be available to offer prevention and education about disease to all members of the workforce. The current epidemic of chronic diseases and the costs associated with these diseases provide an opportunity for an expansion of public health expertise regarding these same diseases in the workplace.

This opportunity could include an expansion in workplace safety and health programs to include surveillance programs for high-risk health behaviors that usually result in chronic diseases as workers grow older. These chronic diseases, including heart disease, lung cancer, and diabetes, cause morbidity and mortality in the same way that exposure to chemicals, dangerous machinery, or injuries in the workplace cause morbidity and mortality. In other words, if we already have OSHA programs established in the workplace to protect against immediate injury, it seems appropriate to also protect workers from expensive chronic diseases caused by personal health behaviors practiced at home and at work. Poor diet, use of tobacco, a sedentary lifestyle, and stress are part of many workplaces. This influence requires greater study in order to protect the worker from acquiring or continuing these behaviors. The CDC calls people from twenty-five to sixty-four years of age the most productive age group in the United States. This is also the age group most likely to be spending time in the workplace. The average worker spends the most productive years of his or her life in the workplace, and if his or her health is damaged, the worker has an overall negative payoff for all his or her hard work. There is nothing more important than personal health.

There is a real need for the expansion of time-tested public health programs, including chronic disease education programs in the workplace. The starting point will include improved gathering of data about workers' health. This should include all health data, including information on the chronic diseases that harm employees and thus their employers.

The law creating OSHA resulted from recognition of the dangers faced by many workers in this country. Over the last several years this nation has made significant improvements in the health of its working people. There is much more work to be accomplished as employers are asked to assume a greater responsibility for their employees' quality of life. Public health expertise needs to be made available to the workers and employers in order to prevent continuing illness and injury from chronic diseases.

HEALTH, DISEASE, AND PREVENTION

If we look at the ways in which health and disease are defined, we can see more clearly why active prevention programs are such an important goal for workplace health and safety. In 1947, the World Health Organization defined health as "physical, mental and social well-being and not merely the absence of disease and infirmity." This definition, now used by governmental bodies worldwide, brings to light many components to be considered in an assessment of personal wellness and illness. The average person, however, defines his or her personal health subjectively, thinking simply about whether he or she feels well or ill, and makes little effort to determine the multitude of components influencing it. Thus the average person also gives little consideration to the likelihood that chronic disease will affect his or her health because most chronic diseases have little recognizable effect on health until they are somewhat advanced.

Turnock (2009) argues that many individuals seem unaware of the fact that wellness can be negatively affected by their own dangerous, high-risk health behaviors. He also points out that the average American still looks at wellness as a function of length of life and not quality of life. Many individuals believe that as one ages one must learn to adapt to poor health as an inevitable consequence of the aging process. They usually are not aware that chronic diseases can be developing while they feel well and can be the cause of long-term illness and premature death. Similarly, McKenzie et al. (2005) point out that illness is often a personal determination of a deviation from one's personal definition of a good state of health. Individuals determine that they are ill because of a temporary or permanent change in their state of health.

At some point the individual who feels ill may seek help from a health professional, who will usually define and name the illness. The individual with a well-defined illness now has a professionally defined disease. The physician can now recommend a course of treatment, which may bring the ill person back to wellness. Unfortunately, it usually costs a great deal more for the cure than it would have cost to prevent the occurrence of illness in the first place.

McKenzie et al. (2005) argue that disease involves a professional definition; it is a construct created by a licensed health professional. It involves tests, medical evaluation, consultation with peers, and an accepted name. The physician and a battery of medical tests can give the individual's illness a name, which leads to the ability to recommend a more precise treatment.

The process of illness developed by CDC is illustrated in Figure 3.1. This epidemiological disease process applies to both communicable and chronic diseases and

FIGURE 3.1. *The disease process.*

Well — Exposure to Agent — Incubation Period — Symptoms — Ill

can also be applied for workplace safety and health issues. If any of the steps in the process are abated, the disease or injury will usually not occur. This sequence of steps is the starting point for a better understanding of how the disease process works and the development of a public health strategy to prevent disease in the community and the workplace. It provides a method to learn more about illness and disease whether the illness is communicable, chronic, or environmental in origin. For example, if we define the parts of this model in terms of salmonella, we find that salmonella is caused by a bacterial pathogen, which is usually present in a food product and ingested by someone. The **incubation period** of this communicable disease is three to seventy-two hours with a median time to symptoms of twenty-four hours. Given the way one is exposed to the agent, prevention methods for this disease include proper handling and preparation and storage of potentially susceptible food products.

The CDC (2009a) points out that the treatment for a chronic disease is usually the same as the prevention recommendations. For example, the recommendations for preventing type 2 diabetes are to eat a healthy diet, lose weight, and engage in physical activity and the treatment for the individual diagnosed with this disease consists of a healthy diet, weight loss, and physical activity. In the case of chronic disease, the disease process model can explain how the disease occurs and, more important, how to prevent the disease or at least prevent the long-term complications from the disease once acquired. Much of this prevention involves modifying the high-risk health behaviors that are known to lead to the development of chronic diseases later in life.

According to Brownlee (2007) the United States spends a large percentage of its gross domestic product (GDP) on a system of health care that is essentially not worth what it costs. That percentage of GDP given to health care delivery is going to continue to rise as the ranks of the elderly increase over the next several years. According to Heffler et al. (2005), health care spending will consume 18.7 percent of GDP by 2014. Therefore, the U.S. health care system is in a state of crisis. According to Sultz and Young (2009), the U.S. health care system has made tremendous advancements in life expectancy over the years but is still a very expensive and wasteful system. A study released by PricewaterhouseCoopers in July 2005 found that 75 percent of large companies may ask employees to pay more for their health insurance and may reduce pay raises for their current employees. Twenty percent of these employers planned to hire fewer workers in 2005 because of rising health insurance costs. This system must undergo radical change in the next few years or what Americans like to think of as the best health care delivery system in the world will go broke.

Chronic disease affects both personal and population health. Almost a trillion dollars is currently being spent on chronic diseases that are usually incurable and for the most part preventable. According to Morewitz (2006), chronic diseases are a major cause of death and disability in this country every year. Over 25 million individuals are affected by these diseases, are unable to work, and experience a decrease in their quality of life. The CDC reports that more than 75 percent of health care costs are due to chronic conditions. These diseases are the most common and costly of all health problems but they are also the most preventable. When public health departments add up the cost of years of potential life lost (YPLL) because of poor health, they discover that the leading causes of death in this country are injuries and chronic diseases. (YPLL is a measure of premature death, usually calculated for the population under sixty-five or seventy-five years of age.) They also discover that injuries and chronic diseases are responsible for much disability and many days lost from work, along with tremendous costs for managing incurable health problems. Finally, employers suffer high financial losses and lose productivity owing to employees' injuries and chronic diseases.

According to former U.S. senator Tom Daschle (2008), the best health care system in the world costs too much, does not allow the sickest members access, and does not place a very high value on preventing illness. When a patient is in crisis he or she may die or may return to better health than he or she enjoyed before becoming ill. Once patients return from illness, they are usually highly motivated to remain well. They start to practice better health behaviors that usually make them healthier. This same transformation needs to occur in the American health care system if it is to survive. In his 1998 book *Who Shall Live,* Fuchs listed the major problems in the health care system as costs, access, and health levels. The most important of these problems, driving the others, seems to be people's level of health. That makes prevention the potential solution to all three problems.

Yet a 2004 national survey conducted by the National Center for Health Statistics shows a pervasive lack of understanding of good health (Adams & Schoenborn, 2006). According to this report, 62 percent of adults (people eighteen years of age or over) reported excellent or very good health. At the same time, however, 62 percent of adults never participated in any type of vigorous leisure-time physical activity, and 15 percent did not have a usual place of health care. Twelve percent of adults had been told by a doctor or health professional that they had heart disease, and 22 percent had been told on two or more physician visits that they had hypertension. Twenty-one percent of all adults were current smokers, and 21 percent were former smokers. Based on estimates of body mass index, 35 percent of adults were overweight and 24 percent were obese.

These statistics indicate that we need to evaluate how we deliver health services and try to understand why the current model of delivery has failed. There are many in public health who believe that we need to refocus the entire health care system on prevention and not on cure. This means that the individual should become the focus of health care reform. This is a major change in the way we as nation think about how health care is delivered and received. There can be no more incremental tinkering with a system that simply does not work. Responsibility for health care needs to become a personal issue and depends on each person practicing healthy behaviors at home and in the workplace. This requires an expansion of health education programs in our schools and workplaces, the ideal locations for providing health information to large segments of the population.

Shifting the focus of health care to the individual should start with the youngest members of the workforce. Defining good health as "I feel well," young people tend to believe that their health will remain good even if they practice one or more high-risk health behaviors. This attitude must change; people need help to understand the value of investing in their future health stock in the present. This is a unique opportunity for public health departments to work with business leaders to educate workers. The incentives for this partnership are that public health departments will be better able to meet their goals for the population and businesses will retain a healthier workforce, reduce medical costs, and increase profits through greater worker productivity.

The high-risk health behaviors practiced by many individuals usually develop very early in life, probably before children enter their teenage years. The development of these health behaviors is usually a result of peer pressure and an individual desire to experiment with danger. The individuals' attitude often seems to be that they are invincible because even though they experiment with high-risk behaviors such as abuse of alcohol, use of tobacco, and unprotected sex, "nothing really bad happens" at the time of their experimentation.

These young people do not realize that they may be incubating a chronic disease that will affect the state of their health in the future. Williams and Torrens (2002) argue that most individuals are unaware of the fact that chronic diseases usually have long incubation periods (twenty to forty years) and, once developed, are usually incurable. Similarly, young adults do not consider the possibility of becoming injured as a result of an accident or violence. They enter the workforce and start or continue unhealthy behaviors, which may increase because of peer pressure, and eventually they develop one or more chronic diseases or injuries. This cycle can be prevented if information about healthy lifestyles is distributed, promoted, and reinforced from the time young people enter the workforce until the time they retire.

THE ROLE FOR PUBLIC HEALTH

If life expectancy is a measure of health, then the last century has witnessed a tremendous improvement in health. Much of this success is due not to medical advances but to the practice of public health concepts. Once we realize that the communicable diseases of the early 1900s in the United States have been replaced as the leading cause of morbidity and mortality by the chronic diseases of today, we may then be able to employ a different model of health care, one that emphasizes prevention and control. Unfortunately, the United States is currently proceeding in this direction only very slowly. And the problem is not only in this country. The World Health Organization's 2005 report *Preventing Chronic Disease: A Vital Investment* predicts that the global epidemic of chronic disease will claim 350 million lives in the next ten years and cost the global community enormous sums of money and lost worker productivity. The report goes on to say that the price to be paid by inaction on this growing epidemic is clear and unacceptable.

However, educating the consumer about personal health is a mammoth task because the current system of health care has no incentives for the individual to be knowledgeable about his or her health. Good health is generally taken for granted in that we are usually healthy when born and remain that way as we grow older. Our mentality regarding illness has developed around our experience with communicable disease occurrences, where we see a doctor, take some medication, and rest until we get better.

Moreover, the quest for good health seems to be surrounded by temptations to practice bad health behaviors, thanks in part to the overwhelming presence of the media in daily life. Television, radio, the Internet, and other media have tremendous influence over the individual's wellness or illness because they influence lifestyle choices through shows and advertising. Billions of dollars each year are spent on exposing audiences to high-fat foods, alcohol, and anything else that brings companies a large profit. These advertisers would not spend all this money on a marketing strategy that was not working. In addition, watching television or any other form of passive entertainment usually replaces physical activity, and while people are watching television or listening to radio they may be more susceptible to the appeal of garbage snack foods and beverages. Advertisers and networks enjoy increased profits while our nation gets heavier and sicker.

The Wellness Council of America (2008) points out that the vast majority of illnesses are preventable if only time were taken to promote wellness. Chronic disease prevention programs show very good results when cost-benefit analysis is applied to the outcomes associated with their prevention efforts. The costs of starting these programs in the workplace can be high in terms of providing a better diet and spending time on physical activity. But as the prevention effort intensifies, a much larger return on the initial investment appears for the individual and the business. For example, Trust for America's Health (2008) argues that if one-tenth of Americans practiced a regular walking program, this action alone would result in a savings of $5.6 billion, money that would otherwise have been spent on the treatment of heart disease. Similarly, Task Force on Community Preventive Services (2005) has recommended that multicomponent interventions that include nutrition and physical activity be employed to control overweight and obesity among individuals as they grow older. These interventions include strategies such as providing nutrition education or a dietary prescription, a physical activity prescription or group activity, and behavioral skills development and training.

The costs of health services can be substantially reduced through the practice of behavioral medicine. This type of medicine requires active participation by the individual who should be attempting to develop and maintain wellness. The health system and the workplace need to move from a secondary prevention model of treating disease (cure) to a primary method of controlling diseases (prevention). The real problem, not disease symptoms, must be properly defined before intervention strategies are developed and implemented. The leading killers in this country are not cancer, heart disease, and stroke but tobacco use, poor dietary habits, and physical inactivity.

As McGinnis and Foege (1993) argue, daily habits such as smoking, drinking alcohol, being physically inactive, and choosing a poor diet are the major contributors to almost all of the chronic diseases in this country.

McGinnis and Foege (1993) argue that after years of devastating the human body, these behaviors manifest themselves in untreatable chronic diseases. In fact, when chronic diseases are evaluated in this context, smoking causes 18 percent of disease, poor diet and physical inactivity contribute another 17 percent, and alcohol causes 4 percent. It seems that our bad behaviors are a greater threat to our health, and contribute more to disability days and premature death, than either our environment or any microbe or toxin. The sad part about these facts is that all we have to do is practice good health behaviors and we most likely will be rewarded with a longer life without disability.

The public health sector could become a catalyst in this process. Public health workers, using the science of epidemiology, are identifying the many risk factors associated with injuries and chronic diseases, and as more information is gathered on these diseases, innovative prevention and control measures are being expanded in educational efforts. This information could easily be shared in the workplace through OSHA. It is the contention of many public health experts that public health strategies can be applied to make the workplace a healthier place to live a large part of our lives. In other words, by using the principles of public health, the workplace can be made safer and can also handle the awesome responsibility of educating workers to avoid practicing high-risk health behaviors after work.

Dedicated public health workers have produced miracles in helping Americans to become healthier. But even the most dedicated public health employees agree that keeping people healthy and teaching them how to avoid chronic diseases and injuries is a mammoth task. There is a limit to what a public health department can accomplish with its limited resources and personnel. This means there is a role for each employee and each employer to play in reducing the individual practice of high-risk health behaviors.

For years, figures such as the 5,524 occupational fatalities and over 4.7 million new, nonfatal injuries and illnesses in the workplace that the National Center for Health Statistics (2005) reported for 2002 were looked at as a price to be paid by working in some hazardous industries. Now the workplace is being seen as an opportunity for public health to use prevention programs not just for the safety and health of employees but to prevent the development of chronic diseases. In recent years there has also been a noticeable change in employers' interest in safety and health issues that might affect their most valuable assets—their employees. Lawsuits, loss of productivity, loss of trained employees to illness and disease, and the costs associated with replacing the sick employee are among the economic issues sparking this interest. For public health this interest offers the chance to develop better plans to deal with not only acute noninfectious health problems but also the chronic noninfectious diseases like heart disease and cancer.

Rowitz (2006), for example, argues that public health leaders must emphasize *best practices* when they attempt to solve public health problems, and he supplies a formula that displays the components of quality improvement in public health programs:

$$\text{Leadership Competency} + \text{High Performance Expectations} + \\ \text{Strategic Capacity Building}$$

Rowitz also argues that individuals need to gain personal mastery over their lives, especially where their health is concerned. They need to obtain a vision of what life could be like if they maintain their wellness as they age and die a natural death without pain. This mental model of wellness does not include: tobacco products, poor dietary habits, or abuse of alcohol and drugs and does include daily physical activity.

Because most individuals spend a majority of their day at work, the workplace seems the ideal location for the use of public health expertise to develop, implement, and evaluate safety and health programs. The use of public health recommendations to prevent disease, illness, and accidents at the workplace needs to become the norm.

Once developed, a chronic disease cannot be cured and because of the long incubation period (also known as the subclinical disease stage), it is unknown when the disease process actually began. It is known that certain high-risk health behaviors are the cause of chronic diseases and that in most cases these diseases' devastating long-term effects result from continued practice of these behaviors after a disease has developed. The key to success with the chronic diseases is found in preventing them from developing or, at the very least, preventing the individual from continued practice of high-risk behaviors once a disease has developed. These public health principles can easily be used to work with safety and health issues in the workplace. Injuries and disease have been studied extensively by epidemiologists, and a great deal of accurate information is available about the cause, effect, and prevention of these health problems.

SUMMARY

Personal lifestyle can lead to morbidity, disability, and eventually premature mortality. Even if one does not die prematurely, quality of life will be affected by the disability associated with injury and chronic disease. Employers are beginning to recognize the value of forming partnerships with public health departments to develop strategies to prevent injury and disease in the workplace. In addition, surveillance for chronic diseases in the workplace should become part of the OSHA mission. The addition of public health strategies to the workplace can provide a major return on investment in terms of improved employee health outcomes, reduced medical and disability costs, reduced absenteeism, and increased productivity and job satisfaction.

An understanding of occupational health and safety goes beyond knowledge about preventing slips, falls, and exposure to toxic substances and complying with minimum Occupational Safety and Health Administration standards. An individual's performance and ability to remain safe and healthy in the workplace are affected by countless factors, many of them known but also others that have not yet been sufficiently explored as crucial components of occupational health.

Stress, drug and alcohol abuse, and violent behavior are major contributors to accidents and injuries. Therefore the psychological component of employee wellness merits increased attention from corporate decision makers. In addition, an understanding of issues that affect employees' everyday lives, such as obesity, proper diabetes management, and smoking cessation, can further enhance a company's commitment to retaining the most efficient workforce. Employers must become aware of widespread health problems at their worksites and prepare to initiate wellness programs as an important and evolving new responsibility that is now being acknowledged as an answer to our burgeoning health care system crisis by major corporations, health care providers, and insurance providers.

KEY TERMS

chronic disease
Healthy People 2010
incubation period

NORA
OSHA
public health

QUESTIONS FOR DISCUSSION

1. Why should employers be concerned about employee wellness and safety?

2. What is the major importance of the Occupational Safety and Health Act of 1970? Explain its importance.

3. How does the Healthy People 2010 initiative deal with worker health and safety?

4. Explain the ramifications of illness and injuries acquired in the workplace on employers' profits.

OCCUPATIONAL INJURIES

After reading this chapter, you should be able to

- Identify the major causes and sources of injuries in the workplace.

- Understand the role epidemiology could play in reducing the total number of these injuries.

- Understand why acting to prevent injuries is a better and more economical choice than waiting for them to happen.

- Discuss the prevalence of workplace violence and what can be done to reduce it.

According to Finkelstein, Corso, and Miller (2006) Injuries are the most serious and deadly public health problem facing the United States today. Twenty years ago, **injury** was a leading cause of death in the United States, causing 143,000 deaths in 1983. Today there are still over 400 deaths each day resulting from injuries, a number of which happen in the workplace. In addition, there are thousands of nonfatal injuries. Such large numbers represent a problem that lends itself to a public health model and the principles of epidemiology for its solution, as we will discuss in this chapter. Table 4.1 offers a comprehensive understanding of the total cost to society resulting from injuries. It considers medical costs and productivity losses so employers can fully understand just how expensive injuries can be to the workplace too.

EPIDEMIOLOGY OF INJURIES

McKenzie, Pinger, and Kotecki (2005) define *injury* as "physical harm or damage resulting from an acute exchange of energy that exceeds the body's tolerance." All types of energy—kinetic, mechanical, chemical, thermal, electrical, and nuclear—are present in American industries and workplaces. Therefore the potential for injuries is present for every worker every day, regardless of occupation.

Injuries are generally classified as *unintentional* or *intentional*. Unintentional injuries result from chance occurrences not intended by anyone to cause harm to another; these injuries are also known as *accidents*. Intentional injuries result from someone intending to cause harm; these injuries are also known as *violence*. Both types of injuries are a major occupational hazard experienced by many workers every day. They represent direct and indirect costs to the employer and to the employee and his or her family.

McKenzie et al. (2005) argue that age-adjusted death rates are the best indicator for examining changes in the risk of death for individuals over a period of time. Accidents, suicides, and homicides represent a significant cause of death in this country.

TABLE 4.1.   **Incidence and costs of injury in the United States**

	Incidence	Medical Costs	Productivity Losses	Total Costs
Fatal	149,075	$1 billion	$142 billion	$143 billion
Hospitalized	1,869,857	$34 billion	$59 billion	$92 billion
Nonhospitalized	48,108,166	$45 billion	$125 billion	$171 billion
Total	50,127,098	$80 billion	$326 billion	$406 billion

Note: Totals rounded.
Source: Finkelstein, Corso, & Miller, 2006.

Although injuries, both intentional and unintentional, cause significant morbidity and mortality in the community and the workplace, we do not have to accept either type of injury as a completely unpredictable, random event. There is a real need for a strong public health presence in the form of better surveillance programs to prevent injuries. The science of epidemiology can lead to the discovery of causes of injuries in the workplace as well as the development of strategies for prevention and control.

The importance of injury control in the U.S. workplace is seen in the document *Healthy People 2010* (U.S. Department of Health and Human Services, 2000). As we noted in Chapter One, Table 1.2, decreasing work-related injuries is represented in five of the eleven occupational safety and health objectives for Goal 20 of the Healthy People 2010 program ("promote the health and safety of people at work through prevention and early intervention"). These five objectives involve

Work-related injury deaths

Work-related injuries

Work-related homicides

Work-related assaults

Needle stick injuries

The goal and objectives of this important program offer a clear starting point for the development, implementation, and evaluation of injury control programs in the workplace.

THE CASE FOR AN EPIDEMIOLOGICAL APPROACH

With stated national objectives for reducing workplace injuries, public health agencies are able to assign responsibility to skilled staff to deal with injuries in the community and the workplace. Injuries fit a case definition; they can be part of an ongoing surveillance system; they can be compared by age, gender, occupation, and geographical location; and most important, they can be prevented. In this way they are similar to disease and therefore lend themselves to an epidemiological approach to discover their cause. They have a societal impact similar to that of a chronic disease in that they can cause long-term medical problems for the individual and they cost a great deal of money. As we come to better understand their epidemiology we should be able to develop and implement better injury prevention programs. Figure 4.1 displays data from a well-developed surveillance system through which injuries are reported with the intent to discover the cause and reduce the incidence of these injuries in the workplace.

The data in this figure allow public health agencies to learn what age group is most affected by fatal injuries. The epidemic of fatal occupational injuries begins with the youngest worker and concludes at the normal age of retirement. In 2002, it peaked in the age range from thirty-five to forty-four, with 25.4 percent, or 1,402 cases, and then slowly dropped again as age and perhaps experience at the job increased. People

FIGURE 4.1. *Distribution of hours worked and occupational injury and illness cases with days away from work in private industry by age of worker, 2001.*

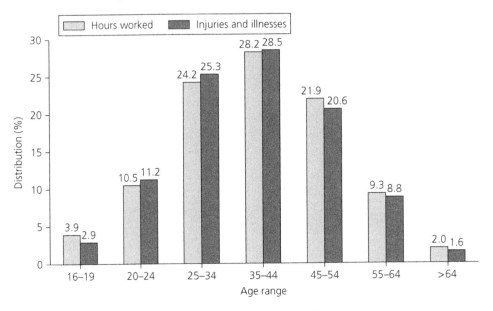

Note: For workers aged 20-44, the percentage of total injuries and illnesses was greater than the percentage of total hours worked. Together, these workers accounted for the majority of injured or ill workers. This surveillance data allows us to now look at potential causes of this injury and illness problem.

Source: NIOSH, 2004, fig. 1-27.

in the twenty-five to forty-four age range suffered a disproportionately high percentage (43.9 percent) of the fatal occupational injuries considering they made up only 35.3 percent of the total workforce. This age group is where greater prevention efforts must be directed. The reasons for this disparity are not clearly known, but among the many contributing factors are experience, family situations, and peer pressure.

Figures 4.2, 4.3, 4.4, 4.5, and 4.6 describe various **demographic characteristics** and **epidemiological characteristics** of U.S. workers in relation to injuries and illnesses. Such data allow public health agencies and businesses to see the absenteeism by occupation, industry sector, nature of health problem, body part affected, and source of injury, giving policymakers and public health officials a better understanding of where the workplace injury and illness problems are occurring. Such data also give employers a better understanding of the value of disease and injury prevention programs developed and implemented in their workplaces.

As injuries were studied over the years by public health departments, it became clear that they were not random events. The more that public health professionals have learned about injuries, whether accidents or the results of violent acts, the more they have become convinced that injuries can be understood and prevented. In 1972, William Haddon, a public health physician for the New York State Health Department,

FIGURE 4.2. *Number of occupational injuries and illnesses with days away from work in private industry for selected occupations, 1992–2001.*

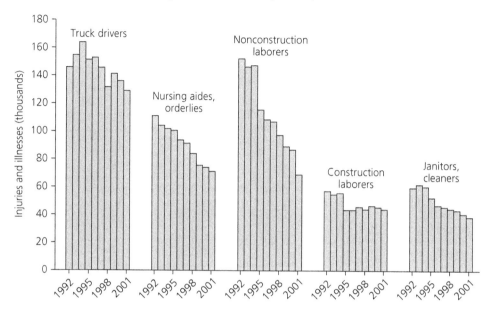

Source: NIOSH, 2004, fig. 1-32.

FIGURE 4.3. *Distribution of nonfatal injury cases with days away from work and nonfatal injury plus illness cases by private industry sector, 2001.*

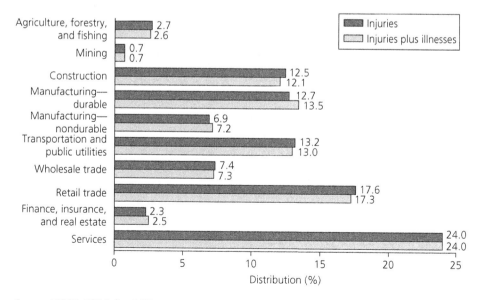

Source: NIOSH, 2004, fig. 1-33.

FIGURE 4.4. *Median days away from work due to occupational injuries or illnesses in private industry by nature of injury or illness, 2001.*

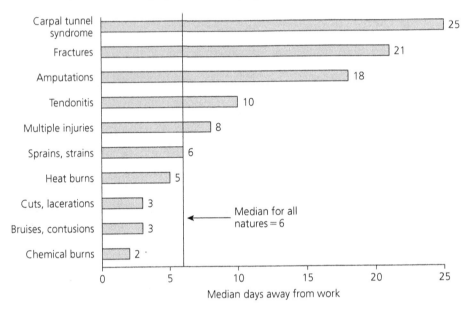

Source: NIOSH, 2004, fig. 1-37.

FIGURE 4.5. *Distribution of occupational injury and illness cases with days away from work in private industry by body part affected, 2001.*

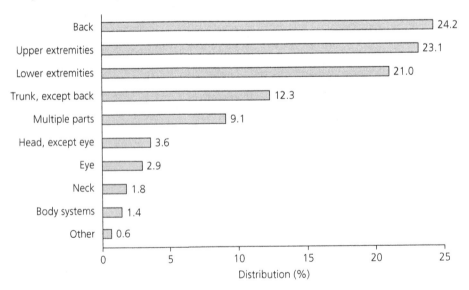

Source: NIOSH, 2004, fig. 1-38.

FIGURE 4.6.   *Distribution of occupational injury and illness cases with days away from work in private industry by source of injury or illness, 2001.*

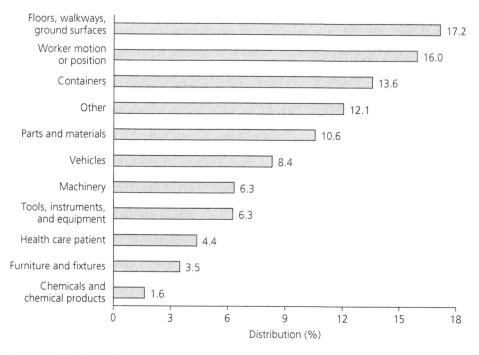

Source: NIOSH, 2004, fig. 1-40.

earned his place in history as the "father of injury epidemiology and injury control" with his publication of "A Logical Framework for Categorizing Highway Safety Phenomena and Activity." This was his study of accidents when he was well aware of the epidemiological dimension of this rapidly developing public health epidemic. His approach, now known as the **Haddon matrix**, organized accidents into three phases:

1. Pre-event

2. Event

3. Post-event

The process of host, agent, and environment; relative risk; and the determinants of the event all play a part in the occurrence of all injuries. At the very least, using epidemiology to confront this public health problem allows us to think about prevention in a new way. The step-by-step process developed by Haddon is very similar to the communicable disease process we discussed in Chapter Three. It allows public health to intervene at an early stage in the injury process in order to effect a change in the outcome.

In the pre-event (or pre-injury) phase, one can introduce focused injury education programs, both in the workplace and the general community, in order to prevent this

FIGURE 4.7.   *The Haddon matrix.*

Factors phases	Human factor	Agent or vehicle	Physical environment	Sociocultural environment
Pre-event				
Event				
Post-event				

Source: Centers for Disease Control and Prevention, 2005.

phase from ever occurring or from continuing into the second phase where the event (injury) actually happens. The Haddon matrix is further developed in Figure 4.7 to include additional variables that may be present in the process of injury occurrence.

Medicine has always been most comfortable dealing with a single cause of disease and illness. In this medical model patients and physicians usually wait until illness occurs to take action. When illness appears, physicians look for a single cause and a single treatment of that cause. This method worked well until medicine was faced with the emerging threat of chronic diseases, which have multiple causes and develop over a long period of time. These diseases also have no cure once discovered in a person. Injuries have presented a similar problem for medicine in that waiting for them to happen opens up the possibility that there can be no cure, just disability or death.

Haddon's matrix offers a model allowing us to think about everything that has led up to an injury and everything that has happened after that injury takes place. It resembles other epidemiological models used for years to help epidemiologists find the causes of other diseases and conditions that were terrorizing populations.

Haddon's matrix clearly placed injuries in the framework of events important to public health and requiring public health solutions. The science of epidemiology, which had been so successful in dealing with communicable diseases, seemed the required tool for dealing with the control of injuries. Using successful methods of public health thinking, employers and agencies can develop ways to limit the damage caused by the injury and at the same time develop approaches to prevention before the injury can take place.

Table 4.2 displays countermeasures that might be applied to reduce the risks of injury caused by handguns and of cancer caused by tobacco use. These countermeasures are focused on the introduction of a *hazard*, defined by McKenzie et al. (2005) as an unsafe act or unsafe condition that increases the probability that an unintentional injury will occur. In Table 4.2, the concept of an unsafe act is expanded to include high-risk behavior that may cause a chronic disease like cancer. Among the ten types of countermeasures are preventing the hazard, reducing the amount of hazard, modifying the qualities of the hazard, and increasing resistance to the hazard. These same ten

TABLE 4.2.   **Application of the Haddon countermeasures to reducing risks of injury by handguns and of cancer associated with smoking**

Countermeasure 1: Prevent the creation of the hazard

Eliminate handguns	Eliminate cigarettes

Countermeasure 2: Reduce the amount of hazard brought into being

Limit the number of handguns allowed to be sold or purchased	Reduce the volume of tobacco production by changing agricultural policy

Countermeasure 3: Prevent the release of the hazard

Install locks on handguns	Limit sales of tobacco to certain age groups

Countermeasure 4: Modify the rate of release of the hazard from its source

Eliminate automatic handguns	Develop cigarettes that burn more slowly

Countermeasure 5: Separate the hazard from that which is to be protected by time and space

Store handguns only at gun clubs rather than at home	Establish shutoff times for vending machines and earlier closings of convenience stores and groceries

Countermeasure 6: Separate the hazard from that which is to be protected by a physical barrier

Keep guns in locked containers	Install filters on cigarettes

Countermeasure 7: Modify relevant basic qualities of the hazard

Personalize guns so they can be fired only by the owner	Reduce the nicotine content of cigarettes

Countermeasure 8: Make what is to be protected more resistant to damage from the hazard

Create and market bullet-proof garments	Limit exposure to other potential synergistic causes of cancer (e.g., environmental carcinogens) among smokers

(continued)

TABLE 4.2.   **Application of the Haddon countermeasures to reducing risks of injury by handguns and of cancer associated with smoking** (*continued*)

Countermeasure 9: Begin to counter damage done by the hazard	
Provide good access to emergency care in the prehospital period	Set up screening to detect cancer in the early stages
Countermeasure 10: Stabilize, repair, and rehabilitate the object of damage	
Provide high-quality trauma care in hospitals	Provide good-quality health care for cancer patients

Source: Runyan, 2003.

types of countermeasures can be used effectively against a whole host of hazards found in the workplace and capable of causing injury and illness to workers. According to Runyan (2003), the Haddon model is applicable to any health problem because of its ability to add a conceptual approach to problems through research and intervention.

EPIDEMIOLOGY OF ACCIDENTS

Unintentional injuries (accidents) are the leading cause of death among all individuals aged from one to thirty-four years. Hilgenkamp (2006) looks at unintentional injuries as events that because of errors in judgment, poor health, or physical inability to prevent them, cannot be avoided. This definition supports the labeling of these injuries as accidents, or events that are not deliberate. These types of injuries lend themselves to evaluation by epidemiologists in terms of time, place, and person. By using these tools in a careful evaluation of a worksite, public health agencies can begin to forecast unintentional injuries.

The most prevalent and perhaps the most preventable occupational fatal injuries (NIOSH, 2009) result from falls, motor vehicle accidents, and being struck by objects. Christoffel and Gallagher (2006) found that unintentional injuries constitute over two-thirds of all injury deaths and one-third of all emergency department visits, and they also point out that motor vehicle and fall injuries are very important in the occupational setting.

These most prevalent types of accidents in the workplace (falls, motor vehicle accidents, and being struck by an object) need to be evaluated in order to develop prevention programs that have a good chance of success.

Falls

The BLS (2005a) reports that fatal work injuries involving falls increased 17 percent in 2004, following two years of decline. The 815 falls reported in 2004 constituted the highest annual total ever reported for this injury category. Fatal falls from a roof increased almost 40 percent and fatal falls from a ladder increased 17 percent. Almost 90 percent of the fatal falls from roofs involved construction workers.

The epidemiological implications of these data are supportive of the development of prescreening programs and better education programs for workers concerning the major causes of falls in the workplace. This educational initiative needs to address where and when the falls usually occur and what the worker was typically trying to do at the time of the fall. The equipment available to prevent serious falls must be evaluated, and consideration must be given to limitation of the damage to the person if a fall does occur in the workplace. If employees are not using proper equipment to prevent or limit damage from falls, then consideration must be given to establishing a workplace policy concerning falls and to determining how to best enforce this policy.

Motor Vehicle Accidents

Occupational motor vehicle accidents also increased in 2004 after falling for the previous two years. The BLS (2005a) reported 1,374 fatal highway accidents in 2004, which represented 25 percent of the fatal work injuries in 2004. Almost 40 percent of motor vehicle accidents are a direct result of driving under the influence of alcohol, illegal drugs, or prescription drugs.

A large number of these motor vehicle accidents occurred while traveling to and from work and while traveling as an employee on work-related business. The implications of these data are that driver education is needed and also strong workplace policies concerning using seat belts and not driving under the influence of alcohol or drugs. By applying the Haddon matrix and sound epidemiological principles to these problems, a prevention program can be developed to reduce motor vehicle accidents in the workplace and reduce disability and death if these accidents do occur.

Being Struck by an Object

The number of workers fatally injured by being struck by objects rose 12 percent in 2004, led by a rise in the number of workers who were fatally injured by contact with falling, rolling, or sliding objects (BLS, 2005a). The implications of these data are that being struck by an object has become a dangerous and common occurrence in many workplaces. Again, the Haddon matrix allows an evaluation of the entire process required for this accident to happen so frequently to workers.

The key to preventing accidents in which people are struck by an object is the development of educational programs concerning the causes of such accidents and what the employer and employee need to do to prevent occurrences. This is another example of how important the pre-injury phase is in preventing the accident from happening or at least reducing disability and death when this type of accident does happen.

EPIDEMIOLOGY OF VIOLENCE

According to *Fear and Violence in the Workplace* (Lawless, 1993), 15 percent of workers surveyed said that they had been physically attacked at some time in their working lives. Although violent acts are all around us in society, this report shocked employers into considering the possibility that this serious problem could occur in their workplaces. Increasingly, **workplace violence** is viewed as a major problem that must be dealt with by the employer. The major categories of intentional injuries in the general population are the following:

- Homicide
- Suicide
- Assault
- Sexual assault
- Child abuse

In the workplace the major areas of concern are homicide, suicide, and assault. These problems of serious intentional injury of fellow workers lend themselves to epidemiological interpretation and public health resolution. Christoffel and Gallagher (2006) point out the patterns and risk factors common to all these categories: "access to firearms, alcohol abuse, maleness, certain childhood experiences (such as a personal history of abuse or violence, or of a parent or caregiver having committed suicide), and—most important—income disparity and poverty." Once the patterns of risk are discovered, education programs and workplace policies can be developed to prevent the problem.

Homicides

According to the BLS (2005c), homicides in the workplace were down sharply in 2004 to their lowest level ever recorded by the fatality census. Overall, workplace homicides are down almost 50 percent since 1994. These violent acts lend themselves very well to the regulatory approach to injury prevention, and these data indicate that since the 1990s, employers have taken the workplace homicide issue seriously and responded with programs that seem to have worked. Workplaces have provided education and anger management programs to workers to avoid this type of violent behavior both in and out of the workplace. The success in reducing workplace homicides, as cited by the Critical Incident Response Group, National Center for the Analysis of Violent Crime (2002), is a clear indication that the worker education process and strong antiviolence programs can make a difference in workplace violence.

Suicides

Suicide is death from an intentionally self-inflicted injury. It may happen anywhere, including home, school, or place of work. Christoffel and Gallagher (2006) report that it is the third leading cause of death among the age groups fifteen to twenty-four and twenty-five to thirty-four. The epidemiological characteristics of suicide are essentially the same whether the act occurs at home, school, or work.

The implications of these data are that this topic requires employers' serious attention in the form of pre-event education and counseling. Epidemiological study of suicide can be conducted in the hope of determining underlying causes for this personal form of violence.

Assaults

Most researchers in the area of injury by assault define *assault* as the use of physical force to cause harm to another person. Assault, which may be verbal as well as physical, happens often in the workplace. Many cases of assault go unreported, according to the Critical Incident Response Group (2002), because of fear of retribution and a feeling that nothing will be done about them anyway.

The implications of these data are that a better-developed surveillance system is needed to record assaults in the workplace. It is well known that the incidence of assaults in the workplace is much higher than formal reports indicate. More attention needs to be paid to this form of intentional violence committed in the workplace. Once the real numbers are discovered then employers need to make resources available to expand education and anger management programs for employees. Workers also need to be made aware that this type of behavior will not be tolerated in the workplace.

SURVEILLANCE SYSTEMS FOR OCCUPATIONAL INJURIES

Well-developed surveillance systems are a prerequisite to the development of public health programs and a requirement for determining the impact of any proposed intervention strategy. In order for public health principles to work in the areas of understanding injuries and, ultimately, preventing them, workplaces need extremely accurate surveillance systems.

Christoffel and Gallagher (2006) state that the death certificate is one of the most important tools for monitoring the health of the U.S. population. The form has been revised in recent years in order to improve the data quality for work-related injuries, because better accuracy in occupational injury reporting is a prerequisite to a better understanding of the true causes of these injuries. Nevertheless, the information derived from death certificates is only as accurate as the information provided by the certifier. The medical examiner is usually charged with this responsibility. According to Miniño, Anderson, Fingerhut, Boudreault, & Warner (2006), little is in fact known regarding the accuracy of the reported circumstances and causes of injury mortality. Lack of specificity is also an issue when researchers are trying to analyze injury diagnoses.

Moreover, Rosenman et al. (2006) believe that the National Electronic Injury Surveillance System may miss two-thirds of the total number of occupational injuries. This level of inaccuracy would of course make it nearly impossible to design a sound epidemiological intervention for this public health problem that is expensive in terms of both human life and workplace productivity. A complete evaluation of the current data collection process is justified, as are improvements in data reporting and accuracy.

SURVEILLANCE RESULTS

Good data concerning occupational injuries are a prerequisite to the development, implementation, and evaluation of injury prevention programs in the workplace. Without reputable data it will be impossible to gain the support of employers in offering injury prevention programs to their employees. This section presents examples of current surveillance results.

Surveillance data on fatal injuries in the workplace have been gathered by the Bureau of Labor Statistics since 1992, and the BLS (2005a) reports that a total of 5,703 fatal work injuries were recorded in the United States in 2004, an increase of 2 percent from work injuries reported in 2003. (See Figure 4.8 for some historical data on fatal injuries in the workplace.) The Census of Fatal Occupational Injuries (CFOI) that the BLS conducts categorizes fatal injuries in many different ways: by manner, by industry, by demographic characteristics, and so forth.

In an effort to better understand both fatal and nonfatal occupational injuries and illnesses, NIOSH collects data on them through the National Electronic Injury Surveillance System (NEISS), the emergency department–based surveillance system.

FIGURE 4.8. *Number and rate of fatal occupational injuries, 1992–2002.*

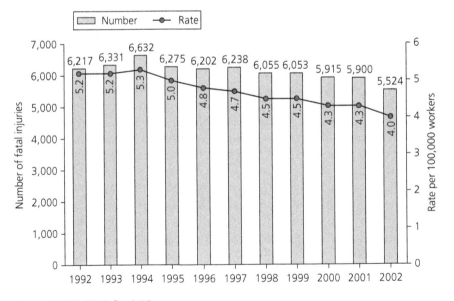

Source: NIOSH, 2004, fig. 2-16.

Many of these data are available in the *Worker Health Chartbook, 2004*, compiled by NIOSH along with other important sources of data found at the NIOSH Web site.

A total of 5,524 fatal occupational injuries were recorded in 2002. During the period 1992–2002, fatality rates declined from 5.2 per 100,000 workers to 4.0.

Private industry reported 5.2 million nonfatal occupational injuries and illnesses in 2001, which translated into an overall incidence rate of 5.7 cases per 100 full-time workers, representing a decrease of 34 percent since 1992. The durable goods manufacturing industry had the highest rate of nonfatal injuries and illnesses reported in 2001, at 8.8 per 100 workers followed by construction (7.9), and agriculture, forestry, and fishing (7.3). The services industry reported 1.3 million cases, or 25 percent, of all nonfatal occupational injuries and illnesses in 2001.

The number of total recordable occupational injuries reached a high of 6.4 million cases in 1990, then declined to a low of 4.9 million in 2001 (see Figure 4.9).

Data such as these allow us to prioritize industries according to their need for more training and regulation.

The CDC (2009c) reports that the lifetime costs of injuries in a single year in the United States total $408 billion in medical expenses and in productivity losses in the workplace. This includes nearly $82 billion in medical costs; $326 billion is linked to lifetime productivity losses.

FIGURE 4.9.   *Number of occupational injury cases by type of case in private industry, 1976-2001.*

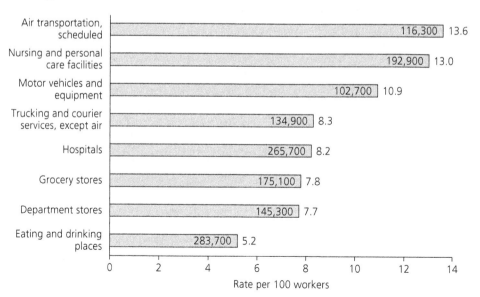

Source: NIOSH, 2004, fig. 2-69.

Occupational Injuries and Illnesses by Demographic Characteristics

According to NIOSH (2009), in 2002 two-thirds of all fatally injured workers were aged twenty-five to fifty-four, with the highest percentage (25 percent) of fatalities reported for workers aged thirty-five to forty-four. Before 1998, black workers had slightly higher fatal occupational injury rates, but after 1998 the rates for white workers were slightly higher than all other races. Male workers held 53.7 percent of the jobs in 2002 and incurred 92 percent of the reported injuries. In 2006, it was reported that younger male workers continued to have the highest overall rates of injury and illness. Male workers in general also had substantially higher hospitalization rates than female workers in general ("Nonfatal Occupational Injuries and Illnesses Among Workers Treated in Hospital Emergency Departments," 2006). These data again allow us to concentrate our attention on the education of those individuals in the high-risk groups in workplaces.

Health Care: A High-Risk Occupation

There are eight million health care workers who may be exposed on a daily basis to occupational bloodborne viral infections that are potentially fatal. These viruses are the hepatitis B and C viruses and the HIV virus, which causes acquired immunodeficiency syndrome (AIDS) (see Figure 4.10). Over 80 percent of the contacts with blood or other potentially infected body fluids occur through percutaneous injuries (injuries

FIGURE 4.10. *Distribution and number of documented cases of occupational transmission of HIV among health care workers by occupation, 1981–2001.*

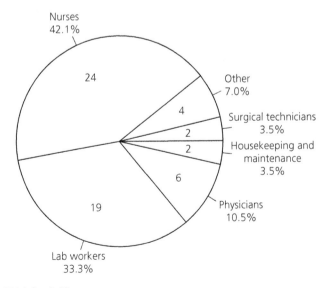

Source: NIOSH, 2004, fig. 2-12.

through the skin) with contaminated sharp instruments such as needles and scalpels. After percutaneous injury with a contaminated sharp instrument, the average risk of infection is 0.3 percent for HIV and ranges from 6 to 30 percent for hepatitis B.

Immunization for health care workers and the practice of universal precautions by those who come in contact with body fluids in their working environment has significantly reduced infections with HIV and hepatitis B and C viruses.

Figures 4.11, 4.12, and 4.13 give us additional valuable information about the dangers associated with working in the health care field. The data also reveal high-risk practices that predispose health workers to infection with dangerous viruses.

INJURY PREVENTION PROGRAMS

Injury prevention has two major components: anticipation of potential hazards and design of the worksite. Well-developed surveillance systems with good data can help the employer anticipate potential injuries, be they accidents or violent acts. Injuries should no longer be considered random acts that result from being in the wrong place at the wrong time. Instead, employers should think of them as high-cost events in terms of medical expenses and lost productivity, costs paid by the worker, the employer, and ultimately the consumer. However, many companies miss the distinction between mere compliance and proactive prevention. In addition, the amount currently being

FIGURE 4.11.   *Estimated number of occupational hepatitis B infections among U.S. health care workers, 1983–2000.*

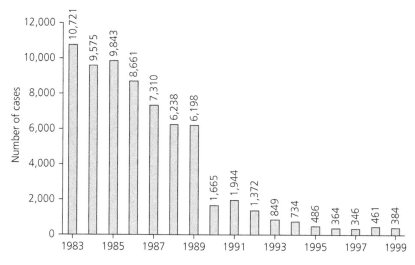

Source: NIOSH, 2004, fig. 2-10.

FIGURE 4.12. *Distribution of 10,378 reported percutaneous injuries among hospital workers by medical device associated with the injury, 1995–2000.*

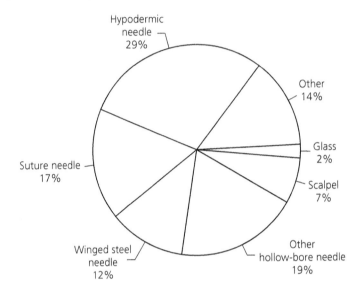

Source: NIOSH, 2004, fig. 2-13.

FIGURE 4.13. *Distribution of 6,212 reported percutaneous injuries involving hollow-bore needles in hospital workers by associated medical procedure, 1995–2000.*

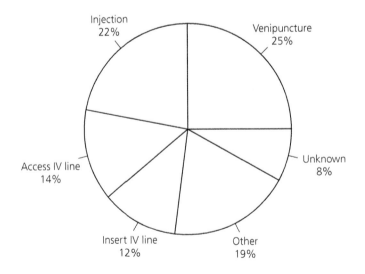

Source: NIOSH, 2004, fig. 2-14.

spent by the federal government on injury prevention is small when compared to the dollars allocated to most chronic diseases. This does not seem to be a wise decision when one considers the years of potential life lost to injuries. It makes economic sense for an employer to have a well-designed injury prevention program in the workplace. Chapter Five examines the case for active prevention in greater detail. Here we will look at constructing a strong prevention program.

McKenzie et al. (2005) discuss the steps necessary to design an injury prevention program, as outlined in the following sections.

Define the Problem, Collect Data, Conduct Surveillance

The epidemiological model can be easily employed in developing injury prevention programs as long as the problem is well understood. That is why the problem definition requires continuous data collection along with accurate surveillance systems. Too often policymakers are defining symptoms of the problem rather than dealing with the real problem that needs to be overcome to solve the public health issue. Good data can help us deal with the definition of the real problem. Once the real problem is better identified, the surveillance systems for that particular problem can become more sensitive and can gather precise data about the problem in question.

One process that can be used in both defining the problem and identifying causes is a **behavior-based safety** (BBS) system. Many of the companies practicing prevention are also using various forms of behavior-based safety programs and processes. A behavior-based safety system looks at actions of people and tries to ensure that individuals do the right things at the right time. There are many BBS variations and numerous consulting companies offering their solution as the best. In the 1990s, behavior-based safety was one of the hottest ideas in the safety world. Many consultants were peddling BBS as the solution to all safety ills, promising that for a large chunk of cash injuries would suddenly go away. The reality of implementing a BBS system is very different. Because BBS did not deliver instant results in most places or sustainable results where some initial results were seen, it got a bad reputation. Nevertheless, many companies with outstanding safety results are still practicing BBS and continue to improve. At a large consumer goods company, of which one of the authors has personal experience, the entire health and safety process is based on BBS and the company's injury and illness rates continue to slowly decline, despite multiple changes in leadership in both direct operational management and safety.

Behavior-based safety is one of the best prevention tools available because when properly implemented, it gets all employees and managers involved in the improvement process by gathering everyone's input and ideas on what the priorities should be. A well-implemented BBS system will take some time to show results, but as it gains traction with employees and managers, it could be a means to continually reduce the frequency and severity of injuries and illnesses. A good BBS system will start by educating managers to the reality that employees will do whatever their leader requires them to do, sometimes at risk of injury to themselves. This then translates to requiring managers to look at themselves and ask what signals they are sending (consciously or subconsciously) to the employees. Next, an analysis of behaviors is conducted to identify the behaviors most likely to result in an injury. Actions are then taken to implement a systemic fix. This fix might be to change the physical layout of equipment, the way the work is done, the procedures followed by employees, or simply employees' bad habits, behaviors, and attitudes.

Identify Causes

After collecting the data, the next step in injury prevention consists of the identification of causes, better known as *risk factor identification*. What places some people at high risk of becoming victims of an injury and allows others to escape the event? Quite often the answer to this question is better education. Those at high risk for injury seem unable to envision the many potential consequences of their risky behavior in the workplace.

Develop and Test Interventions

Once causes are known, the next step is to develop and test interventions to prevent the injury. This involves the use of an injury model such as the matrix developed by William Haddon. This model helps knowledgeable individuals to not just look at the injury as it happens but also to evaluate what preceded the injury and what immediately followed the injury. By looking at injuries in this way one may see, for example, that perhaps an event does not have to be prevented in order to prevent disability or death. The best example of this concept is the use of a seat belt when driving a vehicle. The seat belt does not prevent an accident, but it may reduce the human damage resulting from the accident.

Research Evaluation Techniques

Once appropriate interventions are proposed, evaluation techniques need to be developed that can be used to answer questions such as these: What is the desired impact of the program, and how do we know if we have achieved the objectives leading to this impact? In other words, how do we know if the proposed intervention is worth what it costs, and should we entertain other potential intervention strategies?

Implement Interventions, Measure Prevention Effectiveness

After a thorough evaluation of potential interventions, the one with the best chance of successfully eliminating the pre-event causation or risk factor should be chosen and implemented. The company should have a strong implementation plan in place, with its own evaluation process, in order to have the best chance for a successful launch of the new injury prevention program. Many implementation strategies fail because of unforeseen events. The more individuals (stakeholders) involved in this stage, the better. The timetable for implementation must be agreed on at an early stage so that this step does not get bogged down in personalities, delaying the launch of the new injury prevention program.

Involve the Community

Prior to actual launch of the injury intervention project, the major stakeholders need to be made aware of the new project, including the reasons behind the project and the results the project hopes to attain. A select group of workers and managers needs to see a demonstration of the new program. Effective injury prevention programs also require a tremendous amount of collaboration with local public health departments.

Conduct Demonstration Programs

Demonstrations of the new program need to be given to those responsible for the process. The stakeholders in an industry include members of management, support staff, union members if a union is present, and the employees.

Provide Training

At this point a training program should be established for all employees and supervisors to prepare them to use the new program to prevent injuries in their workplace and to gain their support for the program.

Raise Public Awareness

Successful prevention initiatives will garner public support, which may translate into political and industry support as well. Companies should publicize and reward decreases in injuries and illnesses via public and internal communication efforts and internal rewards processes. This kind of encouragement promotes injury reduction at home and in the workplace.

If all of these steps as outlined by McKenzie et al. (2005) are followed, a new injury prevention program has a good chance of success.

FUTURE CHALLENGES

Many challenges face this country as it attempts to protect employees from unintentional and intentional injuries. Here are five that we consider of particular importance.

Ergonomics

The science of ergonomics deals with making interactions between people and things more efficient. Issues such as repetitive motion, excessive vibration, eye strain, and heavy lifting may require ergonomic solutions to avoid lower-back injuries, carpal tunnel syndrome, and other serious physical problems. According to NIOSH (2006), even though attention paid to ergonomics can have large payoffs in terms of injury reduction and increased productivity, the injuries these workplace physical strains cause do not appear to be decreasing. More will be said about this problem in Chapter Eleven.

Aging Workforce

American workers face stressful demands to be more productive in order to compete with the products and services of cheaper foreign labor. At the same time, the workforce overall is aging, and many individuals are showing signs of disability. If U.S. production continues to rely on the experience of the older worker, health and wellness should be encouraged and rewarded through sponsored wellness and injury prevention programs. The issue of age is discussed again briefly in Chapter Fourteen.

Funding Issues

Because investments in prevention programs do not have immediate payoffs, prevention programs have been experiencing government budget cuts at both the federal and state levels. The fact is that more, not fewer, resources need to be allocated to injury control programs.

Complacency

As the numbers of reported injuries in the workplace decrease, we may tend to become complacent with our success. Public health has a long history of developing successful community health programs and finding that the greater success of these programs causes reduced future funding. Moreover, our victories in decreasing the number of workplace injuries are continually countered by rapidly changing technologies that are creating new health and injury concerns. These changes demand that we continually maintain and increase funding for research on workplace injuries and for implementation of injury prevention programs.

Prevention Versus Limitation of Damage

Many workplace safety programs are referred to as *injury control* programs. This title is indicative of a short-sighted attitude that seeks limitation of injury (control) rather than complete *prevention* of injury. It fails to see the real costs of injuries and the potential dollars that could be saved if these injuries never occurred in the first place. Prevention must be paramount if we are to make the gains in worker health and safety that we know are possible.

SUMMARY

Injuries have always been accepted as an inevitable occurrence in the workplace. Now that public health has largely won the war against most communicable diseases, greater attention and resources are available to concentrate on injury prevention. However, the epidemiology of injuries is not as straightforward as the epidemiology of communicable disease. The political dimensions of workplace regulation to ensure protection from the mere potential for injury or illness require us to muster tremendous amounts of data and more effective awareness efforts so we can demonstrate the potential ramifications of the current epidemic of injuries in the workplace.

Despite these limitations great success has already been achieved by the Occupational Safety and Health Administration (OSHA) and NIOSH in their effort to better define injuries and enforce prevention efforts. The industries most susceptible to fatal and nonfatal injuries are now known, the types of injuries that are most prevalent and the demographics of injuries are now known, and in many instances the best ways to prevent injuries or at least to lessen their impact are also known.

The large number of injuries that occur on a daily basis can be addressed most effectively by a public health model of prevention. Analyzing an injury in terms of the three phases of the Haddon matrix allows us to consider not only the actual injury event but also what happens before and after the injury. The major prerequisite to understanding and preventing injuries is the development and implementation of a good injury surveillance system.

The epidemiological model can easily be used to develop an injury prevention program once the injury is well understood. Very good prevention models are available that have been developed, implemented, and evaluated by public health experts. Between the guidance offered by the Healthy People 2010 program and the use of the Haddon matrix model, the development of workplace injury prevention programs has become much easier. Nevertheless these models need to be expanded and further improved because injuries rank exceptionally high on comparative reports of years of productive life lost (YPLL) and yet injuries are preventable.

Injuries are usually considered easier to deal with than illnesses are, for the following reasons:

- Trauma occurs in real time with no latency period (the sequence of events is immediate)

- Accident or incident outcomes are readily observable (one has to reconstruct only a few minutes or hours)

- Root or basic causes can be more clearly identified

- It is easy to detect cause-and-effect relationships

- Trauma is not difficult to diagnose

- Trauma is highly preventable

Illnesses are more difficult to deal with, for the following reasons:

- They usually have a latency period between the infection or other beginning event and the development of identifiable signs and symptoms.

- Exposures may not be readily observable and may be linked to personal habits and individual encounters with hazards. Multiple exposures and synergistic effects on the job and off the job may be involved.

- It is not always easy to detect cause-and-effect relationships

- They may be difficult to diagnose because symptoms may not be definitive at first.

KEY TERMS

behavior-based safety
demographic characteristics
epidemiological characteristics

Haddon matrix
injury
workplace violence

QUESTIONS FOR DISCUSSION

1. How does the practice of epidemiology procedure assist in determining the causes of workplace injuries and illnesses?

2. What are the various models that can be used to explain injury and illness occurrences? Describe them.

3. Why has workplace violence become a major topic for all employers?

4. How could you take the approaches discussed here and apply them in your workplace?

CHAPTER

COMPLIANCE VERSUS PREVENTION

After reading this chapter, you should be able to

- Understand the difference between prevention of injuries and illnesses and OSHA compliance, and explain why prevention is more valuable.

- Explain the evolution of OSHA and the changes that it has caused in the choices employers make.

- Discuss the OSHA standards development process.

- Discuss some of the costs of workers' compensation.

- Explain the basic OSHA inspection process and what a successful inspection looks like.

A key point many companies miss is whether they are practicing Occupational Safety and Health Administration (OSHA) compliance or using OSHA information as a minimum reference for establishing programs to prevent injury and illness. The mission of OSHA is "to promote the safety and health of America's workers by setting and enforcing standards; providing training, outreach, and education; establishing partnerships; and encouraging continual improvement in workplace safety and health" (OSHA, 2006). This is quite a change from OSHA's original focus, which was understood by most organizations and people to be solely to reduce workplace deaths. The injury statistics shown in Figures 5.1 and 5.2 illustrate the magnitude of the need for prevention and the reason compliance with the minimal OSHA standards is not enough.

As OSHA got started in the 1970s, it began to develop standards and adopted some national consensus standards as ones it would enforce. In those early years OSHA was renowned for its ability to identify minor infractions and turn them into citations and fines. Because a large number of these citations related more to administrative lapses than to actual **employee hazards,** an adversarial relationship developed between businesses and OSHA.

As OSHA has evolved over the last fifteen years, some of its focus has been on cooperation with employers, at least those who actually try to prevent and reduce workplace injuries, illnesses, and deaths. As OSHA has taken on lessons from the

FIGURE 5.1. *Numbers and rates of traumatic occupational fatalities, 1980–2000.*

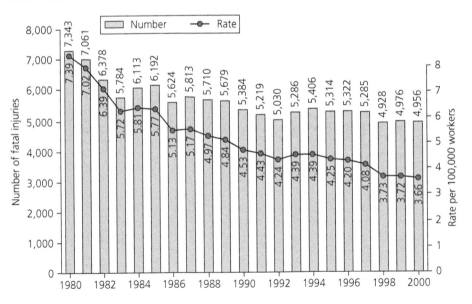

Source: NIOSH, 2004. fig. 2-15.

FIGURE 5.2.   *Number of occupational injury cases by type of case in private industry, 1976–2001.*

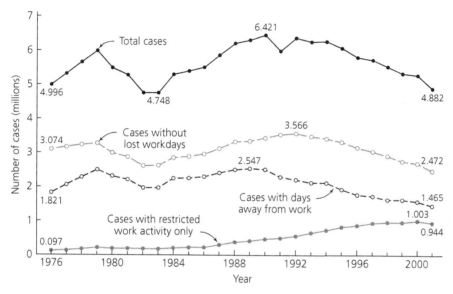

Source: NIOSH, 2004. fig. 2-69.

nation, fewer of its efforts are concentrated on telling employers in detail how to achieve a safe workplace, and more are going to telling them what they need to accomplish. Standards developed and promulgated by OSHA until the late 1980s spelled out exactly what the agency expected every employer to do and how to do it. This was a one-size-fits-all approach that failed to take into account the varied needs, designs, processes, and the like, of the millions of workplaces. After much critiquing by many sources, OSHA started to issue standards that told employers what they must accomplish (**performance-based standards**) rather than exactly what they must do (specification-based standards). From the employers' viewpoint this has been a mixed blessing. The employer can use creativity to meet the requirement but the occurrence of an event such as an injury is judged an obvious failure to meet the requirement. A few employers have lobbied for a return to the old system, but the huge majority prefer the performance approach.

As it has matured, OSHA has also developed cooperative processes, ranging from the **Voluntary Protection Program** (VPP) to alliances with various local, state, and national organizations. These are intended to allow OSHA to use its limited resources to concentrate on the "bad actors." Another part of this evolution has been an increased effort to find the bad actors and hold them accountable. Joining the VPP or an alliance offers some advantages to employers: improvement in safety and health results (which usually means reduced workers' compensation costs), removal from the programmed inspection process, and good publicity. From many employers' perspectives, however, the cooperative process requires too much paperwork and also opens them up to the annual detailed inspections needed to maintain their VPP or alliance status.

OSHA STANDARDS DEVELOPMENT

As part of the examination of the compliance versus prevention choice that employers make, a brief overview of the origin and interpretation of OSHA standards and the process of developing a standard is in order. A standard typically grows out of a workplace problem; a set of injuries, illnesses, or fatalities that gain some attention nationally via the media; OSHA's data analysis; a political leader; or the OSHA secretary. Once this problem is recognized, OSHA may start its rulemaking process.

The actual process is mandated by law and can take years to come to fruition. For example, developing the confined space entry standard took over ten years and still does not apply to the construction industry, and the ergonomics standard has been on the docket for over fourteen years with no final rule in place. (An ergonomics standard was issued in the last days of the Clinton administration but it was negated by a vote in Congress shortly after the change of administrations. Ergonomics are discussed in more detail in Chapter Eleven.)

The process of rulemaking seems to take forever because the process is as much about politics as it is about health and safety. All parties that are interested in the problem addressed by the rule can provide input such as "make changes," "stop it dead," or "hang it up in the bureaucracy." The interested parties include organized labor; the Chamber of Commerce and other associations supporting business; health, safety, industrial hygiene, and fire protection organizations; small business advocates; and politicians; and there are many others. These groups all want the final rule to represent their point of view and their desired level of mandatory actions for employers. Naturally, some of these groups are at extreme opposite ends of the spectrum in terms of how onerous the requirements should be. However, exceptions to this politicized process do occur, as when the steel erection rulemaking committee, which was composed of the major interested parties, developed and issued an updated standard for construction.

OSHA has to walk through the minefields laid by all the interested groups to get even a draft standard distributed. Once this occurs, the real fight begins. Anyone in the United States is allowed to comment on a draft standard, and OSHA must answer every comment. This can be overwhelming. When OSHA published a draft indoor air quality standard, it was viewed as an antismoking standard rather than an attempt to regulate air quality for the workplace and to factor in such newly discovered issues as **sick building syndrome** (SBS), building related illness (BRI), and occupational asthma. OSHA received over 100,000 comments on this standard alone. The OSHA team (these teams typically have two to five members) working on this standard was overwhelmed. The standard languished for several years and then disappeared completely. Even when OSHA gets a standard through to final rule status, parties who are not happy with the final version can and do take the agency to court. The standard may not be stringent enough in the view of some; others may view it as too burdensome on business. The court's decision can range from complete invalidation of the standard (which requires OSHA to start over) to a win for OSHA, with everything imaginable in between. The best way to view an OSHA standard is that it is the "best" requirement OSHA can get through the process it is required to use. It is not the best that it could be for either employees or employers; it is just the amount of regulation that both sides and all other interested parties are willing to live with.

The steps in a typical rulemaking process are

- Advance notice of proposed rulemaking: OSHA asks for information on the extent of the problem and possible solutions.

- Notice of proposed rulemaking: OSHA tells everyone what the agency is thinking of writing about.

- Draft standard: OSHA puts down on paper and issues to the public its proposed standard and requirements.

- Final standard: OSHA has taken all the input from public meetings, written comments, and so forth, and has written what the agency believes to be a good set of requirements.

- **Small business impact review:** the Small Business Administration reviews the rule to ensure it is not excessively burdensome to small businesses.

- Office of Management and Budget review: in this final step before the rule is published in the Federal Register, the White House gets to have the final take and input. This normally does not change the requirements, but it may require significant rework.

For an employer, the consequences of working to ensure only **OSHA compliance** are significant. Doing the bare minimum required by a convoluted, lowest-acceptable-outcome process to provide a safe and healthy workplace for employees results in spending a lot of time checking for items that have little to no bearing on whether or not an employee gets hurt. (Figure 5.3 displays the actual leading causes of fatal injuries from 1980 to 1998.)

Many times a workplace safety leader (such as a safety manager or safety representatives) will inspect an area and pick out all the compliance issues, such as no labels on containers, improper or no labels on exits, and guards that are not securely fastened. These will all get noted as requiring follow-up. Although these issues may lead to injuries or illnesses or in the worst case, fatalities, their likelihood and frequency of being risk factors is relatively low. Meanwhile the safety leader may miss issues whose frequency and likelihood of resulting in an injury is much greater, such as workers adopting an improper body position for lifting, pulling instead of pushing heavy objects across the floor, or failing to use all required personal protective equipment.

FIGURE 5.3. *Annual rate of fatal occupational injuries by leading cause, 1980–1998.*

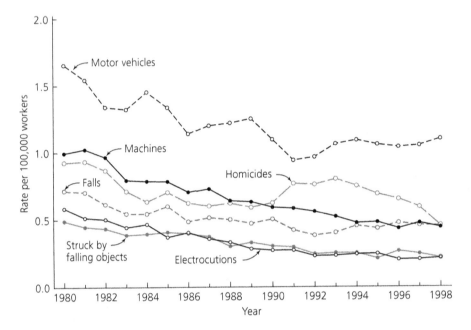

Source: NIOSH, 2004, fig. 2-23.

Concentrating efforts on compliance only does not do much if anything to improve either the workplace or the business. Injuries and illnesses and possibly fatalities may be lower than they would be if nothing at all were done, but they will still occur. Most employers also have a tough time looking for and taking preventive actions against the less likely events that could result in a catastrophe. Nevertheless, an organization that is truly working to prevent injuries, illnesses, and fatalities should use a prioritization process to ensure that it does not overlook these infrequent but extremely severe incidents.

Focusing on only the compliance issues is significant because it ends up costing the employer much more in workers' compensation costs than the employer would pay to implement a proactive, prevention-oriented approach. For example, OSHA, as mentioned earlier, does not have an ergonomics standard, so no manual-lifting requirements formally exist. With no real requirement to assess known lifting issues such as size, shape, grip, configuration, frequency of lifting, and duration of the work in order to ensure employee safety, an employer just complying with OSHA may think it okay to ask employees to lift almost anything. Employees will find ways to get the work done at almost any cost to themselves. The consequence to the employer may be an employee with a back injury. The average medical and indemnity (wage replacement) costs of a back injury in the United States today come to $19,479 (National Safety Council, 2006). This does not include any indirect costs associated with the incident. In a detailed study of costs in Washington State (Washington State Department of Labor and Industries, 2005), it was found that the average direct cost of a back injury claim paid by the state fund was $8,723 and there were 21,486 of these claims per year, which represents 1.6 Washington workers out of every 100 incurring a back injury per year. The cost of finding and installing lifting devices and machines to avoid injuries is much less. These machines do not necessarily cost hundreds of thousands of dollars; some are simple pneumatic lifting devices that can be readily manipulated to replace the human back in lifting requiring a crane-like action. Alternatively, simple process redesign can significantly reduce the risk to employees by factoring in some or all of the known lifting issues to make the work safer. It is an employer's responsibility under OSHA's General Duty Clause to provide a workplace free from recognized hazards. More fundamentally, hard-earned experience tells us that prevention of injuries, illnesses, and fatalities results in an improved business and bottom line.

An issue rarely discussed in business forums is the cost of an injury to the individual worker. Consider this example: at a large consumer products company an individual had his thumb traumatically amputated by a piece of equipment. The machine not only amputated the thumb but ground it up so that no possibility of reattachment existed. This person had returned from service in Vietnam without a scratch despite being in one of the most hazardous military roles there. Now, in an instant, he was maimed for life. After multiple surgeries that included removing the index finger and grafting it to the thumb location to give a semblance of thumb grip, he became addicted to painkillers and alcohol. His behavior nearly drove his family away, but fortunately, his wife was able to help him, and they received counseling. When he returned to work after four years, he could not even walk into the building where the injury had occurred. When asked how things were going, he said, "If I had it to do over again, I would have the whole hand taken off." The company spent approximately $500,000 in medical costs and wage replacement. However, a better question than what was the cost to the company would be what did it cost him and his family? There were other indirect costs associated with this injury. Other members of his workgroup were so upset by the incident that some were unable to continue to work that day. A few required employee assistance program counseling to enable them to work without fear of the same thing happening to them. The psychological costs to both the injured person and others are unknowable but certainly significant.

This operation in which the injury occurred was in compliance with all OSHA requirements but was not designed to be injury free, and it resulted in both direct costs that are known and large indirect costs that will never be quantified because they involved effects on the individual, not the company.

OSHA compliance will provide a set of standards for almost any area of the workplace. However, all of these standards are compromises and thus do not protect employees from death or serious injury or illness as fully as they might. In addition, a slightly different set of requirements exists for construction and for shipbuilding, due to the fact that these industries are very different from general industry. Despite this, a company acting under OSHA compliance will show an improvement over a company that is doing nothing and is relying on random chance to prevent injuries and illnesses to employees. Given this, consider how much greater improvement a company focused on prevention can show.

OSHA standards compliance leaves an employer more vulnerable to OSHA enforcement action than a prevention approach does. This is the case because minimum requirements are pretty easy to overlook and to stop doing in the absence of oversight by OSHA or some other agency. And there is no way to prevent an OSHA inspection once an event occurs that OSHA decides to respond to. Such events range from a formal complaint by an employee (which might include a report on an imminent danger) to a catastrophe (defined by OSHA as the hospitalization of three or more employees as a result of a single incident or as a death), an OSHA-sponsored special emphasis program, or data indicating frequent injuries and illnesses on a worksite. An OSHA inspection is never a pleasant experience, but a well-prepared employer who has an injury prevention program can get through it with minimal pain. Preparing for an inspection requires the employer not only to envision the worst possible scenario but also to develop a well-planned approach for dealing with such cases. Nearly any worst case outcome imaginable has actually occurred somewhere in the workplace being inspected.

THE INSPECTION PROCESS

An inspection starts with the arrival of a compliance officer at the worksite, with or without advance notice. The officer will present her credentials to the first representative of the employer she meets. At this point, the employer will take some control of the inspection. The compliance officer will give the reason(s) for the inspection. As described previously, there are a number of reasons why OSHA may want to conduct an inspection. If this is a formal complaint inspection, the compliance officer will request to see the location where the complaint is alleged to have been or to be occurring. The employer will take a copy of the complaint, review it, and discuss the allegations with the compliance officer for a full understanding of the possible issues. This is typically done in a meeting room or office away from the general traffic flow of the facility. No admission of problems or to the allegations, other than agreeing to go to the location, will be made. At this time the employer's representative will take some time to prepare himself and the organization. He will leave the compliance officer in the room and go to gather any required equipment, documentation, and the like. Depending on the size of the employer, he may contact a higher level of the organization for guidance and coaching.

The OSHA 300 log will be one item the representative brings back to the compliance officer, but it will usually be presented only if it is requested. (On a construction site, it will nearly always be requested, to allow the compliance officer to conduct either a focused inspection or a more general, "wall-to-wall" inspection.) The equipment the representative brings with him will include notepaper and writing implements and any audiovisual equipment needed to parallel any records the compliance officer is making. During this time of preparation, notification of the affected area is made to enable this area to do any last-minute housekeeping to present the most positive image to the compliance officer possible.

Employers typically plan a route to the location that is both direct and that highlights company strengths and does not unnecessarily draw attention to any areas not covered by the inspection at hand. The route can include taking the compliance officer past any recognition items for safety performance the organization has on display. Any issue the compliance officer sees can and will be cited, and additional hazards identified could cause a complaint inspection that is fairly narrowly focused to be expanded into a wall to wall. A wall to wall involves OSHA compliance officers inspecting the entire employer facility, and it can take days, weeks, or months, depending on the size of the facility and the extent of hazards identified or possible.

Compliance officers know that while they are waiting in a meeting room, last-minute preparations are taking place, so the time they are left there needs to be minimized. A good rule of thumb is that ten to fifteen minutes is reasonable and more than that raises suspicions. A suspicious compliance officer is not what the employer wants in what is already by nature an adversarial relationship. Once the route is planned, the company representative takes the compliance officer to the location and stays with her during the entire inspection. The officer has the right to conduct interviews and discussions without the employer's representative present but will not always require this. The nature of the complaint will drive that decision. If the employer is unionized, the union has the right to have a representative accompany the compliance officer along with the employer's representative. If the compliance officer takes any pictures or videos at the scene, the employer's representative should take the same pictures or videos with the audiovisual equipment he obtained previously.

The employer's representative will note the compliance officer's comments throughout but will only acknowledge them and not agree with them, as agreeing means accepting them as fact and this agreement could then become a factor in citations and fines later. If the compliance officer is conducting an industrial hygiene inspection, she may need to conduct formal exposure monitoring. This will normally be scheduled with the employer, and the employer's representative should use identical monitoring equipment placed alongside that of the compliance officer. Once an inspection is completed at the scene, the compliance officer is escorted back, via the same route, to the meeting room. Once there, she will conduct a closing conference, during which time the employer's representative may question her about any problems she saw and citations she may recommend. Again, the employer's representative should not acknowledge any problems or issues even if an issue was obvious. Any admission or formal acknowledgment by the employer's representative is taken as admission of guilt. The employer's representative should escort the compliance officer out the door and then document, in writing, any and all observations he made, comments made by the compliance officer, and any other data that may be pertinent later.

Once back in the office, the compliance officer will compare the information gathered to the OSHA regulations and list any citations. She will make recommendations on the type and severity of citations, ranging from "de minimus" to "willful" and "repeat." She will review the information with the area director, who will decide on proposed penalties for each citation. Penalties can range from $0 to $70,000 per citation. Once this is completed, the compliance officer will formally type up the report and citations and have them signed by the area director and sent to the employer. The employer then has fifteen days to formally contest or accept the citations and the penalties, if any.

The OSHA Review Commission and the courts have been very consistent in supporting OSHA on the fifteen-day rule. Failure to respond within the fifteen days is an admission of guilt. If there are no citations or fines, the file is closed. If there are citations and fines, a prepared employer will request an informal conference with the area director to discuss them. Normally this conference can be set up within the fifteen-day time frame. Discussions with the area director normally include sharing and comparing the compliance officer's observations with the employer's representative's observations. Sometimes significant differences can cause the area director to reduce the severity of a citation and consequently the amount of the fine. Employers who schedule an informal conference usually get a reduction in the proposed fine if they are operating a small business, are a member of an alliance or partnership, or have a good record.

When there is no meeting of minds at the informal conference, the employer can choose to contest the citations and fines. This starts a judicial process that goes to an administrative law judge (ALJ), who can find for either side either in whole or in part. If either side is not satisfied with the ALJ's findings, an appeal can be made to the OSHA Review Commission. The OSHA Review Commission is a three-member panel, appointed by the U.S. president and confirmed by the U.S. Senate to make final decisions on OSHA cases. Of course, in the U.S. system even this process is not truly final as the case can still go to the federal court system. A few cases involving OSHA citations have ended up in the U.S. Supreme Court, whose rulings are final.

The most important point here in the context of this book is that when an employer is doing only compliance, any slight variation from OSHA standards will be readily apparent to the compliance officer. Once a compliance officer sees a deviation from the minimum, he or she can expand the scope of the inspection. Thus a simple response to an employee complaint can turn into an extended wall to wall. There have been cases where OSHA has been in a workplace for weeks doing an inspection due to the compliance officer's initial findings. Conversely, an employer who has gone beyond compliance to proactive prevention is less likely to face such actions.

COMPLIANCE OR PREVENTION

We use the term *prevention* to describe taking action to prevent injuries and illnesses above and beyond the minimum requirements of OSHA compliance. Prevention can also be viewed as *cost avoidance*. The more an employer does to prevent injuries and illnesses, the less likely that employer is to see OSHA take enforcement action. At the same time, the reduction in injuries and illnesses the employer experiences should lead directly to an improved profit margin. This can be a huge amount of money. As an example of the economic benefit of a prevention approach, the following case is presented. There are numerous others, but this illustrates the possibility. In the early 1990s, loggers in Northeast Pennsylvania were paying approximately $58 in workers' compensation costs for every $100 in payroll. Through an initiative led by a consortium of loggers, timber buyers, and Pennsylvania State Forestry personnel, over the next five years this cost was brought down to $38 in workers' compensation cost per $100 in payroll. The initiative consisted largely of training loggers about such things as the safest way to cut, limb, and haul trees; proper personal protective equipment for all persons in the vicinity of the logging operation; proper skidder operation; and proper equipment operation and maintenance. For some work, loggers purchased mechanical fellers (machines to cut and drop trees), in lieu of employing human fellers. Note that with the exception of the mechanical fellers, little of this cost a large sum of money. It cost time away from actual logging but the return was huge. The examples of the economic benefits of this approach are too numerous to attempt to list here; suffice it to say that this approach more than pays for itself.

Another Way to Look at Prevention

Another way to look at the value of injury and illness prevention is to determine how many units of whatever your company produces are required to pay for a workplace injury. (For simplicity we use simple, rounded numbers, without considering taxes or debt service, in the following example.) If, for example, you make a 10 percent profit on every unit sold, with an average selling price of $10, the profit per unit is $1. Thus one "average" back injury at $20,000 requires additional sales of 20,000 units to cover the cost of this one injury. Even if selling 20,000 extra units sounds reasonable, there is more to consider. Although workers' compensation insurance will pay the immediate, direct costs, the insurance carrier will factor that injury cost into the premium for three years, resulting in premium increases for the next three years in your workers' compensation insurance costs. Injury prevention plans focus on identifying equipment, tools, procedures, and people's actions that present an unacceptable level of risk of injury or illness to employees. Employers practicing this process identify all risks and hazards to employees. No organization has the time or resources to reduce all injuries or illnesses at once, so priorities have to be set to determine which risks to reduce first. These employers will usually communicate these priorities to the employees, using this communication process to ensure that the issues the management has identified as priorities match up with what employees know and feel. Often there is a degree of mismatch at first, and an iterative process then takes place to get the right things done at the right time. All of this will also serve to let employees know that the employer cares and is working on issues of concern to employees. Experience in multiple organizations shows that employers who communicate priorities and engage in risk assessment processes receive great support from their employees. Employers who are serious about prevention periodically update their employees on progress made and check to ensure that conditions have not changed enough to warrant changing the priority plan.

Once one hazard is reduced to an acceptable level, another is added to the list. The actions taken to reduce or eliminate risks are not always high cost or slow in implementation. In the personal experience of one of the authors, a hazard that was thought to require over $200,000 per production line to correct—and there were more than twenty lines—could in fact be reduced to an acceptable level on all the lines for less than $40,000 total. Identifying this fix took having an outside set of eyes to analyze the entire process and make some simple suggestions for reducing or eliminating the risks associated with the work. Although this did not completely eliminate all risk from the work, it reduced it sufficiently so that reducing the residual risk could be put on the back burner while other, higher hazards were addressed. In another case the same author was asked to work with a company on a fall protection problem. The management was thinking of putting in properly engineered fall protection tie-off points (that is, the anchorages to which personal protective equipment, or PPE, is attached), purchasing fall protection PPE for all the individuals who might do the work at issue, and providing training for them on fall protection. A simple examination of the workplace showed that modifying the work platform by extending it a few feet eliminated the need for extra PPE, training, enforcement, and extensive reengineering and reinstallation. These are two specific cases where prevention actions were not particularly costly but significantly reduced the risks to employees.

Costs of Injury

The costs of preventing injuries are sometimes difficult to quantify. What is the cost of an eye injury? It depends on the injury, which can range anywhere from simple dust in the eye to the loss of sight or even of the eye itself. Use of safety glasses with side-shields, costing less than $6 per pair, will dramatically reduce the risk. A pair of cut-resistant gloves costs in the neighborhood of $25 per pair. Sutures required to close a laceration are over $200 per suture in most hospitals and clinics, so preventing just one serious laceration requiring sutures is likely to more than pay for enough cut-resistant gloves to be worn by all employees when they use cutting instruments. Training costs also factor into injury and illness prevention. One tool used very effectively by many companies is called the *job safety analysis* (JSA), or *job hazard analysis* (for detailed information on this technique and format see National Safety Council, 2008). This tool breaks work down into jobs, jobs into tasks, and tasks into the discrete steps required to complete the task. Once each step is identified, an assessment is done of the hazards presented by the step, and then actions are developed to eliminate or reduce the risk. Equally as important as identifying the hazards is listing the job steps. Once completed, the JSA serves as an outstanding training tool for new employees and as a refresher for others. Most companies do some annual training in order to comply with OSHA training requirements. Not much more would be required to simply add OSHA-required information or gather information for prevention.

PREVENTION OF CUMULATIVE PROBLEMS

Two areas that employers often do not fully target are hearing conservation and loss and illnesses and injuries resulting from poor ergonomics. The reason they are relatively neglected is that they are cumulative problems. Most health and safety systems target the instantaneous injuries, fractures and lacerations, for example. Many also target and control exposure to hazardous chemicals. These are injuries that are well known and that usually exhibit effects immediately, unlike hearing loss or ergonomic illnesses. Of note, ergonomic illnesses are classified as injuries on the OSHA 300 log so even the government does not fully grasp the long-term nature of these two problem areas. However, both hearing loss and loss of physical function due to poor ergonomics are common and eventually costly. These topics (and also vision problems) are examined in Chapters Eleven and Thirteen.

SUMMARY

This chapter's recurring theme has been that employers have two choices in workplace safety and health: compliance with OSHA regulations or an approach that targets prevention of problems (injuries, illnesses, and catastrophes). The best companies are not just meeting the compliance requirements; they are actively working on preventing problems. The intent of the examples included here has been to illustrate that there are costs and consequences to not going above and beyond the OSHA requirements. These consequences and costs will, over time, far outweigh the costs of prevention. A short-term focus will not show results, but a long-term, planned effort at preventing problems will result in a better, safer, more productive workplace with employees who want to work there and are motivated to improve themselves and the company.

KEY TERMS

employee hazards
OSHA compliance
performance-based standards

sick building syndrome
small business impact review
Voluntary Protection Program

QUESTIONS FOR DISCUSSION

1. What are the practical differences between complying with OSHA standards and having an injury prevention program?

2. What are the steps in the OSHA standard-setting process?

3. From the employer's point of view, what can go wrong with an OSHA inspection at various points of the process?

4. What are the direct costs and what are the hidden costs of workers' compensation?

3

PUBLIC HEALTH ISSUES IN OCCUPATIONAL SAFETY AND HEALTH

CHAPTER

TOXICOLOGY

After reading this chapter, you should be able to

- Understand the need for workplace surveillance for environmental pollutants.
- Describe the value of the science of toxicology.
- Understand the epidemiology of toxins and their public health significance.
- Describe the classification of toxic agents.
- Describe the role of secondhand smoke in the causation of disease.

Toxicology is the science of poisons. Friis (2006) states that toxicology is a corner-stone of environmental health, and he points out that it overlaps the disciplines of pharmacology, pathology, and even epidemiology. Liebler (2006) notes that the poisons of greatest interest to those in public health today include environmental and workplace pollutants including secondhand tobacco smoke. Toxicology is concerned not only with identifying and classifying chemicals that act as **toxins** but also with understanding human and animal dose response mechanisms for chemicals, including chemicals in drugs and food.

The study of toxins and particularly their effects on humans and animals has been going on for centuries, constantly evolving into the science it has become in recent years. Looking back into the history of occupational health, we can note that some of the observations made by Paracelsus, a sixteenth-century physician who is considered one of the very first toxicologists, concerned **environmental pollutants** as a possible cause of several forms of cancer. Today, through extensive research, it has been proven that some natural and manmade poisons can indeed cause undesirable effects such as cancer in living organisms. Liebler (2006) believes that the field of toxicology has had two major goals over the last half century: assessing the effects of environmental pollutants on health and determining the levels at which drugs and other chemicals become toxic to humans and animals, or to put it another way, ensuring drug and chemical safety. The goal of chemical safety is of course important in the prevention of workplace illness, disease, and death.

APPLICATION TO OCCUPATIONAL EPIDEMIOLOGY

Occupational epidemiology relies on current and extensive research in toxicology to provide vital information on toxic agents, means of harmful exposure and transmission, and methods of mitigating the negative effects of toxic substances in the workplace. Toxins in the environment are also a particular concern of occupational epidemiology. Toxicity depends on dose, duration, and route of exposure to the toxin. Toxins' serious and even deadly effects on the body can come from inhalation, ingestion, absorption, or other direct toxin contact. Understanding these cause-effect relationships is important to protecting the many workers who encounter toxins in their workplaces.

According to Liebler (2006), toxicology has evolved into the only discipline that studies the mechanism of chemical injury. He points out that we need a better understanding of this mechanism in order to protect workers from chemical injury that produces toxicity. Knowing how toxicity varies with a varying dose of the chemical (the amount the worker comes in contact with) is extremely important when determining how toxic a particular exposure is. Thousands of new chemicals are made and used in workplaces every year. These new chemicals will be added to the thousands of chemicals already in existence. They are all available for use and misuse by workers in the workplace.

Let's look more closely at the concept of dose and **dose response**, which is important anytime one is dealing with the epidemiology of a chemical entering a living organism and the resulting symptoms. The Agency for Toxic Substances and Disease

Registry (ATSDR) (2006), an agency of the Centers for Disease Control and Prevention (CDC), explains that the *dose* is the actual amount of chemical that enters the body. This dose may result from an acute or a chronic (long-term) exposure. The amount of exposure and the type of toxin will determine the toxic effect, the *response*, in people and animals. Thus one key question that toxicologists try to answer for employers and workers is how much of any given chemical is needed for an exposure to become harmful to a worker? That is, what is the *threshold dose*, the minimum amount needed, either in a single exposure or in exposure over time, to cause an effect (a response) in the exposed person? Levels below the threshold may be considered "safe." Note, however, that for carcinogens no safe level of exposure exists because any exposure to these substances is capable of causing cancer.

It is very important to understand the difference between acute and chronic exposure to chemicals. Acute toxicity is what happens when one is exposed over a short period of time to a dose sufficient to trigger a response. Chronic toxicity occurs when one is exposed to chemicals for a relatively long period of time before displaying a response. Both types of exposures can and do happen in the workplace. Hilgenkamp (2006) finds that in chronic exposures, worker characteristics such as age, gender, current nutritional state, lifestyle, and immune system health will affect the response to a toxic dose as well.

SUBDISCIPLINES IN TOXICOLOGY

The ATSDR (2006) lists the subdisciplines found within the science of toxicology. The following are the areas of particular use in dealing with workplace chemical problems.

Environmental Toxicology

This field of toxicology works to understand chemicals that contaminate food, water, soil, or the atmosphere. It seems obvious that chemical exposure in the workplace may arise from a number of different sources, including environmental sources. Friis (2006) notes that this field overlaps the concerns of reproductive and developmental toxicology.

Food Toxicology

Food toxicology is concerned with the delivery of a safe and edible food supply to consumers. During the process of preparing food many substances may be added to it for various reasons, but some of these additives may cause illness. Many foods may also produce allergies in people, causing them to become ill. In addition, foods can become contaminated with **pesticides** and other environmental chemicals, such as arsenic and cadmium, that are naturally present in soil and water. Food toxicologists determine the acceptable daily limits for these substances. Protection of the food supply from chemicals is important for workers who grow, pack, prepare, or consume food in their workplace.

Descriptive Toxicology

Descriptive toxicology is the product of studies, particularly animal experimentation studies, used to determine how much of a chemical exposure is required to cause illness or death. This information is then used by the Environmental Protection Agency (EPA), the Occupational Safety and Health Administration (OSHA), and the Food and Drug Administration (FDA) to set regulatory exposure limits.

Occupational Toxicology

Occupational toxicology is concerned with the health effects of chemicals for workers. According to the Bureau of Labor Statistics (2006), occupational diseases caused by industrial chemicals account for an estimated 50,000 to 70,000 deaths and 350,000 new cases of illness each year in this country.

CLASSIFICATION OF TOXIC AGENTS

The Agency for Toxic Substances and Disease Research (2006) classifies toxic chemicals into these major categories: heavy metals, solvents and vapors, radiation and radioactive materials, dioxins and furans, pesticides, plant toxins, and animal toxins.

Heavy Metals

Major toxic heavy metals include arsenic, beryllium, cadmium, chromium, lead, mercury, and nickel. The ATSDR reports that heavy metals differ from other toxic substances in that they are neither created nor destroyed by humans, but they are capable of affecting the health of humans through the air, water, soil, and food they are found in.

Occupational exposure to these heavy metals seems likely to be a risk factor in a considerable number of workplace environments. There are many examples of workers who have been exposed to one or more of these heavy metals for years in the workplace and who have subsequently developed cancer or another serious illness. Clapp, Howe, and Jacobs (2006) argue that recent research has proven that unequal workplace exposures among different worker populations provides evidence that chemical exposure at certain workplaces has been the cause of harm. Toxicologists are only in recent years beginning to understand the major health effects of exposure to these heavy metals.

For example, occupational exposure to cadmium can be the result of the production of cadmium batteries, zinc smelting, and employment in metal factories. The metal particulates are inhaled by the worker, potentially causing a wide range of medical problems affecting the bones, the renal and respiratory systems, the prostate gland, and the reproductive organs of the body. Some forms of cancer are also a result of this type of heavy metal exposure. Another metal, chromium, can be inhaled by workers in metal factories and has been implicated as the cause of lung cancer in exposed workers several years after their first exposure.

Solvents and Vapors

Almost everyone has been exposed to solvents, which can range from the correction fluid used by administrative personnel to the chemicals employed in a nail salon. A solvent is a liquid substance that is capable of dissolving other substances. As a solvent evaporates, the vapors may pose a threat to the exposed population.

Friis (2006) explains that there are several types of exposure to solvents, including breathing their vapors, ingesting them from contaminated foods and water, using certain items packed in plastic, and of course smoking cigarettes. Some of the solvents capable of producing acute effects are tetrachloroethylene, trichloroethane, trichloroethylene, toluene, acetone, and benzene. However, for many of the solvents people are exposed to, long-term health effects, such as cancer, are unknown at this time.

Radiation and Radioactive Materials

Radiation is the release and propagation of energy in space or through a material medium in the form of waves, the transfer of heat or light by waves of energy, or the stream of particles from a nuclear reactor. Radioactive contamination and radiation exposure can occur when radioactive materials are released into the environment as a result of an accident or an act of terrorism. The effect of this radiation on human health depends on the amount of radiation and the length of exposure.

According to the U.S. Environmental Protection Agency (2009), radiation cannot be eliminated from our environment, but we can reduce the health effects by controlling exposure to it. Radiation can be inhaled or ingested, or one can have a direct exposure by being near a radiation source. The different types of radiation include alpha, beta, gamma, and neutron radiation, with each having different potential health effects.

The potential hazards of radiation can be found in many occupational settings. For example, radiation exposure is an ongoing concern for workers in health care facilities in this country, who may be exposed to ionizing radiation from sources such as radionuclide and X-ray machines (Friis, 2006). Other areas of potential workplace radiation exposure include research facilities using radioactive materials, nuclear power facilities, and plants producing nuclear weapons.

The CDC (2002) reports that 80 percent of human exposure to radiation comes from natural sources, such as cosmic radiation from the sun, radon gas from the soil, or uranium in rocks and soil. Over 50 percent of that natural exposure is due to radon gas.

The more radiation one is exposed to, either with short-term exposure or with long-term exposure, the greater the chance for serious health consequences. The chance of cancer increases with repeated exposures to radiation over time.

Dioxins and Furans

Dioxins and furans are chemical compounds that are very similar (Chiras, 2006). At high levels dioxins are thought to be carcinogenic. The ATSDR (2006) reports that dioxin, or TCDD, was originally discovered as a contaminant in the herbicide Agent Orange. In addition to being found in some herbicides, dioxin is a by-product of chlorine processing in paper-producing industries and a product of combustion when tobacco products are burned. In general, dioxins and furans are an unwanted by-product of the process of combustion, are released into the air during combustion, and therefore can be found anywhere.

Friis (2006) argues that dioxins are the most toxic chemicals ever used, according to animal research experiments. They can cause chloracne, rashes, growth of excessive body hair, and liver damage, and they can have several negative effects on the reproductive system. Once produced these chemicals take several years to completely decompose.

Pesticides

The EPA defines a pesticide as any substance or mixture of substances intended to prevent, destroy, repel, or mitigate any pest. Pesticides may also be described as any physical, chemical, or biological agent that will kill an undesirable plant or animal pest. A pest is defined as a living organism that appears when and where it is not wanted; pests can include insects, mice, unwanted plants, fungi, bacteria, viruses, and prions. Many household products are pesticides and by their very nature create risk because they are designed to kill living things. Most of these chemicals are made and also used in the workplace and carry a certain risk for employees.

The broad category of pesticides includes herbicides, fungicides, and various other substances to control pests. Biologically based pesticides are very popular and are somewhat safer than traditional chemical pesticides.

Plant Toxins

Some chemicals made by plants will sicken people and animals, and some are lethal. For example, taxol, used in chemotherapy to kill cancer cells, is produced by a species of the yew plant. This plant is considered toxic because it causes chemical injury to a person who either touches or swallows it or breathes its scent. Different portions of a toxic plant may contain different concentrations of its toxic chemical, making some parts poisonous and other parts safe to ingest.

Animal Toxins

Animal toxins usually take the form of venoms that are secreted and released by an animal. Venomous animals are capable of producing a poison in a highly developed gland or a group of cells, and can deliver it through biting or stinging.

All the toxins described here are ones that workers in certain occupations can be exposed to, and they need to be a topic in workforce training programs.

ENVIRONMENTAL TOBACCO SMOKE

Another very dangerous chemical is starting to receive greater attention in the workplace. The chemicals contained in secondhand tobacco smoke are some of the most dangerous chemicals to ever enter the home or workplace. According to the surgeon general's 2006 report (U.S. Department of Health and Human Services, 2006a), **secondhand smoke**, also known as environmental tobacco smoke (ETS), carries at least 250 chemicals known to be toxic and about 50 of these are also carcinogenic. There is no risk-free level of exposure to secondhand smoke; even a brief exposure to it is extremely dangerous to one's health. Yet more than 126 million nonsmoking Americans are exposed to secondhand smoke in their homes, vehicles, workplaces, and public places almost every day. The CDC also reports that the use of tobacco products in buildings exposes nonsmoking occupants to combustion by-products under conditions where removal of airborne contaminants is slow. Inhaling secondhand smoke causes nonsmokers to suffer many of the same diseases that active smokers experience.

The CDC review found 4,000 compounds in mainstream tobacco smoke and also found that the qualitative composition of these components is nearly identical in mainstream smoke (smoke exhaled by the smoker), sidestream smoke (smoke from the burning tip of the tobacco product), and secondhand smoke (mainstream and sidestream smoke combined). With 250 of these compounds known to be toxic, there is no question that this tobacco smoke produces more poisons for human ingestion than any other chemical known to science.

There has been a definite movement toward a smoke-free workplace since the publication of the 1986 U.S. surgeon general's report titled *The Health Consequences of Involuntary Smoking* (U.S. Public Health Service, Office of the Surgeon General, 1986). But even with the mounting evidence about the dangers associated with secondhand smoke, many workplaces are still not smoke-free. Even when there is a smoke-free policy in place, it does not assure workers that they will not be exposed to secondhand smoke. The results of the most recent surgeon general's report on secondhand smoke (U.S. Department of Health and Human Services, 2006a) revealed the following essential information:

- Involuntary smoking is a cause of disease, including lung cancer, in healthy nonsmokers.

- Separation of smokers and nonsmokers within the same airspace may reduce, but does not eliminate, exposure of nonsmokers to environmental tobacco smoke.

- The home and the workplace remain the predominant locations for exposure to secondhand smoke.

- Exposure to secondhand smoke tends to be greater for persons with lower incomes.

- Smoke-free workplace policies are the only effective way to eliminate secondhand smoke exposure in the workplace. Simply separating smokers from nonsmokers, cleaning the air, and ventilating buildings cannot eliminate exposures.

RISK ASSESSMENT

When dealing with chemicals in the workplace, regulators are constantly concerned about the question of exposure risk. Risk usually involves a potential negative impact on something, an impact arising from some present process or future event. In the case of toxic risk, the concern is the possibility of detrimental health effects arising from exposure to a chemical in an individual's work environment.

Friis (2006) describes risk assessment as the process of determining adverse risks to health attributable to environmental or other hazards. One difficulty in making this determination is that many health effects resulting from chemical exposure have a long latency or incubation period between exposure and illness or disability. Another factor to be considered is the dose response information for known hazards and the effects of multiple chemical exposures incurred by an individual over time.

In addition, both the occupational environment and the home environment play a significant role in health through the specific risks associated with noxious agents and general working and living conditions. Some of these conditions result from personal choices that may have profound effects on a person's future health. As a result, surveillance data on lifestyle both at home and at work is very important in the determination of risk and the development of programs to abate this risk. According to Dever (2006), lifestyle behaviors can be divided into three critical types of risks: leisure activity risks, consumption patterns risks, and employment participation and occupational risks. Poor decisions concerning these elements of lifestyle can result in illness and even death. At the very least, they can reduce a person's quality of life as he or she grows older.

- The ATSDR (2006) offers definitions of the elements that must be addressed in assessing risk exposure: A *hazard* is a source of potential harm from past, current, or future exposures.

- A *dose response relationship* is the relationship between the amount of exposure to a substance and the resulting health effect.

- An *exposure assessment* is the process of discovering how people come into contact with a hazardous substance and how long and how much of the substance they are in contact with on a continuous basis.

- A *risk characterization* allows the decision makers to assess the nature of the risk and act accordingly.

A risk assessment should of course lead to the action of *risk reduction or elimination*, in which the employer implements policies that decrease the chance that workers will experience injury, illness, or disease from a chemical exposure.

TOXICOLOGY CASE STUDIES

It is helpful to look at a few case studies to better understand how easy it is for toxic chemicals to become a major public health problem affecting workers and also the general public. Exhibit 6.1 presents summaries of a sampling of reports from around the country that appeared in the *Morbidity and Mortality Weekly Report.*

TOXIN REGULATION AND RESEARCH

According to Chiras (2006), the United States produces 280 billion pounds of synthetic chemicals each year. In addition, we use many chemical compounds that occur naturally. In order to protect Americans, especially workers, from the release of these chemicals in their workplaces and homes and elsewhere, many laws have been passed requiring those who produce and use these chemicals to comply with strict regulations.

One of the most important laws is the Toxic Substances Control Act (TSCA), enacted by Congress in 1976. This legislation authorized the EPA to track industrial chemicals produced in or imported into this country. This act has two major components.

Premanufacture Notification

The first component of the law requires all companies to notify the EPA ninety days before they import or manufacture a new chemical substance not currently being used commercially. Scientists at the EPA then have ninety days to evaluate the product. If within that time the new chemical is not found to pose significant risk, it is approved for use.

Chemicals in Use Before TSCA

This second major component of TSCA requires examination by the EPA of chemicals in use prior to the enactment of this law. Those chemicals thought to be hazardous are tested for toxicity. If risk is considered to be present, use of the chemical is restricted. The final part of the law requires controls and restrictions on chemicals considered to be hazardous to humans and the environment.

Although this law has been in place for three decades, there is still much that we can learn about the interactions of human beings, chemicals, and the environment. Again, information is the key ingredient that needs to be used in policies and programs to protect workers from the toxic effects of the chemicals they use to get their jobs done and earn a living.

EXHIBIT 6.1. Toxicology case studies

Occupational Exposure to Formaldehyde

A company in Illinois that operated three dialysis centers became concerned about the occupational exposure of its employees to formaldehyde. This chemical germicide was being used to control bacterial contamination in water distribution systems for dialysis fluid pathways of artificial kidney machines. Investigators from the National Institute for Occupational Safety and Health (NIOSH) investigated the report and found that workers from two of the three facilities were exposed to formaldehyde concentrations of 0.50 and 0.57 parts per million, which is a very high concentration. Following NIOSH recommendations, the company changed the system used to deliver the formaldehyde by incorporating an automatic metering system so that the operation did not have to be performed manually ("Occupational Exposure to Formaldehyde in Dialysis Units," 1986).

Although this report dates from 1986, it demonstrates that the exposures had to happen before proper protection of workers occurred. It was known before the exposure that the possibility of environmental contamination of patients and workers by formaldehyde was relatively high. The CDC now recommends that employees working in dialysis units be informed about the potential adverse health effects of formaldehyde and wear proper protective equipment whenever handling concentrated formaldehyde or preparing diluted formaldehyde solutions. The protective equipment should include rubber gloves, protective aprons, and eye and face protection.

Flavorings-Related Lung Disease

In August of 2000, the Missouri Department of Health and Senior Services requested technical services from NIOSH in an investigation of bronchiolitis obliterans in former workers of a microwave popcorn plant in Jasper, Missouri. Bronchiolitis obliterans is a serious lung disease that is irreversible. The investigation connected these disease cases with making or using microwave popcorn flavorings. NIOSH recommended limiting job exposures to food flavorings ("Flavorings-Related Lung Disease," 2000).

The main respiratory symptoms experienced by workers affected by bronchiolitis obliterans include cough and shortness of breath on exertion. These symptoms do not improve when the worker goes home at the end of the workday or on weekends or vacations. Workers should be promptly referred for medical evaluation if they have persistent cough; persistent shortness of breath on exertion; frequent or persistent symptoms of eye, nose, throat, or skin irritation; or abnormal lung function studies.

The final recommendations included the use of engineering controls such as closed systems, isolation, or ventilation. Education of employers and employees to raise their awareness of the potential hazards of the flavorings and the controls was also a recommendation in the final report.

Nicotine Poisoning from Contaminated Ground Beef

In a recall of 1,700 pounds of ground beef in Michigan due to customer complaints of illness after consuming the product, the contaminant was identified as nicotine. It sickened over one hundred individuals before the recall was issued. The high nicotine concentrations found in the tested meat prompted concerns that there had been intentional contamination with a pesticide that sometimes contains nicotine as an additive. On February 12, 2003, a grand jury returned an indictment charging a person with poisoning two hundred pounds of meat with an insecticide, Black Leaf 40, which has nicotine as a main ingredient ("Nicotine Poisoning After Ingestion of Contaminated Ground Beef—Michigan, 2003," 2003).

Contamination of food by chemicals occurs sporadically. This investigation underscores the necessity of ensuring that our food supplies are safe from chemical contamination. Surveillance for chemical attacks on our food supply should be increased, and primary care providers need to become more aware of the possible deliberate use of chemicals to make people sick.

Testicular Cancer in Leather Workers

In a two-year time period, three cases of testicular cancer were diagnosed in a leather tannery in New York. The occurrence of clustered cases in association with an exposure to a suspected etiological agent prompted an investigation by NIOSH and the CDC.

In the finishing process, hides on a series of conveyors pass under bands of nozzles that spray the hides with coating materials consisting of solvents and pigments. The three individuals who developed cancer worked alongside the conveyors directly beyond the spray nozzles, and they smoothed the coating materials onto the leather with handheld applicators. The solvent dimethylformamide (DMF) had been used in the finishing line of this tannery until a few weeks before the reports. Other clusters of cases of testicular cancer and the same type of cancer in animal studies had forced the stoppage of the use of DMF even though no definitive causative exposure had been linked to DMF. The New York State Health Department supported the decision to eliminate the use of DMF and urged the improvement of work processes to reduce exposures to all hazardous chemical substances ("Testicular Cancer in Leather Workers— Fulton County, New York," 1989).

Illness Associated with Pesticides

On May 12, 2005, a commercial pesticide application team was spraying in a citrus orchard to control thrips, small insects that can feed on oranges. The pesticide contained pyrethroid, spinosad, and petroleum. In a neighboring vineyard, twenty-seven farmworkers were working. Shortly after the spraying, some of these workers noticed a chemical odor, began feeling ill, and stopped working. All twenty-three of the female workers were decontaminated on site by a hazmat team. They were then transported to local hospitals. Illness symptoms were not reported by the initial applicators, who were wearing appropriate protective equipment

(continued)

EXHIBIT 6.1. Toxicology case studies (*continued*)

("Worker Illness Related to Ground Application of Pesticide—Kern County, California, 2005," 2005).

This incident highlights two potential occupational hazards in agriculture: pyrethroid toxicity and pesticide drift. In high concentrations pyrethroids act on sodium channels to affect the nerves, skin, and other organs. There will usually be profuse salivation and pulmonary edema, clonic seizures, and opisthotonos (the spine is bent forward so that a supine body rests on its head and heels). Again, it is important that evaluating physicians become knowledgeable regarding the potential for occupational illness caused by pesticide exposures.

Respiratory Illness Associated with Sealants

Between February 2005 and February 2006, six regional poison control centers in five states were consulted regarding 172 human and 19 animal exposures to shoe or boot leather protection or sealant products resulting in respiratory illnesses. One product was associated with 126 cases of human illness and another product with 7 cases. A case was defined as a report to a poison control center of illness after exposure to an aerosol agent used for waterproofing boots or shoes. Investigators determined that sprayed shoes and boots brought into the home from garages or outdoors continued to be a source of exposure to both humans and pets as the product evaporated. Five occupational exposures occurred, four while spraying clothing items at work and one while demonstrating a product to a customer ("Respiratory Illness Associated with Boot Sealant Products—2005–2006," 2006).

Two products were primarily associated with the 150 cases of human illness. These products contained 45 percent heptane, 20 to 30 percent petroleum distillates, 25 to 30 percent isobutene propellant, 5 to 10 percent propane propellant, 0.33 percent fluoropolymer, and 0.33 percent silicone. Consumers and workers need to be encouraged to use all products for waterproofing shoes or boots as directed, to apply them outdoors, and to leave the sprayed boots and shoes and any contaminated clothing outdoors until all fumes have dissipated.

SUMMARY

The toxins, or poisons, of greatest interest today include environmental and workplace pollutants and toxic elements that may be present in drugs, dietary products, and certain natural products. Those responsible for workplace safety and health need to have a general understanding of the science of toxicology and its relevant subdisciplines and knowledge of where to get the requisite information to prevent chemical exposures to their workers.

Identifying the dose response is the most important component in the epidemiology of chemical illness. With thousands of new chemicals being developed every year in addition to the many chemicals already in use, employers need to know the exposures that are safe and acceptable for their workers for the chemicals used in their workplaces.

Published reports from governmental agencies such as the CDC and its divisions about chemical exposures in the workplace should be considered tools to prevent occurrences of the same chemical exposures in the future. The key to preventing chemical exposures is the establishment of good surveillance systems and continuous training programs in the workplace. One of the most dangerous chemical exposures that can still happen in many workplaces is exposure to secondhand smoke. Employers should join the strong movement to eliminate all secondhand smoke and offer workers a truly smoke-free workplace.

Toxic chemicals are capable of playing a major role in workplace illnesses that may cause long-term disability or death for employees. Several laws have been passed and enforced by OSHA, NIOSH, and other federal agencies to ensure that workers are not exposed to toxins in the workplace, yet it is very clear that more needs to be done to protect workers from harmful chemical exposures.

KEY TERMS

dose response
environmental pollutants
toxins

pesticides
secondhand smoke
toxicology

QUESTIONS FOR DISCUSSION

1. Why is toxicology such an important part of workplace safety and health?

2. Why is development of an active surveillance system so important in the prevention of workplace chemical exposures?

3. Name and explain some of the important disciplines used in toxicology.

4. What role does secondhand tobacco smoke play in disease in the workplace? What needs to be done to prevent this type of exposure?

7

STRESS

After reading this chapter, you should be able to

- Describe the major problems associated with stress in the workplace.
- Discuss the effects of stress on worker productivity.
- Understand the need for stress counseling programs.
- Explain the epidemiology of stress in the workplace.

Stress at work has been found to be increasing in most of the developed and developing world (Cooper, Dewe, & O'Driscoll, 2001). The drive toward cutting both the workforce and costs has resulted in fewer people doing more work and feeling more insecure in their jobs. In addition, the rapid expansion of information technology through the Internet, cellular phones, and other wireless technology, like BlackBerrys, has accelerated the pace of work and created demands for immediate response to work demands twenty-four hours a day.

The hours people spend on site at the workplace have also increased, which has had negative effects on the two-earner family, which is now in many countries the most common family unit. In fact the number of anxiety, stress, and neurotic disorder cases involving days away from work has increased since the late 1990s. Consequently, Worrall and Cooper (2001) found that lack of work-life balance has moved up the agenda of work-related sources of stress in many employee surveys.

Job stress can be defined as the harmful physical and emotional responses that occur when the requirements of the job do not match the capabilities, resources, or needs of the worker. The individuals charged with supervising occupational health and safety monitor stress because it can lead to poor health and injury as well as decreased productivity that may be tied to the psychological effects of stress.

STRESS BASICS

The most recent report on stress from the National Institute for Occupational Safety and Health (NIOSH) cites the following findings from various surveys of workers on the extent of workplace stress:

- 40 percent reported their job was "very" or "extremely" stressful.

- 25 percent viewed their jobs as the number one stressor in their lives.

- 75 percent believed that workers have more on-the-job stress now than they did a generation ago.

- 29 percent felt "quite a bit" or "extremely" stressed at work.

- 26 percent said they were "often" or "very often" burned out or stressed by their work.

- Job stress was more strongly associated with health complaints than financial or family problems were.

The Effects of Stress

According to the *Encyclopaedia of Occupational Health and Safety* (Sauter, Hurrell, Murphy, & Levi, 1997), stress has been linked to a variety of physical and psychological problems, including the following:

- *Cardiovascular disease.* Many studies suggest that psychologically demanding jobs that allow employees little control over the work process increase the risk of cardiovascular disease.

▪ *Musculoskeletal disorders.* On the basis of research by NIOSH and many other organizations, it is widely believed that job stress increases the risk for development of back and upper-extremity musculoskeletal disorders.

▪ *Psychological disorders.* Several studies suggest that differences in rates of mental health problems such as depression and burnout for different occupations are due partly to differences in job stress levels. However, economic and lifestyle differences between occupations may also contribute to some of these problems.

▪ *Workplace injuries.* Although more study is needed, there is a growing concern that stressful working conditions interfere with safe work practices and set the stage for injuries at work.

▪ *Ulcers, cancer, impaired immune function, suicide.* Some studies suggest a relationship between stressful working conditions and suicide, cancer, ulcers, or impaired immune function. However, more research is needed before firm conclusions can be drawn about these hypothesized connections.

Three Stages of Stress

Physician Hans Selye was one of the first to write about stress, with an article in the British journal *Nature* in the summer of 1936. At that time stress symptoms were referred to as general adaptation syndrome (GAS). Selye later started referring to GAS as "the stress syndrome," and set out to investigate the ways in which the body deals with this syndrome and what he referred to as the "noxious agents" that were present in the body as a result of it. Selye explained that the body goes through three universal stages of **coping**. He determined that first there is an "alarm reaction," in which the body prepares itself for "fight or flight." No being can sustain this condition of excitement, however, and a second stage of adaptation must happen if the organism survives the first stage. In the second stage, a resistance to the stress is built. Finally, if the duration of the stress is sufficiently long, the body eventually enters a stage of exhaustion, which results in a sort of aging "due to wear and tear."

Research built on Selye's early work has determined that stress produces physiological reactions within the body as the body experiences the three stages of reaction to stress. During the first stage, the alarm reaction, the body prepares to cope, and the hormones epinephrine (adrenaline) and norepinephrine (noradrenaline) are secreted in large quantities. They move into the bloodstream to prepare an individual for action. When these hormones are secreted, activity in the sympathetic nervous system steps up, and this can lead to an increase in blood pressure, heart rate, blood sugar, and blood flow to the muscles (Blascovitch et al., 1992).

In the second stage, the **resistance stage**, as the body begins to recover from the initial stress and tries to start coping, the epinephrine secretion decreases, as do the other body responses.

In the third stage, exhaustion, the body's resources are depleted, and the body starts to break down.

Negatives and Positives of Stress

Stress can provide both positive and negative benefits to individuals (Quick, Murphy, & Hurrell, 1992). Positive stress is known as **eustress**, whereas negative stress is referred to as **distress**. Eustress can be defined as a pleasant or curative stress that is healthy or gives one a feeling of fulfillment. Eustress can give a person a competitive edge in performance-related activities such as athletics or giving a presentation on the job. This is an optimal amount of stress. Evidence also exists that stress can improve work performance by raising the level of arousal and enabling a person to accomplish more in a shorter amount of time (Quick, Quick, Nelson, & Hurrell, 1997). And stress can increase work productivity by altering a person's psychological state (Seyle, 1975). In short, by increasing an individual's level of arousal it is possible to increase work productivity and maximize efficiency of both the individual and the workforce. However, when stress increases beyond an individual's ability to cope, it causes the experience of distress, and, consequently, a decrease in performance (Seyle, 1975). Performance under such conditions is usually described as following an inverted U-shaped pattern (Koob, 1991). This means that as performance begins to decline under increasing amounts of stress, the transformation of stress into distress is likely to occur (Quick et al., 1997).

Distress has consistently been shown to be a factor in the development of both mental and physical illness. Sometimes conceptualized as the overload of stressful events or stimuli, distress is "pain or suffering affecting the body, a bodily part, or the mind." Distress can be viewed as the overloading of a person's capacity to handle his or her current stress load. The experience of distress has been linked to lower levels of job satisfaction and perceptions of limited social support (Kaplan, 1990). In addition, the experience of distress has been linked to lower productivity and poor work performance (Seyle, 1975).

Gruen, Folkman, and Lazarus (1988) state that "the conviction that psychological stress is a causal factor in mental and physical illness underlies much current theory and research in the biological and behavior sciences." Understanding the relationship between eustress and distress can allow vocational personnel to work with consumers in finding job positions that maximize productivity and minimize the experience of distress (Steinfeld & Danford, 1999).

The Importance of Job Fit

Job fit is an important determinant of the amount of stress a person will experience on the job. The **integrated stress response** (ISR) person-environment fit model suggests that work stress results when workers and work environments are misfits (Harrison, 1978). In contrast, people who like their jobs are less likely to experience job-related stress. Liking one's job is closely tied to having a work environment that provides opportunities to use one's talents and skills and that can provide status, recognition, and pleasant associations. Therefore it follows that managers may be able to reduce stress among their employees by using more extensive career-testing tools prior to making job offers. Two of the most widely used career tests are those developed by John Holland and by Katharine Briggs and Isabel Myers.

John Holland saw career choice as an extension of personality. He believed that people express their values and interests through career choice. His theory specifies how the individual and his or her environment interact with each other and identifies six personality types—*realistic, investigative, artistic, social, enterprising,* and *conventional*—that can be matched with an environment. When this matchup happens, congruence is achieved (Holland, 1997).

Some jobs within each of the six types are as follows:

- Realistic occupations include mechanic, carpenter, surveyor, farmer, and other occupations requiring mechanical abilities.

- Investigative occupations include scientific occupations such as chemist, physicist, biologist, anthropologist, and other occupations requiring mathematical and scientific abilities.

- Artistic occupations include musician, writer, interior decorator, actor, and other occupations requiring ability in writing, music, fine arts, and other creative areas.

- Social occupations include counselor, psychologist, social worker, teacher, clergyman or clergywoman, speech therapist, and other occupations requiring social and interpersonal abilities.

- Enterprising occupations include salesperson, politician, buyer, sportscaster, television reporter, and other occupations requiring leadership and speaking abilities.

- Conventional occupations include accountant, banker, analyst, bookkeeper, executive assistant, industrial engineer, and other occupations requiring clerical and arithmetical abilities.

Holland arranged these types graphically, in a hexagon with similarity or dissimilarity between types demonstrated by closeness. For example, social and artistic types are considered similar.

Career counselors and human resources professionals can use the Self-Directed Search (SDS), a test Holland developed to determine an individual's type and match him or her to jobs that fall into the corresponding list of suitable occupations. Another test developed by Holland that is often used to determine person-environment fit is the Vocational Preference Inventory (VPI).

Katharine Briggs and Isabel Myers developed another type of test, the Myers-Briggs Type Indicator (MBTI), in the 1940s. The concepts behind this tool were developed in relation to psychology rather than career development and are based on the work of analytical psychologist and philosopher Carl Gustav Jung, who viewed some people as being primarily concerned with what is going on around them and others as more concerned with what is happening with their own views and ideas. Myers-Briggs theory is also known as trait and factor theory. It is concerned with integrating information about an individual with information about the world of work for a particular occupation. The MBTI assesses four dimensions: extraversion-introversion (E-I), sensing-intuition (S-I), thinking-feeling (T-F), and judgment-perception (J-P). The manual that accompanies the MBTI lists the different types of environments in which people may prefer to work based on type.

The Ability to Cope

Differences in individual characteristics such as personality and coping style have been linked to predicting whether certain job conditions will result in stress. This means that what is stressful for one person may not be a problem for someone else. This viewpoint has led to prevention strategies that focus on workers' individuality and ways to foster coping skills in the face of demanding job conditions. *Coping* can be defined as responding to an externally imposed life strain in a way that serves to control or reduce emotional distress. There are two types of coping: active and avoidant. Active coping involves the use of strategies that directly affect the stressor. This can be done behaviorally (doing something to eliminate the problem) or cognitively (thinking about the problem in a new way). Avoidant coping consists of behaviors and thoughts that are designed to draw attention away from the stressor. Active coping strategies have been linked to much more positive psychological outcomes (Preston & Mansfield, 1984).

However, Giga, Cooper, and Faragher (2003) concluded that individual stress management programs—those that attempt to empower workers to deal with demanding situations by developing their own coping skills and abilities—are unlikely to maintain employee health and well-being in the long term without procedures in place within the organization to reduce or prevent environmental stressors. This is because situational factors can often render certain attempts at coping ineffective.

Organizational commitment has been defined as "the strength of an individual's identification with and involvement in a particular organization" (Porter, Steers, Mowday, & Boulian, 1974). A person who is high in organizational commitment wants to stay with his or her organization, work for the good of the organization, and adhere to the prominent values of the organization (Mowday, Steers, & Porter, 1979). Brown and Peterson (1993) determined that when an organization provides support and the employee feels organizational commitment, that helps with the employee's ability to cope with stressors. However, when such support is not available and employees feel a lack of commitment to the organization, that lack of support and commitment becomes an additional stressor. When it is experienced as a stressor, it affects and reduces performance.

WORKPLACE CHARACTERISTICS AND STRESS

The National Institute for Occupational Safety and Health has identified organizational characteristics associated with both healthy, low-stress work and high levels of productivity. For example, the organization can provide

- Recognition of employees for good work performance

- Opportunities for career development

- An organizational culture that values the individual worker

- Management actions that are consistent with organizational values

In addition, according to the NIOSH publication *Stress at Work* (n.d.), several types of job conditions may lead to stress:

- *The design of tasks:* heavy workloads, infrequent rest breaks, and long work hours and shift work; hectic and routine tasks that have little inherent meaning, do not use workers' skills, and provide little sense of control. For example, one worker, we'll call him David, works to the point of exhaustion. Another worker, Theresa, is tied to a computer program, giving her little room for flexibility, self-initiative, or rest.

- *Management style:* lack of participation by workers in decision making, poor communication within the organization, lack of family-friendly policies. For example, Theresa needs to get the boss's approval for everything, and the company is insensitive to her family needs.

- *Interpersonal relationships:* poor social environment and lack of support or help from coworkers and supervisors. For example, Theresa's physical isolation reduces her opportunities to interact with other workers or receive help from them.

- *Work roles:* conflicting or uncertain job expectations, too much responsibility, too many hats to wear. For example: Theresa is often caught in a difficult situation trying to satisfy both the customer's needs and the company's expectations.

- *Career concerns:* job insecurity and lack of opportunity for growth, advancement, or promotion; rapid changes for which workers are unprepared. For example, since the reorganization at David's plant, everyone is worried about his or her future with the company and what will happen next.

- *Environmental conditions:* unpleasant or dangerous physical conditions such as crowding, noise, air pollution, or ergonomic problems. For example, David is exposed to constant noise at work.

Certain occupations have been linked with high levels of stress. Technical, sales, and administrative support jobs were found by NIOSH to have the highest number of days away from work related to anxiety, stress, and neurotic disorders.

ORGANIZATIONAL RESPONSE TO STRESS

Stress in the workplace is closely linked to worker productivity. Cooper et al. (2003) found that the strongest predictor of productivity was psychological well-being. Conversely, he found that symptoms of stress cause individuals considerable suffering, significantly affect absenteeism and productivity levels within organizations, and in general substantially burden the community. Individual physiological, psychological, and behavioral outcomes that result from stress include lower levels of self-esteem, job satisfaction, and motivation, as well as higher levels of blood pressure and cholesterol, depression, ulcers, and heart disease (Goodspeed & DeLucia, 1990).

The established link between work stressors and employee well-being places an obligation on employers to provide a healthy environment. It has also been argued that employers should be aware of the monetary impact of reduced well-being and ill health. For example, Kessler, DuPont, and Berglund (1999) estimated that in cases of depression, each worker experienced monthly productivity losses of approximately $200 to $400. Earlier, Greenberg, Stiglin, Finkelstein, and Berndt (1993) had estimated that lost productivity due to depression cost U.S. corporations $12.1 billion in 1990 alone. Furthermore, the impact on absenteeism of mental illness among workers has been established in several studies. The established link between stressors, well-being, and productivity should provide another motivation to employers to ensure appropriate working conditions are maintained, and it adds to management's understanding of the role of stress in organizations.

O'Driscoll, Brough, and Kalliath (2004) examined the effect of organizations' family-responsive policies on work and family roles. They concluded that although many organizations may introduce these initiatives as mechanisms to reduce strain among their employees, the policies on their own may not be sufficient to generate significant stress reduction. Instead, the development of an organizational culture that is perceived by employees to be supportive of a work-family balance may be a necessary condition for the alleviation of work-family conflict and related negative effects.

Some specific techniques that have been used by organizations in an effort to reduce stress and at the same time encourage organizational commitment among employees are described in the following sections.

Offer an Occupational Stress Workshop

The **occupational stress workshop** strategy has several advantages. It sends a message to employees that the organization is concerned about them and their stress levels. It helps to educate them so that employees and managers are all speaking a common language about stress. Finally, it can help leaders to identify some of the most important personal and organizational concerns about stress. In fact, for employees to take such a workshop seriously, it is important that discussion of both organizational change strategies and personal stress management be included.

This training can be comfortably done in either a half-day or full-day session. Prior to the end of the training, the facilitator should ask participants to indicate if they are interested in working further on the issue of workplace stress. Most organizations routinely obtain participant evaluations of any training, and this is a particularly good idea for an occupational stress workshop. This feedback will help management judge the quality of the training, and how important a concern stress is to employees. Finally, the feedback may reveal the need for additional programs or activities to reduce stress.

For example, an occupational safety and health training agency in Massachusetts offered a stress-reduction workshop to a diverse group of workers. Agency staff expected the workshop would be of most interest to human service workers as well as other public sector workers. However, a number of workers from the manufacturing sector also came to the workshop and were active participants. One concrete benefit to emerge from the initial workshop was that both the training agency staff and the manufacturing workers realized the extent to which stress on the job was negatively affecting the workers' home lives. This led to additional training on coping skills and family dynamics. Workers participating in this second round of training found it extremely useful. Thanks to the initial occupational stress workshop, a serious problem had been identified, and employees had been motivated to address it.

Organize an Occupational Stress Committee

A reasonable next step might be the formation of an occupational stress committee. This group could meet on an ongoing basis and formulate a strategy for improving the organization's work environment. This group should have a unique identity and focus. Group membership should include both labor and management. If employees are represented by a union or bargaining unit, representatives from this group should be committee members, in order to avoid potential conflicts with the collective bargaining process. If no bargaining unit exists, then a representative group of employees and administrators should attend meetings. Management representatives should include persons with real authority in the organization. Employee members should represent various departments, divisions, shifts, and workgroups. Because this committee is examining issues of the work environment, everyone involved in that work environment should be represented, including clerical, support, and maintenance staff.

It is also essential that employee representatives be protected from discrimination resulting from their participation on the committee. The committee should be provided with adequate resources to make a serious and sustained effort. These resources might include access to relevant consultants, training materials, relevant records, and release time.

An effective committee needs an effective set of rules and guidelines. What should the committee discuss? What limitations are there? What topics are off limits because they are part of the collective bargaining agreement? How confidential should the meetings be?

Social scientists have written many volumes defining effective group process and how to achieve it, but here are a few, brief commonsense guidelines to start with:

- Every member of the group should be valued and have a chance to speak.

- There should be no negative consequences for opinions expressed in the meetings.

- The group should be given clear instructions and the authority to make specific recommendations. Where a bargaining unit exists, instructions need to include a thorough understanding of what issues the group may not address because of collective bargaining restraints. One example is that discussing salary levels and job categories would not be allowed outside of a collective bargaining process.

- Meetings should have a clear starting and ending time. Participants should understand that their time is valuable.

- The role of chairperson should be rotated between managers and employees.

- The committee needs to be distinguished from other ongoing committees. This is not a training committee or a productivity committee. This is an occupational stress committee and reducing stress levels and enhancing coping strategies should be its focus.

Conduct Individual Interventions

Individual interventions that may help employees reduce stress can range from those performed by supervisors or human resource professionals to those done by mental health professionals. A workplace intervention to reduce an individual's stress may be as simple as a change in hours or the hiring of additional staff. But when the stressor cannot be so easily corrected or when it is combined with additional mental health issues or drug or alcohol use, it is best to have a professional from the company's employee assistance program (EAP) oversee the intervention.

An EAP program can be a crucial tool in reducing employee stress. In an ideal situation, an employee can contact the EAP on his or her own by just picking up the phone or going to see an EAP coordinator. The service is confidential, and coordinators will usually arrange to meet the employee away from the workplace to further guarantee confidentiality. Supervisors, union representatives, and personnel officers should be trained on how best to use and suggest the program.

Consider Stress Management Techniques

Yoga Yoga is a form of relaxation training that can relax the body as a means of combating stress. The practice of yoga involves stretching the body and forming different poses while keeping breathing slow and controlled. The body becomes relaxed and energized at the same time. There are various styles of yoga; some involve moving through the poses more quickly and others encourage relaxing deeply into each pose. Some types of yoga have a spiritual focus, whereas others are used purely as a form of exercise.

Sleep Although there are many things a person can do to reduce stress, the first line of defense against stress is to get enough sleep. Sleep restores the body systems and provides rejuvenation. Sleep-deprived bodies will be too depleted to perform the important stress-reducing physical and mental activities we are describing.

Cardiovascular Exercise Exercise is good for the mind, not just the body. Exercise can help with stress relief because it provides a way for the body to release tension and pent-up frustration. It can also help stave off the depression that can set in when stress levels become too high. It does this by raising the output of endorphins, one of the "feel good" chemicals in the brain. Any form of exercise can combat stress, but it is important that the activity be enjoyable, vigorous enough to discharge energy, and produce a relaxing effect when one is finished.

Spending Time in Nature Psychology researchers have recognized the mental health benefits of spending time in the natural world. Activities done in nature can calm the mind and emotions and can bring greater body awareness as a way to let go of mental stress. From taking walks in one's neighborhood to observing animals in the wild to planting a garden, there are many different ways for people to connect with the grounding and nurturing energy in nature.

Massage Therapy A professional massage from a trained therapist can provide soothing, deep relaxation and can improve physiological processes such as circulation. A stress-relieving massage targets specific muscles that may be tense and painful. As the tense muscles relax, so does the person's entire body as well as his or her over-stressed mind. According to the American Massage Therapy Association, the most common type of massage is a Swedish massage, which is specifically meant to relax and energize.

Recognize Special Circumstances

A special type of intervention is often required in response to what is known as a *critical incident*. A critical incident is any event that causes an unusually intense stress reaction. The distress people experience after a critical incident limits their ability to cope, impairs their ability to adjust, and negatively affects the work environment. Here are some examples of traumatic events that can produce such reactions:

- A coworker's death or serious illness

- A coworker's suicide

- A violent or threatening incident in the work setting

- A natural or manmade disaster that affects workers' ability to function in the workplace

The intervention most often used in response to a critical incident is the critical incident stress debriefing (CISD), a process that prevents or limits the development of posttraumatic stress in people exposed to the incident. Professionally conducted CISD helps people cope with and recover from an incident's aftereffects. It enables participants to understand that they are not alone in their reactions to a distressing event and provides them with an opportunity to discuss their thoughts and feelings in a controlled, safe environment. Ideally, CISD occurs within twenty-four to seventy-two hours of an incident. Such interventions are used most often with rescue and police personnel and health care workers, those most likely to encounter critical incidents.

WHEN TO GET HELP

Stressors such as being constantly worried about being laid off or doing the job of two people can cause serious problems for workers. In an employee's personal life, circumstances such as going through a divorce, caring for elderly parents, or dealing with a serious illness can test that person's coping abilities. Employers should know the following American Psychological Association (2004) indicators that it is time for a person, including a worker, to seek professional help:

- He feels trapped, as if there's nowhere to turn.

- She worries excessively and can't concentrate.

- The way he feels affects his sleep, eating habits, job, relationships, and everyday life.

SUMMARY

Stress is a constant presence in many people's lives and has been increasing in workplaces over the last several years. The push toward increasing productivity at work coupled with reductions in the number of workers has produced insecurity along with the resulting stress. Information technology has forced workers into a job structure where the work never ends.

This stressful workplace has resulted in reductions in productivity and more important, negative health effects on the worker. If nothing is done by employers, this epidemic of stress is going to result in an escalation of health care costs along with the loss of some very productive employees.

The answer to this problem is to, first, recognize that stress, especially in the workplace, has become an epidemic. As with any other workplace epidemic, it is the responsibility of management to find the cause of the stress. This will require talking to employees to find the stressful areas in the workplace and to deal together with the issue. This can be the starting point for gaining employees' trust and trying to help them to live healthier lives.

There are several effective therapies for stress that can be offered, beginning with stress counseling. This should result in healthier, happier employees and an overall increase in productivity, which in turn will affect the profitability of the company.

KEY TERMS

coping
distress
eustress
integrated stress response

job stress
occupational stress workshop
resistance stage

QUESTIONS FOR DISCUSSION

1. What is job stress?
2. Why has stress increased in the workplace over the last ten years?
3. What are the three stages of the stress?
4. What is the function of an occupational stress workshop?
5. What are some of the techniques individuals can use to reduce stress?
6. What is management's role in helping workers to reduce stress?

CHAPTER

THE IMPAIRED EMPLOYEE

After reading this chapter, you should be able to

- Identify the workplace costs associated with an impaired employee.

- Understand the major problems associated with employee addiction in the workplace.

- Understand that addiction has become a chronic disease with no cure, only control.

- Describe the benefits of establishing an employee assistance program in the workplace.

According to the National Institute on Drug Abuse (NIDA) (2006b), a part of the National Institutes of Health, **drug abuse** is a public health issue affecting society through both the direct costs related to medical care and the indirect costs associated with lost earnings, crime, and accidents related to misuse of substances. In recent years agencies and employers have become very aware of the extent of substance use and abuse in the workplace, and now they must develop strategies to deal with this significant behavioral health issue. Moreover, a number of reports issued by governmental and other health agencies indicate that the drug abuse problem in this country is not only growing but is beginning at an earlier age. The problem of drug abuse will not be left at home when these younger individuals go to work to earn a living.

The Occupational Safety and Health Administration (OSHA) (1998) points out that the majority of people who abuse drugs are employed, and they cost their employers about twice as much in medical and workers' compensation as their drug-free coworkers. The number of injuries and the rate of absenteeism among impaired employees are also causing considerable employer concern. Moreover, over 60 percent of the unintentional injuries at work are a result of substance abuse. Employees who abuse drugs file six times more workers' compensation claims than those who do not abuse drugs. OSHA (1998) also reports that employee health benefit utilization is 84 percent greater in dollar terms and work absences are sixteen times greater for those who abuse drugs. According to the Office of National Drug Control Policy (2001), the majority of the costs associated with drug abuse come from productivity losses, incarceration of those involved with drugs, and drug abuse–related illnesses and premature death.

The Substance Abuse and Mental Health Services Administration (SAMHSA), an agency of the U.S. Department of Health and Human Services, points out that current drug use is responsible for employees missing one or more days each month from work, making frequent changes in employment, and incurring a significantly higher rate of injuries than other employees while at work. In addition, impaired employees also affect coworkers in that they may have to cover for a person who abuses drugs or work harder to make up for the impaired person's reduced productivity. The use and abuse of drugs has become a family, community, and workplace public health epidemic. An entire family can be destroyed by one member's drug abuse.

Substance abuse has a considerable impact on health. According to SAMHSA, alcohol and illicit drug use are associated with child and spousal abuse, sexually transmitted diseases including HIV infection, teen pregnancy, school failure, motor vehicle crashes, escalation of health care costs, low worker productivity, and homelessness. Alcohol abuse alone is associated with motor vehicle crashes, homicides, suicides, and drowning—leading causes of death among youths. Long-term heavy drinking can lead to heart disease, cancer, alcohol-related liver disease, and pancreatitis. Alcohol use during pregnancy is known to cause fetal alcohol syndrome, a leading cause of preventable mental retardation.

Having workers with drug problems is nothing new for American businesses. Employers have always had to deal with employees who bring their drug addiction problems with them when they come to work. In fact, a survey on substance use dependency or abuse among full-time workers (SAMHSA, 2002) found that among full-time workers aged eighteen to forty-nine in 2000, 8.1 percent reported past month heavy alcohol use, and 7.8 percent reported past month illicit drug use. This same survey discovered that occupations and industries with more male employees, such as construction and mining, had higher rates of substance use than other occupations and industries did.

The impaired employee is of great concern to businesses in this country. Despite all the employers' efforts to keep the workplace free of drugs and impaired employees, the real world does not guarantee total compliance with these efforts. Therefore employers need to have employee assistance programs in place to help these problem employees, as we will discuss in this chapter.

Taking into account its widespread negative impact on society, the workplace, and the mental and physical well-being of the individual, substance abuse can be seen to have the characteristics of a disease. Using epidemiological methods we can analyze this disease to find causes, trends, contributing factors, and other information necessary to recommend ways of preventing and mitigating it. Although there is currently no cure for addiction, there are several treatment programs that have reported successful outcomes in managing it. Goetzel (2004) argues that improvements in employee health are intertwined with reducing medical care costs and enhancing worker safety, productivity, and organizational competitiveness. Nowhere is this argument more pertinent than in encouraging employer efforts to deal effectively with impaired employees. These efforts can save money and provide a positive return on investment. The problem of substance use and abuse in the workplace also lends itself to a public health approach to disease. If American workers are to remain productive and reduce the costs of health insurance for themselves and their employers, the drug abuse issue has to be dealt with now, both in the workplace and in the community.

DRUG USE FREQUENCY AND DEMOGRAPHICS

SAMHSA's survey on drug use and health conducted in 2005 revealed the following major results (SAMHSA, 2006b):

- An estimated 19.7 million Americans aged twelve or older were current (past month) illicit drug users, meaning they had used an illicit drug during the month prior to the survey interview. The estimate represents 8.1 percent of the population.

- Marijuana was the most commonly used illicit drug (14.6 million past month users).

- About 6.4 million (2.6 percent) persons aged twelve or older used prescription psychotherapeutic drugs nonmedically in the past month.

FIGURE 8.1.   *Past month illicit drug use among persons aged twelve or older, by age, 2005.*

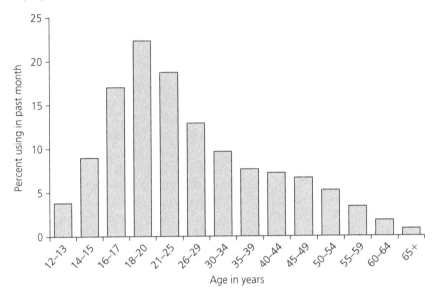

Source: SAMHSA, 2006b, fig. 2.4.

- Past month nonmedical use of prescription-type drugs among young adults aged eighteen to twenty-five increased from 5.4 percent in 2002 to 6.3 percent in 2005. This was primarily due to an increase in pain reliever use.

- Among Americans aged twelve or older, 51.8 percent reported being current drinkers of alcohol. This translated to an estimated 126 million people, which was higher than the 2004 estimate of 121 million people (50.3 percent).

- More than one-fifth (22.7 percent) of persons aged twelve or older participated in binge drinking (having five or more drinks on the same occasion on at least one day in the thirty days prior to the survey).

Substance abuse has clearly become a national concern. Age is one factor in drug and alcohol use. Figure 8.1 shows that the 2005 rate of illicit drug use was 18.7 percent among those aged twenty-one to twenty-five and that it declined among older adults. Figure 8.2 shows the rates of binge drinking. The combined rate of binge drinking was 41.9 percent for young adults aged eighteen to twenty-five and heavy alcohol use was reported by 15.3 percent of persons in that same age group. Driving under the influence of alcohol was also clearly associated with age in 2005, as illustrated in Figure 8.3. Figure 8.4 displays the overall use of a number of specific illicit drugs in 2005. There were no significant changes between 2002 and 2005 in the percentage of persons with dependence on or abuse of illicit drugs (3.0 percent in 2002, 2.9 percent in 2003, 3.0 percent in 2004, and 2.8 percent in 2005; SAMHSA, 2006b).

FIGURE 8.2.   *Current, binge, and heavy alcohol use among persons aged twelve or older, by age, 2005.*

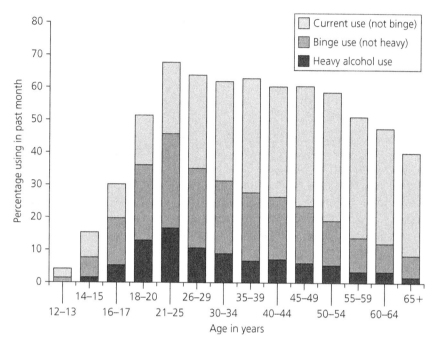

Note: Rates of binge alcohol use in 2005 were 2.0 percent among 12- or 13-year-olds, 8.0 percent among 14- or 15-year-olds, 19.7 percent among 16- or 17-year-olds, 36.1 percent among persons aged 18 to 20, and 45.7 percent among those aged 21 to 25. The rate peaked at ages 21 to 23 (49.9 percent at age 21, 46.6 percent at age 22, and 47.7 percent at age 23), then decreased beyond young adulthood from 32.9 percent of 26- to 34-year-olds to 18.3 percent of persons aged 35 or older. The rate of binge drinking was 41.9 percent for young adults aged 18 to 25. Heavy alcohol use was reported by 15.3 percent of persons aged 18 to 25.

Source: SAMHSA, 2006b, fig. 3.1.

The Healthy People 2010 program addresses the toll taken by substance abuse. Its goal for substance abuse states: "Reduce substance abuse to protect the health, safety, and quality of life for all, especially children." Table 8.1 summarizes the focus of the objectives associated with this goal.

EPIDEMIOLOGY OF ADDICTION

Epidemiological principles can be employed to study the process of drug addiction. Indeed, the epidemiology of drug addiction is very similar to that of many other chronic diseases, such as diabetes, heart disease, and cancer.

FIGURE 8.3. *Driving under the influence of alcohol in the past year among persons aged sixteen or older, by age, 2005.*

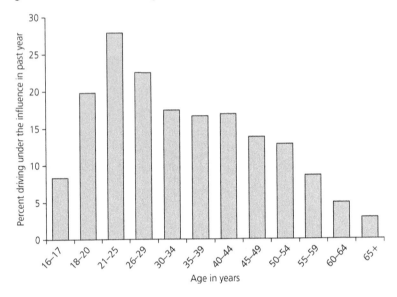

Source: SAMHSA, 2006b, fig. 3.6.

FIGURE 8.4. *Dependence on or abuse of specific illicit drugs in the past year among persons aged twelve or older, 2005.*

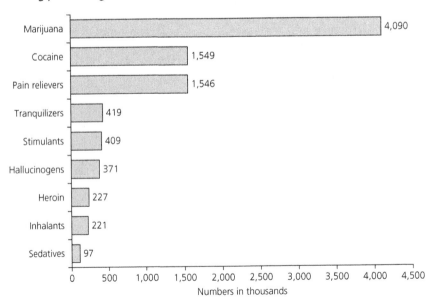

Source: SAMHSA, 2006b, fig. 7.2.

TABLE 8.1.   **Healthy People 2010: short titles of substance abuse objectives**

Number	Objective Short Title
Adverse Consequences of Substance Use and Abuse	
26-1	Motor vehicle crash deaths and injuries
26-2	Cirrhosis deaths
26-3	Drug-induced deaths
26-4	Drug-related hospital emergency department visits
26-5	Alcohol-related hospital emergency department visits
26-6	Adolescents riding with a driver who has been drinking
26-7	Alcohol- and drug-related violence
26-8	Lost productivity
Substance Use and Abuse	
26-9	Substance-free youth
26-10	Adolescent and adult use of illicit substances
26-11	Binge drinking
26-12	Average annual alcohol consumption
26-13	Low-risk drinking among adults
26-14	Steroid use among adolescents
26-15	Inhalant use among adolescents

(continued)

TABLE 8.1.   **Healthy People 2010: short titles of substance abuse objectives (*continued*)**

Number	Objective Short Title
Risk of Substance Use and Abuse	
26-16	Peer disapproval of substance abuse
26-17	Perception of risk associated with substance abuse
Treatment for Substance Abuse	
26-18	Treatment gap for illicit drugs
26-19	Treatment in correctional institutions
26-20	Treatment for injection drug use
26-21	Treatment gap for problem alcohol use
State and Local Efforts	
26-22	Hospital emergency department referrals
26-23	Community partnerships and coalitions
26-24	Administrative license revocation laws
26-25	(BAC) levels for motor vehicle drivers

Source: U.S. Department of Health and Human Services, 2000.

Process of Addiction

Addiction is a chronic, progressive dependence on a substance the user requires to be able to cope with daily activities. The stages of addiction are introduction, experimentation, incubation period, dependency, and withdrawal. According to NIDA (2006b), the first time a drug of abuse such as nicotine, alcohol, marijuana, cocaine, or heroin is used it results in a very pleasurable effect because it causes the release of certain chemicals into the brain. Addiction is actually a disease of the brain, and it is a chronic, relapsing disease, characterized by compulsive, often uncontrollable, drug seeking and use in the face of negative consequences.

Once using starts, the brain begins to change almost immediately. Therefore just experimenting with a drug of abuse changes the way the brain functions. There is also a noticeable craving for the new drug, which is the same effect as the desire for food, water, or friendship. There is no established norm for the number of drug episodes that are necessary to move the individual to addiction to a particular drug. However, the most frightening part about addiction is the relatively short incubation period from exposure to the drug until addiction to the drug, and then the much longer incubation period usually present from addiction to long-term morbidity and mortality. It is during the time period between addiction and disease that the substance abuse usually produces a negative impact on the person's family, community, and workplace.

Although treatments are readily available, the addicted individual does not usually want to be treated. Substance abuse has become a normal way of living for the addicted person. Life without the drug has actually become an abnormal way of living. Addiction is characterized by a desire to continue and to expand the use of a substance despite its harmful and dangerous effects. The predominant factors present in substance abuse that indicate addiction are tolerance for the drug, withdrawal symptoms as a dose is wearing off, and dependency.

One study (National Institute on Alcohol Abuse and Alcoholism, 2006) has found that if individuals become alcohol dependent before age twenty-five they are less likely to ever seek treatment than are those who become alcohol dependent at age thirty or older. The study also discovered that these younger individuals are more likely to have multiple dependence episodes of longer duration. This study helps us to understand the need for education at an early age.

Addiction Potential

Different drugs have different levels of addictive capabilities and therefore pose different levels of dangers for individuals. However, when addiction does occur, it usually is at a young age and it persists; to reiterate, it is a chronic disease. By classifying addiction to drugs as a chronic illness, we can employ the time-tested skills of the epidemiologist and the concepts of incubation periods, surveillance data, risk factors, years of potential life lost, and more elaborate analytical studies to better understand the process of addiction.

The **addiction process** is complicated because it involves human behaviors that are driven by changes in brain processes. *Healthy People 2010* (U.S. Department of Health and Human Services, 2000) explains that behaviors are individual responses or reactions to internal stimuli or external conditions. These behaviors can have a reciprocal, biological relationship: in other words, each can react to another. Personal choices and the social and physical environments surrounding individuals can shape their behaviors. The social and physical environments include most factors that affect the lives of individuals, positively or negatively, many of which may not be under an individual's immediate or direct control.

According to SAMHSA (2001), addiction begins with the act of taking drugs that may lead to a compulsive drug craving and this craving continues even in the face of negative consequences. The drug begins to affect brain functioning, which in turn affects behavior. Most drugs of abuse activate a part of the brain colloquially called the reward system, and that makes the drug user feel good (NIDA, 2006b). The prolonged use of a drug changes the brain in fundamental and long-lasting ways. Scientists have linked the release of dopamine in the brain to most drugs of abuse, including cocaine, marijuana, heroin, alcohol, and nicotine. All these drugs activate the reward system and cause neurons to release large amounts of dopamine. Over time, drug use damages this part of the brain.

Merrill and Timmreck (2006) identify four common stages of the **disease process**: stage of susceptibility; stage of presymptomatic disease; stage of clinical disease; and the stage of recovery, disability, or death. Each disease follows its own unique route as the host progresses from exposure to the disease agent to the manifestation of disease and disease complications. The model of addiction also begins with a susceptible host. We are all susceptible to drug addiction, but some are predisposed to it because of heredity and family and peer modeling of drug use. Then the individual is confronted with a point of exposure to drugs, typically during the early adolescent years. Many drugs do not need a high level of exposure; addiction may be the price of even minimal use. The chance for a cure for drug use ends when the addiction phase of the drug abuse actually begins.

Once addiction to the drug begins, the abuse becomes a chronic disease with no cure and only treatment, if the addicted person is willing to pursue it.

Model of Causation

Merrill and Timmreck (2006) point out that many behavioral, environmental, and genetic factors contribute to the development of noninfectious diseases, and therefore noninfectious and infectious diseases need to be studied in different ways. This is especially true when dealing with drug abuse, which presents epidemiologists with difficulty in the identification of causative factors.

A model of causation involving risk factors is an interesting method of studying chronic disease that may allow epidemiologists to obtain an accurate diagnosis of the causes of a number of these diseases. In this model the disease is the central focus, and the investigation works its way through a web of epidemiological factors that may be causes. These factors include but are not limited to the variables of time, place, person, agents, and exposures. Once a web of causation for a specific disease has been defined, the investigation can progress to using a causation decision tree, which guides brainstorming to identify the best way to prevent or at least control the noninfectious and chronic disease.

SUBSTANCES OFTEN ABUSED

The misuse and abuse of two categories of addictive drugs in particular have become epidemic in both the workplace and society over the last several years. These misused and abused drugs are alcohol and prescription drugs. Addictions to these and other drugs are having profound effects inside businesses and on individuals' family members.

Alcohol

SAMHSA (2006c) defines alcohol dependence or abuse using the criteria specified in the *Diagnostic and Statistical Manual of Mental Disorders* (*DSM-IV*). These criteria include experiencing withdrawal symptoms, developing tolerance, using alcohol in dangerous situations, having trouble with the law because of alcohol, and having alcohol interfere with major obligations at work, school, or home during the last year.

Alcoholism was once thought to be simply a human weakness, but as evidence of its disease-like characteristics grew, it was finally classified as a disease by the American Psychiatric Association in the early 1970s. According to SAMHSA (2002), the prevalence of alcohol consumption is higher for men (62.4 percent) than for women (47.9 percent). This drug alone is responsible for a very large part of rising health care costs, decreasing productivity, and family misery in this country.

Alcohol affects every organ in the body, especially the brain, and is responsible for a number of chronic diseases, including chronic liver disease and cirrhosis, gastro-intestinal cancers, heart disease, stroke, pancreatitis, depression, and a variety of social problems (Centers for Disease Control and Prevention, National Center for Chronic Disease Prevention and Health Promotion, 2005). Alcohol is also responsible for over one hundred thousand deaths each year, making it the fourth leading cause of death in this country (Brownson, Remington, & Davis, 1998). This disease is also a contributing factor to a whole host of other morbidity and mortality statistics, including years of potential life lost at an early age.

Alcohol use and abuse is a major contributing factor to injuries, especially in the workplace. Alcohol has pronounced negative effects on motor skills, judgment, and reaction time, making driving an automobile or operating machinery after consumption of alcohol very dangerous. This problem can be especially threatening in the workplace for both the impaired employee and those who work with him or her. Alcohol contributes to arguments, violence, employee absenteeism, and lost jobs (Eldin & Golanty, 2006). All these results of alcohol abuse have a tremendous effect on the productivity of the American workforce.

Binge drinking seems to be a catalyst for incidences of serious problems in the workplace. Naimi, Brewer, Mokdad, Denny, & Marks (2003) define binge drinking as having five or more drinks on one occasion and notes that one in three adult drinkers has reported past month binge drinking. Naimi et al. also finds that binge drinkers are fourteen times more likely to drive automobiles while intoxicated than nonbinge drinkers are. Binge drinking is also associated with unintentional and intentional injuries while on and off the job. According to SAMHSA (2006b), binge drinking occurs most often in young adults, with a prevalence rate of 38.7 percent. Fortunately, the problem of binge drinking decreases with age and becomes relatively rare after age sixty-five (see Figure 8.2).

The National Highway Traffic Safety Administration (NHTSA) (2006) reports that in 2005, 16,694 people in this country died in motor vehicle crashes involving alcohol, 39 percent of all traffic deaths in that year. These fatal accidents also represented a monetary cost to the nation of $51 billion. The CDC's National Center for Injury Prevention and Control (2002), reports that 4 percent of individuals who consume alcohol admitted to driving while impaired at least once during the past month. These individuals were usually male and single.

Prescription Drugs

The nonmedical use and abuse of prescription drugs in the United States is increasing (NIDA, 2006a). The three primary classes of prescription drugs that have been abused in recent years are opioids, central nervous system (CNS) depressants, and stimulants.

- *Opioids*. These drugs are used to relieve pain. Some of the more familiar opioids are OxyContin, Percodan, Percocet, Vicodin, and Darvon. They act on the brain to eliminate the perception of pain. These drugs are also capable of producing a sense of euphoria in the brain.

- *CNS depressants*. These drugs are prescribed to treat anxiety and sleep disorders. Among these drugs are barbiturates, such as mephobarbital, Valium, and Librium.

- *Stimulants*. These drugs include Dexedrine, Ritalin, and Concerta, which are used to treat attention deficit disorder and narcolepsy. Stimulants can cause hypertension, increased heart rate, and elevated blood glucose levels.

Simoni-Wastila and Strickler (2004) report that 1.3 million Americans aged twelve and over have become addicted to the use of prescription drugs. Their study also found those who abuse prescription drugs to be mostly female, older, and in poor health, and many of them are also using alcohol. Many of these individuals are still working and bringing their addiction to the workplace with them.

Prescription drugs provide great value to society by allowing individuals suffering with pain, depression, or other health problems to continue to be valuable members of their community and place of work. However, using these sometimes very dangerous drugs inappropriately or mixing them with alcohol can have dangerous effects on the individual and those around him or her. Making matters worse, the person misusing prescription drugs can easily become addicted to their use.

DRUG-FREE WORKPLACES AND EAPS

The **drug-free workplace** is an employment setting in which employees are discouraged from alcohol and drug abuse and encouraged to seek treatment and complete recovery if they have a drug abuse problem. The concept of a drug-free workplace has been around for years, and most businesses in this country have seriously addressed this issue. These companies are all well aware of the human and economic costs associated with an impaired employee. One way to encourage treatment is to have an **employee assistance program** available.

Employee Assistance Programs

Businesses across America have realized that they have a responsibility to help their employees who are experiencing difficulties in life. It has become a corporate responsibility to aid troubled employees, and it makes good economic sense to do so. The development of an **employee assistance program** (EAP) can help an employer to identify employees with problems and attempt to get them the help that they need.

An EAP usually includes many employee services such as financial counseling, marriage counseling, wellness programs, and drug and alcohol assistance programs. They are usually strongly supported by supervisors because they offer a supervisor one additional tool to deal with an employee with a performance problem. These programs have a preventive component in that they can help employees early on in their problems through educational initiatives conducted at the workplace. The problem with asking companies to offer prevention is that it is hard to measure the success of a program that prevents something from ever happening in the first place.

Employee assistance programs are paid for by the employer, so the costs are very visible before anything visible is accomplished. To understand the value of an EAP, employers need to be aware of all the costs associated with an impaired employee. In addition to the higher medical costs and costs of lower productivity already mentioned, if the company finally has to terminate employment with the employee, there will be costs associated with conducting the termination and then recruiting and training and acculturating a new employee. This can be a very expensive process, with no guarantee of obtaining a more productive employee. There may also be costs from losing the terminated employee's contacts and experience and from morale problems among that employee's former coworkers.

An employer can ignore the problem of drug abuse or be proactive and deal with potential problems arising from drug abuse before they happen. There were 3.9 million persons aged twelve or older (1.6 percent of the population) who received some kind of treatment for a problem related to the use of alcohol or illicit drugs in 2005. Of these, 1.5 million received treatment for the use of both alcohol and illicit drugs, 0.7 million received treatment for the use of illicit drugs but not alcohol, and 1.3 million received treatment for the use of alcohol but not illicit drugs (SAMHSA, 2006b).

Among these 3.9 million persons aged twelve or older who received treatment for alcohol or illicit drugs, more than half (2.1 million) received treatment at a self-help group. there were 1.5 million persons who received treatment at a rehabilitation facility as an outpatient, 1.1 million at a rehabilitation facility as an inpatient, 1.0 million at a mental health center as an outpatient, 773,000 at a hospital as an inpatient, 460,000 at a private doctor's office, 399,000 at an emergency room, and 344,000 at a prison or jail. None of these estimates changed significantly between 2004 and 2005.

Persons who did not receive treatment even though they made an effort to get it and felt they needed it cited such access barriers as cost or insurance issues, not being ready to stop using alcohol or illicit drugs, and stigma (see Figure 8.5).

Once the decision is made to establish an employee assistance program, the next issue is whether to operate the program internally or contract the process out. The most important components of a well-developed program that will support a drug-free workplace are described in Exhibit 8.1.

FIGURE 8.5. *Reasons for not receiving substance use treatment among persons aged twelve or older who needed and made an effort to get treatment but did not receive treatment and felt they needed treatment, 2004–2005.*

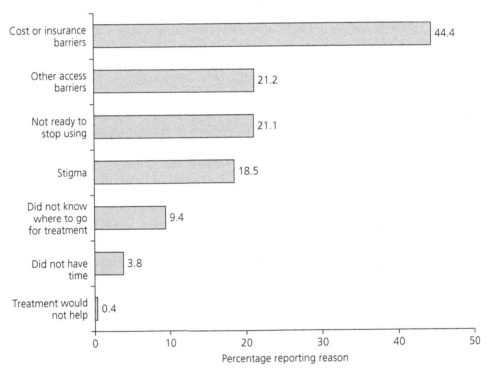

Note: Persons who made no effort to receive treatment were more likely to report that they were not ready to stop using (45.3 percent) as a reason for not receiving treatment than persons who made an effort to receive treatment (21.1 percent) (2004–2005 combined data). Among those who made no effort to receive treatment, 26.3 percent reported stigma and 31.0 percent reported cost and insurance barriers as reasons for not receiving treatment.

Source: SAMHSA, 2006b, fig. 7.8.

EXHIBIT 8.1.   **Important components of an EAP that supports a drug-free workplace**

A Written Policy

The most important thing for an employer to do in dealing with workplace drug abuse is to develop a written policy informing all employees about the company position on drug and alcohol use in the workplace. This policy needs to be completely clear and applied to everyone in a clear and consistent manner. It needs to explain the consequences for an employee using, selling, or possessing drugs or alcohol in the workplace. Finally, all employees need to acknowledge, in writing, that they have read or heard the provisions of the policy and that they accept them.

Access to Assistance

The assistance to which employees have access needs to be a professionally managed assistance program with certified professionals capable of helping the troubled employee. The majority of health insurance plans offer some coverage for drug and alcohol treatment programs to help with this part of the workplace problem.

Employee Education

Educational programs concerning drugs, drug abuse, and drug addiction need to be offered to all employees of the business. These programs need to be developed, implemented, and evaluated by staff with a health education background.

Supervisor Training

The supervisors of the business need to receive the same training as the employees, with an additional component consisting of advanced training on how to deal with an impaired employee. The supervisor should learn to always concentrate on performance when disciplining and terminating employees, in order to avoid discrimination charges. This training should also emphasize how to properly document the actions taken by employers and the reasons for these actions.

Drug Testing

If drug testing is to be done, company administrators and human resource managers need to determine the type of drug testing needed and when it should be done, and they need to develop and evaluate a process for it. The only method of drug testing approved by the U.S. Department of Health and Human Services is urinalysis. Most employers look for an approved contractor to handle this part of the employee assistance program because the test must be performed by certified technicians. The company needs to be very careful not to violate employee rights when doing employee drug testing.

Source: SAMHSA (2006a).

Companies that decide not to participate in an EAP program can still offer their employees a choice between their continued use of drugs and loss of their employment with the company. If employers do not stop drug abuse among employees they are supporting the addiction process.

EAP Cost Effectiveness

NIDA (2006a) reports that treatment of addicted employees is less expensive than incarceration. Every dollar invested in treatment programs results in a reduction of up to seven dollars in crime-related costs. When the costs of health care resulting from addiction are included in the equation, the savings increase to twelve dollars saved for every dollar invested in treatment programs. Businesses also experience a reduction in interpersonal conflicts, improved worker productivity, and fewer drug-related accidents, making investment in workplace drug reduction programs a very successful and cost-effective decision for employers and our society.

SUMMARY

Drug abuse in the workplace has become a major safety and occupational health issue for employers to resolve. The costs of doing nothing are enormous and include lost productivity, higher health insurance premiums, declines in worker morale, increases in injuries, and more disability claims.

An epidemiological approach can determine how to best prevent and control the complications of substance abuse in the workplace. When this chronic disease is looked at as an economic cost for the business as well as the society in which the business functions, there is a much better chance of gaining the attention of administrators and managers and developing, implementing, and evaluat-

ing workplace programs that have a chance of success.

Because abuse of drugs is also a community health problem, a great many resources are available to businesses to help them establish a drug-free workplace. There are also numerous governmental agencies available to help small and large businesses in the development, implementation, and evaluation of an employee assistance program.

Programs developed to prevent and control drug abuse in the workplace do very well when evaluated through cost-effectiveness analyses. Money spent on assisting employees through drug abuse problems will show a positive return on investment for the employer.

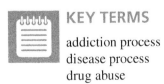

KEY TERMS

addiction process
disease process
drug abuse

drug-free workplace
employee assistance program

QUESTIONS FOR DISCUSSION

1. What does the designation *impaired employee* mean?

2. What are the health impacts of substance abuse?

3. What are the stages in the process of addiction?

4. How does drug abuse impact the employer? How does drug abuse result in increased costs for the employer?

CHAPTER

9

WELLNESS PROGRAMS

After reading this chapter, you should be able to

- Understand the value of workplace wellness programs.

- Identify high-risk behaviors responsible for worker illness and injury.

- Describe the stages of developing a workplace health promotion program.

- Discuss the value of programs to improve workers' nutrition and physical activity.

Public health departments throughout the country recommend that establishing health promotion efforts in the workplace, especially at smaller worksites, should continue to be an important goal. Healthy People 2010 objectives call for at least 75 percent of worksites to offer comprehensive health promotion programs, but only about 7 percent of workplaces currently offer these programs, according to a recent survey. This number must become higher, because for the employer health promotion just makes good economic sense.

One of the most important studies ever conducted involved an epidemiological evaluation of heart disease in Framingham, Massachusetts. This cohort study, which began in 1947 and which we have described in Chapters One and Two, found that smoking, a sedentary lifestyle, and poor nutrition were causes of heart disease and other **chronic diseases.** The people of Framingham gave all of us some very valuable information about how to improve our quality of life and live a longer life by making a few simple adjustments in our health behaviors. These high-risk health behaviors, if prevented or changed, can free us from many potential health problems as we grow older. The catalyst required for this behavioral change is nothing more than well-developed health promotion efforts (Centers for Disease Control and Prevention, 2009a) and health information that is provided frequently to large groups of people in order to convince them of the value of behavioral change. Two of the best places to provide this information to the vast majority of Americans are the school and the workplace.

The Institute of Medicine (2003) points out that a majority of employers have several reasons to take an interest in the health of their employees. Compared to their healthy coworkers, injured or ill employees consume more health resources, make more disability claims, and receive more workers' compensation; they are also less productive. However, leadership is required if **workplace wellness programs** are to become a reality for most businesses. This leadership can be provided by the public health sector of our health care system.

David Satcher (2006), the former surgeon general of the United States, sums up what individuals need to do in order to remain healthy:

- Practice moderate physical activity on a daily basis.

- Consume at least five servings of fruits and vegetables per day.

- Avoid toxins like tobacco, alcohol, and illicit drugs.

- Practice responsible sexual behavior.

These simple activities can go a long way toward reducing the current epidemic of chronic diseases and protecting those who already have chronic diseases from developing complications from those diseases. Satcher calls this list a prescription for good health in the age of an escalating epidemic of chronic diseases. It is sad that we know so much about how to prevent chronic diseases and their complications and yet are still struggling with the development of health promotion programs that will be successful. The development of chronic diseases is not the result of a lack of access to health care; it results from a lack of good information about high-risk health behaviors, information that could easily be provided in schools and workplaces.

There is mounting evidence in the medical literature of a clear relationship between the reduction of a few **modifiable risk factors** and the later development of chronic diseases. These behaviors involve the use of tobacco, the use of alcohol, a sedentary lifestyle, and poor nutrition. Because workplace wellness programs are usually limited in scope and available resources, this chapter will concentrate on the prevention of chronic diseases through **evidence-based prevention programs** made available to all employees in the workplace and focusing on behaviors involving tobacco use, alcohol use, physical inactivity, and poor nutrition. (Injury prevention is discussed in Chapters Four, Eleven, and Thirteen, and alcohol abuse is addressed in Chapter Eight.)

CHRONIC DISEASES IN THE WORKPLACE

The epidemiology and control of chronic diseases is a rapidly growing field in this new century. The leading cause of morbidity and mortality in this country has changed from communicable diseases such as tuberculosis and influenza to chronic diseases, especially heart disease, cancer, and diabetes. Long-term exposures to behavioral and environmental risk factors at home and at work are the cause of these chronic diseases. These noninfectious diseases are much different from communicable diseases in having a much longer incubation period, in lacking a cure, and in producing long-term, negative effects on the quality of life.

According to Morewitz (2006), there are 25 million Americans with chronic diseases; many are unable to work and most have a decreased quality of life because of their disease. These diseases are bad enough, but the real cost occurs after the complications that can result from these diseases develop later in life. These complications persist when individuals continue to practice the same modifiable risk factors that caused their diseases in the first place. As we have discussed, these diseases do not lend themselves to cure, only to prevention. (Additional information about chronic diseases is discussed in Chapters One and Three.) The prevention of chronic diseases requires us to change our idea that disease is an inevitable consequence of the aging process. It also requires that an intervention to prevent a disease occurs before the disease begins to develop; ideally this will be even before the high-risk behaviors for that chronic disease begin or when these behaviors have been practiced for only a short period of time.

Recent surveillance data from the Centers for Disease Control and Prevention indicate that 21 percent of all adults are current smokers, and 21 percent are former smokers. Using estimates of body mass index, analysts have determined that 35 percent of U.S. adults are overweight and 24 percent are obese. These statistics do not make one optimistic about the success of helping people to understand the long-term ramifications of chronic diseases. It does indicate that we need to evaluate how we deliver health services and try to understand why our current model of delivery has failed. Many in public health believe the entire U.S. health care system should be restructured to focus on prevention and not on cure.

Workplaces in the United States are experiencing one of the largest epidemics of chronic disease in the world, and it is growing in numbers of victims. The chronic disease incubation period can be as long as forty years. Compared to other diseases, chronic diseases produce the greatest burden in terms of disability, death, and financial cost. The ironic part is that these diseases are almost totally preventable and yet they are being ignored by employers and employees. The Occupational Safety and Health Administration (OSHA) and the National Institute for Occupational Safety and Health (NIOSH) care a great deal about environmental risk factors for occupational disease, but they too seem to ignore the behavioral risk factors that employees practice. There seems to be a real need for the leadership that can effectively advocate for well-constructed chronic disease prevention programs in the workplace.

THE VALUE OF WELLNESS PROGRAMS

Illness and injuries are having a tremendous impact on U.S. workplaces. Employee health has become a major concern for employers because, as we have discussed in previous chapters, healthy employees benefit employers in two important ways. First, healthy employees have higher productivity than unhealthy employees because they come to work more often and they feel well while they are participating in work. Second, unhealthy employees use more medical services and drive up health insurance costs. Expansion of health care programs with the goal of prevention can make the individual healthier and, in the long run, reduce health care costs and increase productivity.

Most companies in the United States think nothing of training workers in order to increase their productivity if this transfers into increased company profits. Yet they have been reluctant to develop workplace wellness programs, which could increase productivity and reduce health costs while making employees healthier through the practice of behavioral medicine. This type of medicine requires active participation by the individual who is attempting to develop and maintain wellness. It is to both employees' and employers' advantage to use the workplace as a catalyst for the development and practice of good health habits. In order to achieve this win-win situation, trust must be built between workers and managers. Wellness programs to prevent chronic disease also require good planning and evaluation in order to show success. The leadership role in this venture must be assumed by management.

Cost-benefit analyses of outcomes typically show that chronic disease prevention programs are financially worthwhile. The costs of starting health promotion and disease prevention programs can be quite high in their initial stage of development. But as the prevention effort intensifies, a much larger return on the initial investment is realized. What businesses need to do is consult with public health experts who have established successful worksite programs and know how to reduce program start-up costs. The participation rate in a voluntary worksite health promotion and disease prevention program is usually quite low in the beginning, making the program cost quite high for each employee who uses the program. Therefore the key to success seems to be the addition of some type of incentive, so that a greater number of employees become involved in the program earlier rather than later. Discussion between management and workers about the value of wellness programs needs to happen long before the new initiative is put in place, and this can also aid participation.

One way to reduce wellness program costs is to first survey the company employees in order to discover their overall health status. In other words, separate the symptoms from the real problems. Successful programs have hired consulting companies to develop ways to increase employees' health literacy and to devise a marketing approach to increase program participation. The expertise of local and state health departments can also be called upon when developing a worksite wellness program. Because participation is usually not mandatory, such programs must be promoted as a voluntary employee choice that will help the employee reduce health costs in the long run for both employer and employee and at the same time help the employee to feel healthier now and avoid major health problems later.

ADDRESSING OBESITY AND NUTRITION

One component of an overall workplace wellness program focused on prevention must address reducing **obesity** and improving nutrition.

Understanding Obesity in the Workplace

Overweight and obesity are a leading cause of the development of many chronic diseases, including heart disease, hypertension, diabetes, arthritis, and some cancers, and overweight and obesity are now epidemic in the United States. In the past thirty years the prevalence of overweight and obesity has increased dramatically for both children and adults, more than doubling in the last few years alone. More specifically, 66 percent of Americans are reported to be overweight, and 33 percent are obese. Many of these individuals are members of the workforce.

Generally speaking, individuals whose weight is 20 percent over their desirable weight in relation to their height are considered obese. More precisely, obesity in an adult is defined as having a body mass index (BMI) over 30, whereas overweight in an adult means having a BMI between 25 and 29.9. But whether people are overweight or obese, the added body weight is going to make them more susceptible to chronic diseases the longer that they carry the weight around with them.

It is not that individual Americans are unaware of their weight gain. At any given time, over 50 percent of the men and women in this country are attempting to lose weight. They spend a great deal of money on fad diets and useless food supplements attempting to lose weight and improve their body image. Some of these people are successful in their weight loss only to gain the weight back in a short period of time. The original weight gain probably took years and the loss of this weight is going to take time. There is no easy fix; losing weight is hard work. It requires a reduction of calories and an increase in physical activity.

This epidemic of being overweight or obese has a direct and negative effect on employers. The total cost of obesity in this country in 2000 was about $117 billion (Centers for Disease Control and Prevention, 2009d), with a good proportion of that money coming directly from employers' profits. But the workplace is also the ideal location in which to provide individuals with the motivation to reduce their weight. The worksite can promote regular physical activity and good nutrition and can create an environment that supports these behaviors. The starting point for dealing with this epidemic in the workplace is to begin a workplace discussion about the problem and entertain potential solutions to address the issue.

The CDC is conducting extensive research into how employers can best prevent and control obesity among their workers. The research data will be shared with employers to help them deal with this epidemic. It has become very clear from the Framingham Heart Study and recent research on obesity that the answer to reducing weight or preventing weight gain lies in good nutrition and daily moderate physical activity. It has also become clear that nutrition and physical activity can become part of the workplace daily habits.

William Dietz, director of the CDC's Division of Nutrition, Physical Activity and Obesity, believes that the answer to the obesity epidemic lies in encouraging individuals to eat more fruits and vegetables, engage in more physical activity, and reduce their consumption of high-calorie foods and sugar-sweetened beverages. This does not seem like too hard a task given the need to reduce people's weight and help them avoid chronic diseases. Better diet and more physical activity should be promoted by all worksites in this country.

Developing a Nutrition Wellness Policy

Dietary factors are associated with four of the ten leading causes of death: coronary heart disease, some types of cancer, stroke, and type 2 diabetes. These and other health conditions related to dietary factors cost society an estimated $200 billion each year in medical expenses and lost productivity (United States Department of Agriculture, 2009). According to the International Labour Organization (2005) of the United Nations, in the United States the annual economic costs of obesity in insurance, paid sick leave, and other related payments alone come to $12.7 billion, and around the world poor diet on the job is costing countries up to 20 percent in lost potential productivity.

The Prevention Institute (2002) points out that eating is a behavior greatly influenced by the workplace. Work is where many people spend the majority of their weekday waking hours. At least one meal is consumed at work, and snacks are often a means to relieve pressure and a way to pass the time during rest breaks throughout the workday. The food available in employee cafeterias, in vending machines, and at work-sponsored events frequently determines what employees eat during their work hours. Many times, food provided by the workplace is not highly nutritious or is high in fat or sugar; for example, snacks and meeting foods typically include cookies, pastries, candy, and other sources of surplus fat, sugar, and calories. The realities of the work environment can overpower the good intentions of workers to eat healthier. Employers should implement workplace policies that require nutritious food options in employee cafeterias and at work-sponsored events.

A 1999 study in health education and behavior found that "the majority of programs in the U.S. designed to improve workplace health have focused specifically on changing individual behavior without making much effort to make institutional changes in the work environment" (Prevention Institute, 2002). The implementation of wellness policies that require nutritious food options in the workplace can establish a healthy workplace environment and demonstrate employer commitment to employee health.

Food recommendations included in nutrition wellness policies should be based on *Dietary Guidelines for Americans 2005*, a joint publication of the U.S. Department of Health and Human Services and the U.S. Department of Agriculture (2005), and on MyPyramid, a food guide pyramid maintained by the U.S. Department of Agriculture (2009). The dietary guidelines for Americans are science-based recommendations for healthy Americans aged two years and over about food choices that will promote health and prevent disease. The MyPyramid resource helps individual consumers personalize these recommendations to fit their unique nutrition needs.

Nutrition research has found that American diets are low in fruits, vegetables, low-fat dairy products, and whole grains and are high in refined carbohydrates, total fat, and saturated fat. Given the strong relationship between diet and health and the increasing rates of obesity, guidelines can and should be developed to facilitate employees' selection of low-fat and low-calorie food and beverage options in workplace cafeterias and vending machines and also at meetings, seminars, and catered events.

Here are four general areas to consider when developing nutrition wellness policies:

- Healthy meeting policies

- Vending machine nutrition standards

- Healthy dining menu guidelines

- An employee wellness program

Implement Healthy Meeting Policies   Many meetings and seminars during the workday provide food, often high in fat and sugar. A healthier approach is to promote bottled water, diet soda, and low-calorie food options for snacks during company meetings, or consider not offering food at mid-morning or mid-afternoon meetings, presentations, and seminars. In America we are surrounded by food all day, everyday; it is important to consider whether it is necessary to provide food at every event, especially ones that do not take place during people's regular meal times. Companies should try to create an environment where food does not have to be omnipresent and is not used to try to motivate people to attend certain events. Meeting sponsors might consider offering only beverages. If they decide to provide food, they can offer only fruits, vegetables, and other healthy options. (See, for example, University of Minnesota, School of Public Health (2003), for general guidelines and specific food suggestions.)

Set Vending Machine Nutrition Standards   A Fit City initiative in San Antonio, Texas, reports that many employees choose to get food regularly from vending machines. Vending machines and company stores can employ variable pricing to encourage the purchase of foods with higher nutritional values or the less healthy choices they carry can be limited. This initiative developed some vending machine guidelines, including recommendations for healthy snacks and beverages. Items that met "healthiest" and "healthier" criteria were identified and marketed as such. Exhibit 9.1 displays these criteria.

EXHIBIT 9.1.   Criteria for healthy vending machine items

Snacks

Healthiest—must meet both criteria

- 3 grams of Total Fat or fewer per serving (Nuts and seeds exempt from restrictions.)
- 30 grams of Carbohydrates or fewer per serving (All candies are considered unhealthy. Fruit in any form is permitted, regardless of carbohydrate count.)

Healthier—must meet both criteria

- 5 grams of Total Fat or fewer per serving (Nuts and seeds exempt from restrictions.)
- 30 grams of Carbohydrates or fewer per serving (All candies are considered unhealthy. Fruit in any form is permitted, regardless of carbohydrate count.)

Portion Size—portion size is not defined for any items, but smaller portion sizes are preferred.

Beverages

Healthiest

- Milk—Lowfat (1%) or nonfat preferred, any flavor
- Water—Pure
- Juice—At least 50% fruit or vegetable juice

Healthier

- Water—Flavored or vitamin enhanced
- Low-calorie beverage—<50 calories per 12 oz serving

Source: Fit City, San Antonio, Texas, 2002.

This Fit City initiative also offers these suggestions for organizations looking to improve vending machine options (adapted from Fit City, San Antonio, Texas, 2002):

1. Identify a representative to meet with or contact the vending machine provider and arrange a meeting to discuss healthy vending options

2. Decide how many healthy items you would like in your vending machines. For many organizations, 100 percent healthy is too high. If this is the first health initiative in your organization, you might decide to try for 50 percent. Decide what makes sense for your organization.

3. Talk to employees about the initiative: send out memos; put articles on your Web site or in newsletters. Promote the good stuff and publicize your success stories. Try to be positive and nonjudgmental.

4. Promote healthy options in vending machines with window clings or price tags that identify "healthiest" and "healthier" choices.

5. Monitor sales of healthy options to determine reordering needs and track success.

Create a Healthy Dining Menu   If in-house dining is available offer healthy food choices at breakfasts, lunches, dinners, and receptions. There are many options for tasty foods and beverages that are also nutritious. Fruits and vegetables should always be emphasized, along with low-fat dairy products and whole grains. Portion sizes have increased substantially in the United States in recent years and can contribute to unnecessary calories. Consider offering smaller portions of foods; this can greatly reduce the total calories consumed. Cafeterias may also institute variable pricing based on the nutritional and caloric values of foods served.

Make Nutrition Part of the Wellness Program   Nutrition education should be a key component of a successful workplace wellness program. A registered dietitian serves as a valuable team member in this program and can provide counseling and in-house services to address employees' specific nutrition concerns. A dietitian can also evaluate the cafeteria and vending machines to determine healthy food options. He or she may even work with local food services to ensure regular healthy choices on the menu and in vending machines. Dietitians can also provide weight management classes or support groups. Exhibit 9.2 provides some examples of organizations that encourage healthy eating in the workplace.

ADDRESSING PHYSICAL INACTIVITY

The United States is also experiencing an epidemic of **physical inactivity**, a behavior defined as getting less than the recommended amount of regular physical activity. The Framingham study uncovered the relationship between regular physical activity and the avoidance of the majority of chronic diseases. Unfortunately, the vast majority of Americans do not receive enough physical activity to aid them in the prevention of coronary heart disease, diabetes, and colon cancer. Indeed, a sedentary lifestyle affects

EXHIBIT 9.2. **Examples of successful nutrition wellness programs**

The companies in the following examples were winners of the 2004/2005 Fit Business Award.

Dole Food Company (More than 1,000 Employees)
Dole has created a healthy food and fitness environment that encourages employees to make healthier choices. Dole's "Model Cafeteria" has eliminated all saturated fat in most foods, sugar sodas, unhealthy food, and expanded offerings of fish entrees, vegetarian and vegan selections, and healthy desserts. In addition, free fruit and vegetable snacks are available to employees in the morning and afternoon.

Mammoth Hospital, Mammoth Lakes, California (100–299 Employees)
Mammoth Hospital also provides an environment for healthy eating at the worksite. There are healthy choices in vending machines and a cafeteria with a calendar of daily menu items that are healthy. The company uses three symbols to help its employees make healthy choices in the cafeteria. A heart symbol is for healthy heart low-calorie meal days, the stop sign symbol signifies that the meal may be high fat, and the triangle symbol tells employees to watch their portion sizes and side dish options.

Source: California Task Force on Youth and Workplace Wellness, 2005.

virtually all dimensions of health—physiological, psychological, and societal. And as Satcher (2006) points out, poor nutrition, overweight and obesity, and physical inactivity feed off each other, increasing individuals' chances of developing a chronic disease, becoming disabled, reducing their quality of life, and dying prematurely. Physical inactivity is another high-risk health behavior that has a major economic impact in terms of health care costs and reduced worker productivity. It is also another example of how the changing of a lifestyle behavior can have a major effect on one's overall health.

The CDC and the American College of Sports recommend that individuals get thirty minutes of moderate intensity physical activity most days of the week ("Trends in Leisure-Time Physical Inactivity . . . ," 2005), and this can even be broken down into two fifteen-minute segments. This physical activity can come in the form of cardio or aerobic activities and resistance, strength building, and weight-bearing activity. This type of exercise affects most parts of the body and is an appropriate activity no matter what one's age.

Two objectives of the Healthy People 2010 program are to increase the proportion of adults who engage in regular moderate or vigorous activity to at least 50 percent and to decrease the proportion of adults who engage in no leisure-time physical activity to no more than 20 percent ("Trends in Leisure-Time Physical Inactivity . . . ," 2005). These goals can be achieved during leisure time at home or in the workplace. It does not matter where the physical activity occurs; it only matters that it occurs almost every day. Daily physical activity helps to reduce anxiety and depression. This can go a long way toward improving self-esteem and increasing feelings of well-being. It also raises the good cholesterol in the arteries along with increasing blood flow.

There is also evidence that daily physical activity improves people's chances of getting a good night's sleep. Nationally, 50 to 70 million people suffer from chronic sleep loss and sleep disorders. This loss of sleep has been associated with obesity, depression, and some high-risk health behaviors such as cigarette smoking, heavy drinking, abuse of sleep medications, and physical inactivity,

It does seem that the negative outcomes from the health behaviors first uncovered by the Framingham study and supported by most studies since point to the need to change a few lifestyle choices to improve our quality of life and reduce our chances of premature death. These findings about physical activity are also important for the workplace if it is to reduce health care costs and increase worker productivity.

Some of the major barriers to physical activity include

- Time constraints

- Lack of self-motivation

- A feeling that exercise is boring and not enjoyable

- Lack of confidence in one's ability to be physically active

- Lack of encouragement, support, or companionship from family and friends

All of these barriers can be reduced or eliminated in the workplace that has a physical activity program. Moreover these programs can have tremendous cost-benefit results from a small investment. A recent cost-benefit analysis concluded that over $4 billion per year could be saved in health care spending if all sedentary adults participated in a walking program at home or at the workplace (Jones & Eaton, 1994). The barriers to participating in physical activity on a daily basis can be removed by the employer who encourages physical activity at work. Another major advantage of workplace physical activity programs is that they could potentially act as a surveillance system to report progress and further evaluate the cost-benefit effects offered by this type of employee wellness program.

ADDRESSING TOBACCO USE

We have known about the relationship between the use of tobacco and lung cancer since the early 1950s. We know that tobacco is far more dangerous than originally thought now that it has been linked with other forms of cancer and other chronic diseases as well. We also know that use of tobacco is addictive because of a drug in tobacco called nicotine. This one modifiable behavior is responsible for 430,000 deaths each year, which represents 20 percent of the total yearly mortality in the United

States. A recent CDC report states that about 2.4 million cancers were diagnosed in the United States from 1999 to 2004, with lung and bronchial cancers accounting for almost half of these diagnoses. According to the study's lead author, "The data in this report provides additional, strong evidence of the serious harm related to tobacco. We've long known tobacco was associated with lung and laryngeal cancer, but this study gives us even greater clarity. The rates for these two cancers were highest in areas with the highest prevalence of tobacco use (CDC, 2008a).

According to the CDC (2008a), tobacco use is the number one cause of preventable morbidity and mortality in the United States. This is a significant finding for employers across our country. Smoking affects every organ in the body, causing many diseases and negatively affecting smokers' overall health. Many of the diseases caused by tobacco have a very long incubation period, perhaps twenty to thirty years, making it probable that using tobacco in the workplace is helping the development of these deadly diseases.

In spite of the dangers of tobacco, it is still used by far too many Americans. Approximately 45 million adults use tobacco on a daily basis. This epidemic of tobacco use costs $96 billion per year in direct medical expenses and $97 billion in lost productivity in the workplace (CDC, 2008b).

In addition, the workplace is still a major source of **secondhand smoke** exposure for adults. As discussed in Chapter Six, the smoke exhaled by smokers is involuntarily inhaled by those who do not smoke, and this secondhand smoke can cause adverse health effects including cancer, respiratory infections, and asthma. This environmental carcinogen remains in the air hours after the cigarette is gone, emitting hundreds of chemicals including formaldehyde, benzene, vinyl chloride, arsenic ammonia, and hydrogen cyanide. Thirty percent of workers are exposed to passive smoking in the workplace.

Secondhand smoke has been designated a known human carcinogen by the U.S. Environmental Protection Agency, the National Toxicology Program, and the International Agency for Research on Cancer. The surgeon general calls smoking the single greatest avoidable cause of death for the smoker and all those around him or her. Yet, despite knowing all this scientific evidence, many employers have been reluctant to prohibit use of tobacco in the workplace or to offer their workers smoking cessation programs in the workplace. This means that although many states have instituted laws making workplaces smoke free, we still have a long way to go in freeing all workers from secondhand smoke. Those at highest risk are blue-collar and service workers, who quite often have to choose between their current job in a workplace where people smoke and a lower-paying job in a smoke-free environment. This must change.

The 22.5 percent of Americans who smoke cigarettes and are unable to quit need assistance. Smoking is an addictive behavior and stopping this habit is probably the most difficult thing many people will ever attempt to do. In many workplaces in America the use of cigarettes has become part of the culture. Employers should have a strong interest in helping their employees to stop this deadly habit. In order to be effective in helping employees to quit smoking, employers need to develop and implement smoke-free policies for the workplace and help employees quit smoking through funding tobacco cessation programs.

The American Legacy Foundation (2006) reports that smoking cessation efforts in the workplace are very inexpensive, costing less than $0.50 per member per month. The benefit from such a program is a reduction in medical and life insurance costs of at least $210 each year almost immediately. The CDC estimates that smoking contributes $92 billion dollars each year in lost productivity that results from smoking-related diseases ("Annual Smoking-Attributable Mortality . . . ," 2005). Many managed health care programs are very responsive to helping employers develop and implement workplace tobacco cessation programs.

DEVELOPING COMPREHENSIVE HEALTH PROGRAMS

Employers need to know the value of health promotion programs and, more important, which programs offer the greatest value. Fortunately, research over the last few years is available to help employers decide which health promotion programs offer the greatest values in terms of costs and benefits to both employers and employees.

Health promotion programs have been developed in many businesses in a methodical way over the last several years. Wilson, Holman, and Hammock (1996) find that these programs have usually progressed through four generations. First-generation programs were not really offered to improve health in the short term. Second-generation programs were developed around a single intervention. Third-generation programs usually offered many interventions designed for several risk factors. Now, in the latest generation, these programs have taken a comprehensive approach, fulfilling several organizational policies, providing many interventions, and offering help with decisions that affect employees' health.

A comprehensive workplace health promotion program, as defined in *Healthy People 2010,* contains five elements, outlined in Exhibit 9.3.

The first element, health education, should be a learning experience that facilitates voluntary adoption of positive health behaviors designed to facilitate a state of good health. Such health promotion should also be designed to decrease exposure to harmful factors that can affect health. Development of a comprehensive workplace health promotion program begins by understanding the need for both these factors.

The second element, a supportive environment for the development and practice of these positive health behaviors, comes into being in the workplace when the vast majority of participating workers are attempting to implement positive changes in their lives.

The third and fourth elements both encourage worksite wellness programs to become part of the structure of the business, giving health promotion new credibility among employees.

The Partnership for Prevention (2001) recommends the following ten-step process when developing a comprehensive worksite health promotion program, with employers making whatever variations are needed to accommodate a particular workplace and its specific health goals. These steps have been used by many employers to develop wellness programs. The first seven steps constitute the planning phase, and it

EXHIBIT 9.3. Elements of a comprehensive worksite health promotion program

1. *Health education,* including a focus on skill development for health behavior change, and information dissemination and awareness building, preferably tailored to employees' interests and needs.

2. *Supportive social and physical environments,* including implementation of policies that promote health and reduce risk of disease.

3. *Integration of the worksite program* into your organization's structure.

4. *Linkage to related programs,* like employee assistance programs (EAPs) and programs to help employees balance work and family.

5. *Worksite screening programs,* ideally linked to medical care to ensure follow-up and appropriate treatment as necessary.

Source: U.S. Department of Health and Human Services, 2000.

is during this time that support from management is especially critical and that consultation with public health professionals can go a long way toward making the process easier and successful.

1. Establish a planning committee.

2. Complete a needs assessment of management and employees.

3. Complete a formal mission statement, including goals and objectives for the wellness program.

4. Establish a time line for measurement of success and develop a budget for the program.

5. Select incentives.

6. Acquire resources.

7. Develop a marketing plan for the program.

8. Implement the program.

9. Complete an evaluation of the success or failure of the program.

10. If necessary, change the program on a continuous basis.

Employers should be encouraged to contact their local or state health department before starting the process of developing a comprehensive health promotion program, to help ensure that they will develop a successful program that can improve the health of their employees.

The Role for OSHA and NIOSH

There is a tremendous role to be played by OSHA and NIOSH in workplace wellness programs. What is the difference between asbestosis, silicosis, pneumoconiosis, and byssinosis on the one hand and lung cancer and heart disease on the other? The answer is that the first four are lung diseases caused largely by inhaling specific workplace dusts and irritants and are regulated by governmental agencies. The last two are chronic diseases caused largely by tobacco use (including passive smoking) and other risky behaviors and are not currently regulated. They are not regulated and not reported in the workplace, yet they are leading causes of death and disability in our country.

There is a tremendous opportunity present for NIOSH to help workplaces develop sophisticated surveillance systems that can track chronic diseases in the workplace. Data from such a system could be an essential tool for developing and implementing programs to reduce or eliminate these health problems. Chronic disease surveillance systems ought to be developed and implemented in every business in this country.

In 1878, the U.S. Marine Hospital Service was authorized by Congress to begin collecting disease data on cholera, plague, smallpox, and yellow fever for use in quarantine measures. It is as true now as it was then that the epidemiology of disease is only as good as the accuracy of the surveillance systems in the places of concern. Chronic diseases have an occupational disease component. If we wish to identify all the causes of chronic diseases and successfully prevent and perhaps one day cure them, we need to track them in the workplace.

In recent years, governmental agencies have held meetings across the country in an attempt to get all stakeholders involved in better reporting of occupational illnesses and diseases together. In particular, these discussions have involved how public health agencies can promote surveillance in workplaces and also fill gaps not met by that surveillance. Surveillance is dependent on the occupational health expertise of the provider of health care. Therefore there is a real need to educate all health care providers about occupational health. There is also a need to take advantage of innovative information technologies, already being used by businesses for other purposes. The most important component of good epidemiology and chronic disease surveillance systems in the workplace is collaboration. All areas of public health need to be represented, and they must all beware of the importance of not isolating occupational health. In fact, NIOSH already has established goals for surveillance of occupational injuries and diseases. Exhibit 9.4 displays NIOSH's goals. The same sophisticated systems required by these goals could be used for chronic illnesses. Once all the real problems are identified for chronic diseases, workplace wellness programs can become the catalysts and provide the tools for abating these diseases.

THE ROLE FOR PUBLIC HEALTH

Many organizations and agencies have a role to play in the achievement of a healthy population. One of the roles that public health departments in this country have been

EXHIBIT 9.4. NIOSH surveillance: strategic goals

1. Advance the usefulness of surveillance information at the federal level for prevention of occupational illnesses, injuries, and hazards.

2. Strengthen the capacity of state health departments and other state agencies to conduct occupational surveillance.

3. Strengthen surveillance of high-risk industries and occupations, and of populations at high risk, including special populations.

4. Promote effective occupational safety and health surveillance conducted by employers, unions, and other nongovernmental organizations.

5. Increase research to improve occupational surveillance.

Source: NIOSH, 2001.

charged with is being the catalyst for the achievement of the goals and objectives put forth in *Healthy People 2010*. And what better place to concentrate some of the public health talent fulfilling this role than at the place most Americans visit every weekday, the workplace.

Wilson et al. (1996) have found that most of the research evidence supports the effectiveness of workplace wellness programs in keeping employees healthy. The employer already has the incentive to keep workers healthy in order to avoid increases in health insurance premiums and loss of productivity when a worker becomes ill and cannot come to work or goes on disability. Public health departments are experienced in dealing with population health and thus in working with large numbers of people to achieve goals, and workplaces offer those large numbers. The employer and public health agency partnership seems like a mutually beneficial collaborative opportunity, requiring only public health leadership to make it happen.

In addition, incentives to remain healthy abound in the workplace. The employer desires a well-trained, healthy workforce that is capable of producing profits. The employee desires a fair wage and a benefit package that includes health insurance paid predominantly by the employer. Most employees also desire to remain healthy as they grow older so they can enjoy life to its fullest. These incentives at all levels of the organization offer a unique opportunity for employer and employee to join forces in the focus on good health for everyone in the place of employment.

Both strong leadership and dedicated followership will be needed in the workplace in order to achieve and maintain wellness. One or more individuals in top management need to become convinced that workplace wellness programs are worth the investment of time and money necessary to develop fertile ground in the company and to seize this opportunity to keep workers well. Workplace leaders of the future will be involved in building health promotion cultures that guide others.

Public health departments need to work with the senior managers of a company and share with them the vision of preventing disease rather than trying to cure disease after it happens. Then the followers need to form a working group, such as a commission on health care costs, that can become educated about the cultural change the leaders are attempting to implement and can pass that education along to everyone in the workplace.

The last two decades have witnessed significant interest in and growth of health promotion and disease prevention programs offered in the workplace, with an emphasis on chronic disease states and conditions such as tobacco use and exposure to secondhand smoke, obesity, diabetes, and cardiovascular diseases. Dishman, Oldenburg, O'Neal, and Shephard (1998) argue that the workplace has great potential for health promotion and education because of the hours most adults spend there and because behavioral interventions there are thought to be potentially more substantial than interventions in other community settings. Moreover, the Task Force on Community Preventive Services has recommended multicomponent interventions that include nutrition assistance and physical activity (with strategies such as providing nutrition education or dietary prescriptions, physical activity prescriptions or group activity, and development and training of better health behaviors) to control overweight and obesity among adults in worksite settings.

Finally, Rowitz (2006) points out that public health leaders must emphasize *best practices* when they attempt to solve public health problems. He notes the importance of quality improvement in public health programs, adding the right ingredients to both old and new programs to improve chances of success. These ingredients or components of quality improvement include leadership competency, high performance expectations, and strategic capacity building.

SUMMARY

The incentives are present for public health departments to focus on the expansion of workplace health promotion programs. Employers know they have good economic reasons to do a better job of keeping their most important resource healthy and free from disease. Employees know they have economic and quality-of-life reasons for improving their health. The necessary knowledge is present as well. The medical literature shows a clear relationship between the reduction of a few modifiable risk factors (tobacco use, alcohol use, sedentary behavior, and poor nutrition) and the prevention of chronic, expensive, and incurable diseases later in life. The only way to avoid these costs is to mount prevention efforts that stop these diseases from occurring in the first place. And reliable information for developing and implementing viable and comprehensive health promotion programs in the workplace is readily available.

What is lacking now is mostly leadership. It is sad to see that the opportunity present for employers and public health departments to cooperate to improve the health of employees has not been used to any great extent. For whatever reason, these individuals with similar goals for the health of large numbers of individuals seem to avoid working together. That has to change, because there is so much to be gained by the formation of a strong partnership designed to improve employee wellness.

KEY TERMS

chronic diseases
evidence-based prevention programs
modifiable risk factors
obesity

physical inactivity
secondhand smoke
workplace wellness programs

QUESTIONS FOR DISCUSSION

1. What are the multiple reasons why employers should have a great interest in offering their employees a wellness program in the workplace?

2. What are multiple factors that go into developing a comprehensive health promotion program for the workplace?

3. What are the major high-risk health behaviors that pose the greatest risk for employees? Explain why they are risks.

4. Why have public health departments not made any great effort to work with employers to improve the health of employees?

CHAPTER

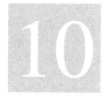

EMERGENCY RESPONSE PLANNING

After reading this chapter, you should be able to

- Describe the role of the workplace emergency and disaster planning team.
- Discuss the value of workplace emergency management.
- Understand the need for workplace preparation for bioterrorism.
- Develop an emergency and bioterrorism response planning document for the workplace.

The devastating loss of life in the 2001 World Trade Center attack shocked the business community into facing serious deficiencies in its ability to prevent and respond to disasters and emergencies and thus protect the most important asset of any business: the workers. This is another example of the value of well-developed **surveillance systems**—in this case systems that can warn people in the workplace of impending emergencies and disasters. The more information the business has immediately available and the better its plan to deal with a catastrophic event, the better able it will be to prevent or reduce the damage from the event.

Emergency response planning is extremely important for the business community and a requirement of doing business in the twenty-first century. McDade's 1999 discussion of bioterrorism shows that it was known even before the World Trade Center attack in 2001 that our nation's capabilities for responding to a terrorist attack had many serious deficiencies. Unfortunately, these problem areas were ignored, with devastating results.

DEFINITIONS

According to Novick, Morrow, and Mays (2008) **disasters** are ecological disruptions or emergencies capable of producing deaths, injuries, illnesses, and property damage that cannot be handled by routine procedures. Although disasters are normally thought of as affecting communities and families, they are also a concern for businesses. Disasters are capable of destroying a workplace and making it impossible for an employer to produce goods or services ever again.

Emergencies are events that require an immediate response, including disasters, nuclear accidents, terrorist attacks (such as bombings), and **bioterrorism**. The life cycle of an emergency is known as the *disaster continuum* or *emergency management cycle*. All business organizations need an emergency services component that is capable of handling extreme situations, but it is common knowledge that most workplaces are not prepared to handle a number of twenty-first-century emergencies, events that can include disasters and bioterrorism incidents.

FEMA (1993) defines **emergency management** as "the process of preparing for, mitigating, responding to, and recovering from an emergency." This definition has taken on new meaning since the disasters and terrorism events of the last several years. In the workplace, this process should involve a top management–backed emergency management planning team that coordinates training and drills and other planning activities. The initial members of this team should include someone who is already familiar with planning for emergencies.

EMERGENCY MANAGEMENT PLANNING STEPS

The focal point of the development of an emergency preparedness plan for business should be the formation of an emergency planning team. This team consists of the following key players: members from upper management, labor, and human resource management; a consultant with public health experience; a person with responsibility for communicating with the public; representatives of community emergency responders; representatives of key support areas such as data maintenance, engineering, and finance; and representatives of functions directly involved in emergency response such as security, safety, and medical services. This team needs authority, a mission statement with appropriate goals, and a yearly budget.

The next step in workplace emergency preparedness should include working with Occupational Safety and Health Administration (OSHA) and National Institute for Safety and Health (NIOSH) officials to complete an internal and external analysis. During the internal analysis, the planning team would do well to complete a SWOT analysis to identify workplace strengths, weaknesses, opportunities, and threats, with the objective of developing better surveillance systems for identifying potential threats to the team's workplace. (For a general discussion of SWOT analyses, see, for example, Kotler, Shalowitz, & Stevens, 2008.) During the external analysis, the team should identify external resources that may be available to its workplace. Hospital and health care executives, public health professionals, media representatives, and other community stakeholders can be invited to participate in the business's planning process. These individuals may also be suppliers of critical resources if an emergency occurs in the workplace.

An effort also needs to be made to evaluate potential emergencies, paying particular attention to the very real possibility of disasters or bioterrorism events. An inventory of possible events and the potential damage if these events occur in the workplace also needs to be completed. Another issue the planning team ought to examine is whether the workplace should stockpile emergency supplies such as food and water. Exhibit 10.1 contains a comprehensive list of emergency supplies that should be available at home or work.

Public health agencies also have major responsibilities to the workplace before and after disasters occur. These agencies have a wealth of information about prevention and control of the effects of both natural and man-made disasters, and therefore they can help businesses learn from many organizations' past experiences and do an excellent job of preparing their own workplaces and employees for future disasters. Again, there is a major role for NIOSH in preparing and disseminating relevant data and conducting employee training programs.

Disasters are a fact of life and will occur no matter how careful or lucky people are. Businesses can limit damage and injuries by being proactive and planning for the worst-case scenarios. Such planning is an investment that few businesses wish to make but they also do not want to be caught off guard and to become disaster victims. There is a role for public health departments in helping businesses become prepared for emergencies, terrorism, and bioterrorism, and this chapter focuses largely on the issues of bioterrorism and disease outbreaks where enlisting the skills and knowledge of public health systems and professionals is especially critical.

EXHIBIT 10.1. Recommended emergency supplies

Talk to your coworkers about what emergency supplies the company can feasibly provide, if any, and which ones individuals should consider keeping on hand. Recommended emergency supplies include the following:

Water, amounts for portable (emergency supply) kits will vary. Individuals should determine what amount they are able to both store comfortably and to transport to other locations. If it is feasible, store one gallon of water per person per day, for drinking and sanitation.

Food, at least a three-day supply of nonperishable food

Battery-powered radio and **extra batteries**

Flashlight and **extra batteries**

First aid kit

Whistle to signal for help

Dust or **filter masks,** readily available in hardware stores, which are rated based on how small a particle they filter

Moist towelettes for sanitation

Wrench or **pliers** to turn off utilities

Can opener for food (if kit contains canned food)

Plastic sheeting and **duct tape** to "seal the room"

Garbage bags and **plastic ties** for personal sanitation

Source: Ready Business, 2009.

TERRORISM AND BIOTERRORISM

The most powerful nation in the world was the victim of a set of massive and deeply shocking terrorist attacks on September 11, 2001, the day our country changed forever. The United States was not prepared for these events, and as thousands of American citizens died in the destruction of the World Trade Center, the damage to the Pentagon, and the crash of a hijacked plane in Pennsylvania, millions became terrorized because this disaster was in their own country and could happen again. The age of terrorism had begun with a vengeance in the United States. The goals associated with this attack on America included disruption of our way of life and the replacement of a calm environment with one of fear and distrust. The main terrorist goals are typically to disrupt society, produce panic and terror, and to get as much publicity as possible.

This was not the first time terror had struck in this country, and unfortunately, it will not be the last time that we have to deal with terror on our own soil. There are a number of recorded instances of terrorism over the history of the United States; some have been minor and many have been deadly.

A particularly worrisome form of terrorism is bioterrorism, and the threat of biological warfare has already become a reality for citizens of the United States. The CDC (2007a) defines *bioterrorism* as the deliberate release of bacteria, viruses, or other agents for the purpose of causing illness or death in humans, animals, or plants. Terrorists use these agents because they are often difficult to detect, can be spread among a population easily, and have the potential to produce high levels of morbidity and mortality and to inspire panic in their intended victims. Being constantly prepared to cope with the threat of bioterrorism may seem an impossible task, but the consequences of not planning for this threat could be devastating.

According to Török et al. (2006) the first bioterrorism attack in the United States occurred in 1984 in Texas and Oregon. This particular attack involved a religious cult that used bacteria known as salmonella, which can cause serious gastrointestinal illness in humans, to contaminate food at salad bars. The objective was to prevent individuals from voting in local elections. The resulting large outbreak of foodborne disease demonstrates the ease of using common bacteria and shows the vulnerability of self-service foods to intentional contamination. Over seven hundred people became very ill. No one died, but panic and terror raged

Another outbreak of disease due to intentional food contamination, this time with bacteria known as shigella, was reported by Kolavic et al. (1997). The resulting outbreak of shigellosis involved forty-five laboratory workers who became ill with diarrhea and fever after consuming muffins and doughnuts that had been placed in the laboratory's break room. The interesting part of this investigation was the conclusion that the outbreak had been caused by the deliberate use in food of bacteria obtained from the laboratory itself. The result again included causing mass panic in large numbers of people, at a very low per-victim cost for the perpetrator.

The use of explosives is a feature of many terrorist acts. The 2001 attacks used fuel-laden airliners as explosive devices. An earlier act of terrorism in 1993 had involved an explosion in the parking garage of the World Trade Center in New York City. This act of terrorism claimed seven lives and wounded over one thousand people. A rental truck loaded with 1,200 pounds of explosives was used in this incident that created panic and terror in the entire country.

In April 1995, we were all glued to our television sets watching the results of home-grown terrorism in Oklahoma. The federal office building in Oklahoma City was destroyed by a truck bomb detonated by three Americans. This attack killed 169 people, including 19 children, and injured 500 more people. At the time it was called the deadliest terrorist attack in the United States, but no one knew what was to come.

The common thread running through this brief historical review is how unprepared this country has been for terrorism in any form. This nation cannot let this history continue to repeat itself. The level of preparedness for such events cannot remain so low as to invite terrorist acts to be launched against our vulnerable population. Public health departments need to help businesses prepare for terrorism and particularly bioterrorism in the workplace.

A 2005 report issued by Trust for America's Health (Hearne, Segal, Earls, Juliano, & Stephens, 2005) presented a severe critique of our country's preparedness efforts against bioterrorism since the attacks in September 2001. This report found that both the federal and state readiness for major health emergencies must be improved in order to adequately protect the American people. It was especially critical of hospitals' lack of ability to consult with infection control experts about possible and suspected disease outbreaks, and it pointed out that nearly half of the states do not use national standards to investigate and track disease outbreaks. The report concluded with the sobering fact that hospitals and health care workers are not adequately prepared for major health emergencies like natural disasters and bioterrorism events.

Our country had not paid much attention to bioterrorism until the recent publicity about such events. Indeed, many foodborne and waterborne outbreaks over the years could have been the result of an intentional act of individuals who, for whatever reason, decided to poison our food and water supply. Terrorism using biological agents is very inexpensive for each attack, hard to identify, and because these events now generate widespread publicity, capable of producing mass panic for days to years after each event.

The answer to becoming better prepared to respond to disease outbreaks from any source, including bioterrorism, is a well-developed and maintained surveillance system that will give people at risk an early warning of events so they can prevent or at the very least limit the damage.

After the terrorist attacks of September 11, 2001, state and local health departments initiated various activities to improve surveillance systems and response, ranging from enhancing communications (between state and local health departments and between public health agencies and health care providers) to conducting special surveillance projects. These special projects have included active surveillance for changes in the number of hospital admissions, emergency department visits, and occurrence of specific syndromes. Activities in bioterrorism preparedness and emerging infections over the past few years have better positioned public health agencies to detect and respond to the intentional release of a biological agent. Immediate review of these activities to identify the most useful and practical approaches should help to refine disease surveillance efforts in various clinical situations. At the same time, the Trust for America's Health report summarized earlier suggests that these activities could be considerably improved. The proactive behavior described here must continue to be developed in public health agencies and it must also begin to be developed in U.S. workplaces as soon as possible.

WORKPLACE PREPAREDNESS FOR TERRORISM

American businesses cannot and should not rely solely on the government to protect their property and their workers from bioterrorism. They too must become proactive in protecting their workplaces from home-grown or international terrorists. Preparedness for bioterrorism has become everyone's responsibility. The leadership component for this responsibility should be embedded in the U.S. public health surveillance and response system. The most effective responses to bioterrorism will ultimately come from public health departments and from individuals trained in public health. It seems ironic that almost every federal government administration has attempted to decrease the federal funds flowing to public health departments and that these cuts have grown in recent years even though the war against terrorism and bioterrorism is requiring more and more public health expertise. Complacency began eroding essential components of public health departments as early as the 1970s and continues to do so today.

Deficiencies include inadequate surveillance systems, lack of rapid diagnostic systems, vaccine shortages, inability to rapidly communicate potential health problems, and insufficient public health training of physicians, epidemiologists, and laboratory personnel. Unfortunately, in most cases, by the time a public health epidemic is recognized, it is ending, with large numbers of casualties having already occurred.

Hamburg (2001) offers an unnerving scenario of a potential public health nightmare involving bioterrorism. It is relatively easy to conceal the small quantity of pathogenic material required to produce widespread disease. In Hamburg's scenario thousands of people working in or visiting a particular building are secretly exposed to a biological agent. When they return home and get sick hours, days, or weeks after exposure, no one is equipped to understand that this mass illness resulted from a common source exposure. Making matters worse, if such an agent were communicable person to person, there would most likely be a secondary outbreak of the same illness days after the first cases were reported. If a scenario such as this became a reality, it could produce a medical emergency that would rapidly overwhelm local health care systems.

According to the CDC (Khan & Sage, 2000) acts of biological or chemical terrorism cannot be predicted, and how such an attack would occur is only speculation. That being said, it is still possible to prepare for such an event in the workplace (and the community), and such preparation must become a major priority because it seems inevitable that such attacks will occur. Each business needs to recognize that it is entirely management's responsibility to ensure that surveillance systems to prevent or control bioterrorism in its workplace are present and fully operational. This preparation must include assistance from a strong and flexible public health presence and vigilant primary health care providers. Workplaces cannot count on continuous government presence, however; instead, as outlined in discussing the emergency planning team, they must collaborate with as many other players and stakeholders as possible.

The United States is vulnerable to biological and chemical threats, as has been proven yet again in several incidents in which anthrax spores have been mailed to various victims, with fatal results in some cases. These attacks revealed that instructions for preparing inexpensive bioterrorism substances are readily available. In addition the CDC (Khan & Sage, 2000) notes that covert dissemination of a biological agent in a public place, such as a workplace, will not have an immediate impact, because such agents have an incubation period before illness occurs. Therefore the morbidity and mortality from this type of attack will usually be recognized by physicians or primary care providers only some days after the exposure. These are additional reasons why workplaces have to be prepared for and educated about bioterrorism attacks.

The biological agents that can cause human illness are so numerous that they cannot all be the focus of public health and workplace preventive initiatives. But an effort needs to be made to concentrate on the most likely sources of this type of public terrorism. Workplace preparedness is not yet a reality, and there will be a rush for information once an event does occur.

CDC'S STRATEGIC WORKPLACE PLAN

The CDC has developed a strategic plan for responding to biological and chemical emergencies and attacks (Khan & Sage, 2000). This plan outlines five focus areas for training and research that can also guide the efforts of employers and employees in the workplace. In addition, information and regulations relating to these areas can be developed and enforced by OSHA. These areas are

- Preparedness and prevention

- Detection and surveillance

- Diagnosis and characterization of biological and chemical agents

- Response

- Communication

Exhibit 10.2 displays the desired outcomes of activities to fulfill the CDC's strategic plan for preparedness and response.

The federal government needs to help all workplaces in America to receive the same surveillance systems, public health training, and resources so they can independently protect themselves from bioterrorism. A local response to bioterrorism saves time and lives.

APPLYING EPIDEMIOLOGY TO PREPAREDNESS

Public health professionals are employing multiple models in order to understand emergency management as it relates to preparedness. Barnett et al. (2005) have proposed a model (employed in Table 10.1) that is an extension of the **Haddon matrix** model (described in Chapter Four and Figure 4.7), which was used in injury prevention for years, to better understand and respond to disasters and bioterrorism events. This

EXHIBIT 10.2.   CDC strategic plan outcomes

Implementing CDC's strategic preparedness and response plan by 2004 will ensure the following outcomes:

- U.S. public health agencies and health care providers will be prepared to mitigate illness and injuries that result from acts of biological and chemical terrorism.

- Public health surveillance for infectious diseases and injuries—including events that might indicate terrorist activity—will be timely and complete, and reporting of suspected terrorist events will be integrated with the evolving, comprehensive networks of the national public health surveillance system.

- The national laboratory response network for bioterrorism will be extended to include facilities in all fifty states. The network should include CDC's environmental health laboratory for chemical terrorism and four regional facilities.

- State and federal public health departments will be equipped with state-of-the-art tools for rapid epidemiological investigation and control of suspected or confirmed acts of biological or chemical terrorism, and a designated stock of terrorism-related medical supplies will be available through a national pharmaceutical stockpile.

- A cadre of well-trained health care and public health workers will be available in every state. Their terrorism-related activities will be coordinated through a rapid and efficient communication system that links U.S. public health agencies and their partners.

Source: Khan & Sage, 2000.

model should work very well to guide the development of a workplace response to emergencies. It is much like the communicable disease model used for years by epidemiologists to rapidly identify and find solutions for communicable disease epidemics. A business planning team using this model will initially assess possible hazards, prevention, and preparedness within the immediate infrastructure and the preparedness of the community, in this case the workplace.

Next, the team will evaluate the emergency response to the crisis; the management and communication of the crisis; and treatment, sheltering, and evacuation plans. The final phase, the post-event evaluation, includes mitigation and cleanup, information updates, the community or workplace response post-event communication, and post-event health surveillance activities. In short, this model, as displayed in Table 10.1, gives the user a conceptual overview of public health emergency readiness and response.

TABLE 10.1.   Haddon matrix and public health emergency readiness and response: a conceptual overview

| Phase | Influencing Factors | | | |
	Host	Agent/Vector	Physical Environment	Social Environment/ Organizational Culture
Pre-event	Risk assessment	Properties of biologic, chemical, radiologic, or other agents	Existing clinical infrastructure Vulnerability of food and water supplies	Need for culture of readiness among public health and other first responders
	Pre-event risk communication	Capacity of agent as WMD	Transportation infrastructure	Knowing one's functional role(s) in emergency response*
	Pre-event surveillance	Potential for reengineering of agent to produce unexpected health effects		Demonstrating use of communication equipment*
	Primary prevention (e.g., pre-event vaccination)		Proximity of community to chemical and radiation facilities	Knowing one's communication role(s) in emergency response*

	Preparedness training for public health responders			Identifying key system resources for referring matters that exceed one's personal knowledge and expertise*
	Interagency first response planning			Participation in readiness exercises and drills Baseline community trust in public health and other response agencies Public acceptance of pre-event risk communication Culturally based pre-event risk perception Public awareness of large-scale threats Demographics of community
Event	Crisis risk communication	Emergency response clinic setup and operations	Disease or injury caused by agent	Community responses to crisis risk communication
	Decontamination and treatment	Emergency access to medical supplies (e.g., Strategic National Stockpile)	Response of the agent to decontamination and treatment efforts	Community adherence to public health guidance during event

Note: WMD = weapons of mass destruction.

*Potential targets for public health intervention.

(continued)

TABLE 10.1. Haddon matrix and public health emergency readiness and response: a conceptual overview *(continued)*

Phase	Host	Influencing Factors		
		Agent/Vector	Physical Environment	Social Environment/ Organizational Culture
Event (cont.)	Sheltering	Potential for agent detection	Clinical surge capacity	Culturally based crisis-phase risk perception
	Post-exposure prophylaxis	Psychosocial impact of agent during event	Shelter availability	Access of community to crisis response clinics
	Crisis-phase mental health response Crisis-phase interagency first response collaboration Epidemiological workup (including forensic epidemiology as applicable) Evacuation	Acute health effects of agent	Emergency accessibility of transportation	

Post-event	Consequence-phase risk communication	Long-term psychosocial impact of agent	Application of lessons learned to better safeguard vulnerable infrastructure	Community responses to post-event risk communication
	Application of lessons learned to improve response systems Consequence-phase mental health response	Response of agent to mitigation and cleanup efforts		Willingness of public health responders to embrace lessons learned
				Post-event community trust in public health and other response agencies
Post-event health surveillance Mitigation and cleanup After-action assessment and follow-up				Culturally based consequence-phase risk perception

Barnett et al. (2005) call this an "all hazards approach," one that assists the public and private sectors to prepare for and offer a response to a wide range of emergencies from disease to a weather-related disaster. In addition to using the three-phase approach to understanding emergency readiness and response, it also considers the influencing factors of host, agent, physical environment, and social environment. This is truly a public health approach, one that helps its users to abstract a possible solution to a complex set of public health problems.

This excellent planning tool can become a catalyst in brainstorming sessions among planning team members looking for new ways to deal with disaster and bioterrorism planning for their workplace. Barnett et al. (2005) demonstrate that the Haddon matrix can easily move beyond injury control issues and play a prominent role in disaster and bioterrorism preparedness planning. Their model can and should be used by workplaces all over the country as they continue to make their workers and physical plants less susceptible to disasters and the threat of bioterrorism events. A model based on the Haddon matrix helps emergency planning teams to

- Prioritize tasks.

- Assess their performance in the achievement of preparedness goals.

- Attain a more efficient use of scarce resources.

- Deal with many types of workplace health events.

APPLYING AN INFORMATION MODEL TO PREPAREDNESS

Turnock (2004) offers an information model that could be a valuable component of the assessment function of public health and may be especially useful in evaluating readiness for emergencies in the workplace. The assessment process is a critical piece in planning for disasters and bioterrorism events, especially in the workplace, and Turnock argues that information, especially from surveillance, is the most vital component of public health assessment in at least three ways, becoming the catalyst for planning, intervention activities, and health communication.

1. It helps to monitor community (or workplace) health status.

2. It allows those responsible to become aware of the availability of community (and workplace) resources to address public health problems.

3. As assessment findings, it can then be communicated to decision makers and policymakers so that they are better able to intervene in the health problem area. The more information that is gathered before, during, and after an emergency or disaster, the better we become at being prepared for the next event.

In short, the benefits of using this information model include better monitoring of workplace health status, increased awareness of available workplace and community resources, and better ability to plan for the next emergencies.

INVOLVING OSHA AND NIOSH IN PLANNING

There are obvious leadership roles for OSHA and NIOSH in assisting workplaces to prepare for and respond to disasters and bioterrorism events. OSHA can offer appropriate regulations, and NIOSH can engage in the research, development, and expansion of sensitive surveillance systems.

Regulation

OSHA has both the right and the responsibility to require workplaces to be prepared for disasters and bioterrorism events. Such OSHA regulations could make it mandatory for workplaces to develop a comprehensive plan to deal with disasters and potential bioterrorism threats. The regulations should require the appointment of a planning team and insist on the use of public health consultation as the plan goes through the developmental process. The regulations should also set a timetable for implementation and for mandatory periodic evaluation for compliance by assigned employees.

Surveillance Systems

NIOSH surveillance systems, along with CDC support in the form of that agency's communicable disease surveillance, are already in place and can easily be adapted for use by the individual workplaces. Several new surveillance systems have also been developed and could be made available to assigned members of the workforce. Available systems range from communicable and chronic disease reporting to disaster and bioterrorism event reporting and information.

One of the best examples of a public health surveillance and information system is the Epidemic Information Exchange (Epi-X). This system facilitates Web-based communications among public health professionals. State and local health departments and poison control centers are currently using this system to access and share preliminary health surveillance information. The system supports postings and discussions about disease outbreaks and other public health events that may spread to other parts of the nation or the world. Epi-X allows rapid communications whenever there is a need, and its staff are available twenty-four hours a day seven days a week to provide consultation. Created to provide public health officials with current information and alerts involving the health of the public, the system's primary goal is to inform health officials about important events that may affect the public's health and to help them respond to public health emergencies.

NIOSH could make Epi-X available in a modified form to workplaces to aid them in obtaining up-to-date requisite information to plan for emergency events. This system could also be used to foster growth in expertise and exchange of information among assigned members of workplace emergency management teams.

Information

The most important component of emergency preparedness is the availability of good information concerning the current problem. The specific information required to cope with emergencies is usually readily available from local public health departments. Workplace planning teams need to be able to receive this public health information on a daily basis, rapidly interpret what it means for their businesses, and then be able to immediately communicate the information to those who need to know.

Training Programs

Training programs that help people in the workplace to prepare for and respond to disasters and bioterrorism have never been more important for businesses in this country and the world. This training needs to be offered to managers and employees at the same time by a consultant with a strong public health background and up-to-date reliable information. The training should address basic epidemiological principles, surveillance systems, and computer use in disaster and bioterrorism surveillance activities.

Evaluation Systems

Preparedness evaluation systems should incorporate models based on the Haddon matrix and the Turnock information model for use by the planning team. Case studies and practice drills should be conducted on a routine basis and should be graded by a public health consultant for successful outcome management.

As early as April 2000, the CDC has made recommendations concerning the need for a preparedness and response plan for biological and chemical terrorism in the community and the workplace. They are too important a segment of our country to ignore. Everything is present for successful collaboration between business and governmental public health agencies in order to develop, implement, and continuously evaluate workplace preparedness programs that can function on their own and protect America's workers from harm.

SUMMARY

Workplace disaster and bioterrorism preparedness responsibilities for American businesses are large but essential tasks. These responsibilities must be addressed by a planning team appointed by top management in every workplace in this country. This team requires the help and guidance of public health professionals in the early stages of team development. Disaster planning for business needs to focus on prevention and control of damage before and after the event. Attention also needs to be paid to methods of evaluation, improvement, and communication used by businesses in times of emergency. There are also important roles for OSHA and NIOSH in the preparedness phase of the planning effort. The assumption must be made, however, that after the planning steps are completed, there may not be a great deal of help available from government during the actual response to an emergency.

Workplace disaster and bioterrorism planning requires consultation with public health experts in order to recognize public health threats as early as possible and be able to respond to these threats immediately. Workplace surveillance systems need to be developed, implemented, and constantly evaluated. These systems should track instances of communicable diseases and other health problems that might result from bioterrorism events.

At least two models need to be understood and considered when the workplace develops long-term plans to deal with these serious potential events. The Haddon matrix model, previously used for injury control programs, can be easily adapted to guide emergency preparedness. This model allows planners to brainstorm around events that occur before, during, and after the disaster or bioterrorism event.

The Turnock model is a public health information model that can also be easily adapted to planning for workplace emergencies. It uses surveillance activities performed by the business to recognize potential problems in the workplace and prepare for a rapid response.

Businesses have to be prepared for disasters and bioterrorism events in their workplaces. In order to assure this readiness, OSHA and NIOSH need to work with businesses to plan and provide training for these possibilities, just as they would help these employers with planning and training to respond to and prevent workplace illnesses or injuries.

KEY TERMS

bioterrorism
disasters
emergencies
emergency management

FEMA
Haddon matrix
surveillance system

QUESTIONS FOR DISCUSSION

1. What are the major responsibilities of the workplace emergency planning team?

2. What are the steps for conducting bioterrorism planning in the workplace? (Outline them.)

3. How can the Haddon matrix be adapted to emergency planning in the workplace?

4. What is the value of using public health consultants in the bioterrorism planning process?

CHAPTER

ERGONOMICS

After reading this chapter, you should be able to

▪ Identify the major issues associated with poor ergonomic design.

▪ Understand that there are simple solutions to some ergonomic challenges.

▪ Describe the role each leader can play in reducing ergonomic challenges.

▪ Explain how ergonomic challenges can be addressed either on a small scale or across an entire system.

Ergonomics is a word that has gained a lot of attention over the last fifteen or so years. It has appeared on talk shows, in news magazines, in the press, and in many other forms of public discourse. Throughout this time it has had many different meanings, depending on the speaker and the speaker's agenda. This chapter uses a focused selection of the available meanings, including a pair of dictionary definitions, a definition drawn from the term's root words, and more important than any of these, a practical definition—one that can be used by both professional ergonomists and people who do not have this detailed expertise but who are working to reduce workplace injuries and illnesses.

"The term ergonomics was coined in 1950 by a group of physical, biological, and psychological scientists in the United Kingdom to describe their interdisciplinary efforts to design equipment and work tasks to fit the operator," say Plog, Niland, and Quinlan (1996, p. 347). The 1966 *Random House Dictionary of the English Language* defines *ergonomics* as "biotechnology." The 1967 *World Book Dictionary* describes it as "the study of the relationship between individuals and their work or working environment, especially with regard to fitting jobs to the needs and abilities of workers: The essential nature of ergonomics is the convergence of the disciplines of human biology (especially anatomy, physiology and psychology) on the problems of Man at work." The word has its roots in the Greek words *ergon*, meaning "work," and *nomos*, meaning "law" (Brauer, 1994). Thus it can also be taken to mean "the laws of work."

A more practical definition is this: *making the job fit the people.* This sounds simple, but it can be extremely complex. One needs to consider the full range of human beings' physical and mental capabilities to perform tasks. Some simple examples will begin to explain the complexity of the topic and the potential difficulty of solving ergonomic issues. The average male in North America has a height of approximately 5 feet 8 inches. The average male in Indochina has an average height of approximately 5 feet 3 inches. If you are designing a product to be used standing up and for global use, what height do you design for? If you are designing a workstation for use in North America, do you design it for the 95th percentile (tall) male or the 5th percentile (short) female, knowing that there is about an 18-inch difference in height? How do you design a workstation that can accommodate both fully able individuals and those with physical limitations? What characteristics should a control system have to enable individuals to always do the right thing at the right time when the system is operating 24 hours a day, 7 days a week, 365 days a year, but people are still genetically programmed to sleep when it is dark and be awake when it is light? How do you design control systems with colored lights when approximately 13 percent of males are color-blind (primarily to red)? These are just some simple examples to illustrate that using a simple, universal approach to ergonomics does not help us in reducing the frequency or severity of injuries and illnesses resulting from ergonomic issues.

Because the topic is complex, it is easy to see why media and the general public do not understand what ergonomics really entails or why solutions are not always simple. At the same time, a solution to an ergonomic issue may be fairly simple when the people dealing with it take their "we've always done it that way" blinders off and think differently and creatively. Once they understand that there are alternatives and options that do not necessarily cost a fortune, all kinds of solutions present themselves to make things better.

This chapter provides an overview of ergonomics but does not go deeply into the medical, physiological, psychosocial, or prevention aspects of the topic, as there are multiple books, research papers, articles, and so forth, available to readers interested in pursuing these topics further. Applying public health concepts of identifying the problem trends and sources, isolating them, and then applying solutions to reduce or eliminate these sources can be of significant assistance to the people in the field working to reduce the frequency of ergonomic injuries.

TWO APPROACHES: BROAD AND NARROW

There are two fundamental approaches to ergonomics: holistic and narrow, or macroergonomics and microergonomics. In a way these terms parallel the terms microeconomics and macroeconomics. In macroeconomics, one studies the interrelationships and dependencies among organizations like banks, federal and state regulatory agencies, and similar organizations. In microeconomics, one studies how companies and small-scale organizations function.

Macroergonomics

In the **holistic approach,** or **macroergonomics,** practitioners look to design an entire system to accommodate human performance capability in all its aspects. This used to be called the field of *human factors engineering* (McCormick, 1976). It consists of taking into account human abilities to see, hear, touch, and so forth, over the full range of possibilities, and then designing for "error-free" work. Initially, much of the effort to develop a holistic approach was led by the military in the design of aircraft control systems and was driven by the increasing complexity and speed of aircraft. Today there are Department of Defense (DoD) standards and instructions targeted toward achieving ergonomic design. For example, DoD Instruction Number 6055.1, dated August 19, 1998, includes guidance on establishing and incorporating ergonomic principles and practices into the safety and occupational health programs and processes at all DoD facilities. It lays out responsibilities for safety and occupational health and expectations for reducing injuries, illnesses, and fatalities. Of more direct application to the topic of ergonomics is the Department of Defense Design Criteria Standard for human engineering (DOD, 1999). It is over two hundred pages in length and "establishes general human engineering criteria for design and development of military systems, equipment and facilities. Its purpose is to present human engineering design criteria, principles and practices to be applied in the design of systems, equipment, and facilities so as to

a. Achieve required performance by operator, control and maintenance personnel.

b. Minimize skill and personnel requirements and training time.

c. Achieve required reliability of personnel-equipment combinations.

d. "Foster design standardization within and among systems."

This standard and its criteria setting are driven by hard-earned lessons in improper applications of human factors engineering. For example, during World War II, an experienced pilot climbing into a brand-new P-47 Thunderbolt fighter in response to an air raid warning, suddenly discovered, to his dismay, that the controls were very different from the controls on the P-47s he had been flying. They were so different that he could not even find the fuel gauge. He was able to start and taxi the plane and survive the air raid, but he commented later that he had never understood why someone would redesign a fighter plane's instrument panel in the middle of a war (Casey, 1998). In order to reduce the likelihood of dangers like this occurring in the future, the standard includes both general and specific requirements in a number of areas: for example, standardization, simplicity of design, safety, and functional use of color. There is a growing belief that many incidents and accidents are due to poor ergonomic design of the workspace. Here are two examples of serious events that were at the least exacerbated by poor design.

The National Transportation Safety Board report on the August 27, 2006, crash of Comair Flight 5191 in Lexington, Kentucky, found that several ergonomic factors were major contributors to this fatal crash. Among them were pilot distraction during the taxi, controller sleep deprivation and workload, confusion about airline rules for takeoffs from unlit runways, and confusing taxiway lighting. All of these are examples of failures and issues in the holistic approach to ergonomics.

The nuclear reactor accident at Three Mile Island (TMI) in 1979 is a good example of poor controls design, according to a human factors engineering professor from the University of Tennessee who was called in to be part of the lessons-learned team that assessed the control system. (The chapter author heard this professor's views as a student in the professor's class.) A properly designed alarm system will use different combinations of sounds, lights, and colors to indicate different levels of importance. In a well-designed system the highest level alarm, requiring immediate attention from the operator, is a flashing red beacon. This alarm may be either on a control panel or located remotely from the control panel but will be unmistakable for anything else (the master caution light on military aircraft panels is a great example). Lesser alarms step down from the flashing red light with sound to flashing red to solid red to orange or other patterns. The exact combination is not important as long as operating personnel are well trained in it and understand it. In addition, the controls to respond to the highest levels of alarm should be located immediately adjacent to each alarm indicator. At Three Mile Island little of this good design was present. In the opinion and experience of the human factors engineering professor, the problems at TMI were a disaster waiting to happen. As he described the controls, the alarm that meant the reactor was melting down was a small red light mixed in with a series of other lights and it had no horn or flashing light. The flashing lights were reserved for the signals that it was break time for the operators. In addition, the controls used to respond to the critical alarm were located across the control room from the warning light and were not labeled clearly. Also, at least one of these controls operated opposite to the normal expectation for a control, up being open and down being closed. This was the only control in this set of controls that operated this way. And a number of additional issues were clearly not conducive to either normal or emergency error-free operation. When the issues started to pile up, operators were unable to take the proper steps to mitigate the problems, and this was at least partly due to the nonergonomic design of the control room and control system.

Design for Safety, Quality, and Productivity   The point of these examples is that safety, quality, and productivity can all be negatively affected by a poor ergonomic design. System designers need to consider a multitude of factors in order to avoid problems later. The DoD Design Criteria Standard for human engineering, for example, is intended to help military system designers apply the necessary kinds of thinking. Here is what the standard says about safety, for instance: "Design shall reflect applicable system and personnel safety factors, including minimizing potential human error in the operation and maintenance of the system, particularly under the conditions of alert, battle stress, or other emergency or non-routine conditions. Design of non-military-unique workplaces and equipment shall conform to OSHA standards unless military applications require more stringent limits (e.g., maximum steady-state noise in personnel-occupied areas)" (DoD, 1999). The best way to apply the appropriate kind of thinking to system design is to engage a team of people ranging from operators to engineers and designers to think of all the ways the system could function (or malfunction). The operators will bring expert, firsthand knowledge of how things really work under 24/7 operating pressures. The engineers will bring technical expertise on how to make all the parts of the system fit together to produce the desired outcome. The designers will take the ideas of the operators and engineers and make a layout and design drawings. Once this initial design is developed, one of the several hazard and failure analysis methods available should be used to "fail-safe" the design. Bringing operators into this process will ensure that the people on the front end of the system who will actually have to work with it both have input into the design and share with the design team all their ideas and experiences about the possible misuses of the system and its components. The system designers can then build this information into the design to minimize the chances that these misuses will occur or to mitigate the effects if they do. Moreover, designers need to factor in not just what day-shift workers need but also what night-shift and weekend workers need.

Picture the reduced capability of individuals who have young children at home and are going to work on a Saturday evening for a twelve-hour shift. These workers have probably not gotten a normal amount of sleep, have not had much time with their families, and are thinking of all the things they would rather do on a Saturday night than go to work and make the employer's product. Their mental capacity is not at 100 percent when they start the shift and by the 3:00 to 4:00 A.M. hour, when the state of alertness in human beings is normally at its lowest, this capacity is reduced even more.

The military fully understands this, which is why Operations Desert Storm and Iraqi Freedom were started with air attacks at about 3:00 A.M. local time, to take advantage of this reduced state of alertness. It is inherent in humans after millions of years of evolution that day is awake time and night is sleep time, with peaks and lulls throughout, and the deepest lull is between 3:00 and 4:00 A.M. (Hastings, 1998). Now picture one of these workers running into an emergency in the operation and, for example, having to shut a complex system down to solve the problem. How ready is this worker to function effectively? Can this worker think through all the control schemes and emergency procedures in a timely fashion? Is he or she capable of making good decisions in a complex set of issues? Can he or she effectively interact with others who may be in the same or even worse low state of alertness to accomplish the required steps? A good system will take all this into account and will make it easy for operators, no matter their physical and mental state, to do all the right things at the right times and to avoid doing the wrong things at the wrong times. This is accomplished by designing the alarms so that they cascade from lowest level to highest level in a manner that is obvious to even the least alert (but awake—we have to start somewhere) operator. Tied to this is a set of controls; what each one governs is obvious, and these controls are laid out and function in the manner that an operator would expect. There is also a problem-solving flow chart, either printed out or displayed on a computer screen, that functions as an *expert system* to lead the operator through the problem and to a solution. When controls such as valves that are located remotely from the operator's station need to be manually activated, there are diagrams and labels that make it obvious how to find the valves and how to operate them. All of this helps the operator minimize a problem once it occurs.

Design Mistakes Out   An even better choice is to design the system so that it is virtually impossible for many system failures to occur, or if they do occur, they are minimal, meaning that loss of productivity is limited and that the consequences of a failure are relatively minor. Of course, depending on the type of production process, even a minor failure can be expensive. If a bank teller gets tired from standing all day on a hard floor and does not properly service a customer, what is the loss? It could mean a customer goes to a different bank with all of her money. This could be relatively minor but what if this customer is the richest person in town? What is the cost of this loss to the bank? What would the cost be to supply the teller with a workstation where he could alternate sitting and standing and avoid the tired feeling late in the day that could lead to poor service and a lost customer? Similarly, if a minor leak of water occurs in the cooling system for an operation, it might be nothing to get excited about. However, if the operation is a nuclear power plant, even a minor water leak is a big deal. It probably requires shutting down the reactor, making a report to the federal and local regulatory agencies, sending teams in hazardous materials suits to ensure no radioactivity has escaped and then to repair the leak and restart the reactor. What would all this cost? Most likely somewhere in the millions of dollars. A well-designed operation will have all its pipes in places where preventive maintenance and inspection personnel can visually inspect them and where people do not need to stand on their heads, for example, to look at seams and welds, which are the most likely leak points. Designing this in from the beginning enables a simpler and more effective inspection process and therefore minimizes the risk of failure at an unexpected time.

Microergonomics

The narrow approach to ergonomics, or **microergonomics,** looks at disorders that are primarily due to exposure to a series of risk factors that combine to create issues in the human body. Often this means a focus on the field of **musculoskeletal disorders** (MSDs), also referred to as **cumulative trauma disorders** (CTDs). (This chapter follows Putz-Anderson, 1988, in using the term *cumulative trauma disorders*.) "A useful definition of CTDs can be constructed by combining the separate meanings for each word. *Cumulative* indicates that these injuries develop gradually over periods of weeks, months, or even years as a result of repeated stresses on a particular body part. The cumulative concept is based on the theory that each repetition of an activity produces some trauma or wear and tear on the tissues and joints of the body. The word *trauma* signifies bodily injury from mechanical stresses. And the term *disorders* refers to physical ailments or abnormal conditions" (Putz-Anderson, 1988, p. 4).

In layperson's terms, this means that some activity is done repeatedly in such a manner or frequency that it hurts. If it hurts long enough, it becomes an injury. This is not to imply that work may not hurt sometimes without leading to a CTD. Anytime people do some physical activity that they have not done before or in a long while, they expose their muscles, tendons, and ligaments to stresses they are unused to. This will cause some physical discomfort. After some amount of repetition and recovery time, this discomfort goes away as individuals become hardened to the activity. A CTD is different in that no work hardening is possible; the activity is such that the soft tissues do not recover between times of exposure, and eventually they become chronically irritated. This chronic irritation can lead to various blood flow, range of motion, or nerve function losses. In the worst cases, nerves can be killed due to chronic irritation and pressure on them. The most common CTDs are in the upper body, mostly the hands and wrists, elbows, shoulders, and neck. There are parallels in the lower body to these injuries. Many of the overuse issues associated with the wrist are seen in the ankle, and parallels to shoulder and elbow issues are sometimes seen in the knee. Because the hands and fingers and not the feet are the primary tools used by humans, there are few ergonomic issues with feet or toes. (The examples in this chapter will focus on the upper body.)

Many times microergonomic problems are associated with productivity or quality problems. When performing a job hurts, a worker will find ways to deal with the pain, even if it means a reduction in quality or productivity. An example related to the chapter author in an ergonomics training session illustrates this point. A worker was tasked to fill gearboxes with a defined amount of oil as each gearbox came down the assembly line. When the gearbox was full, a light illuminated to tell the worker to stop the flow of oil. The problem was that the light was located above the worker's head in such a position that the worker had to crane his neck backward during the entire filling cycle. By late in the shift, the worker performing this task was in pain, so on some occasions he would just step back to where he could see the light without craning his neck, which meant that the oil got dumped on the floor. The reader can probably guess what the biggest single warranty claim for this device was. Correct! Gearbox failure due to no lubrication. How many other poorly designed workstations exist that reduce productivity or quality? How many settings where you work, play, or study are user unfriendly and reduce productivity or quality for you? Figure 11.1 displays many of the factors that can lead to accidents.

FIGURE 11.1. *Model of events and behaviors contributing to an accident.*

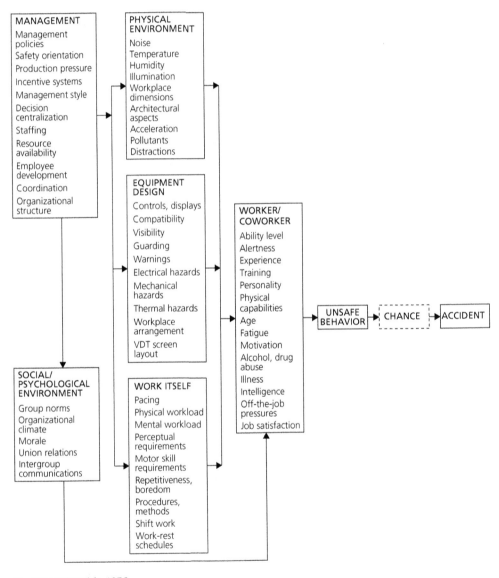

Source: McCormick, 1976.

ERGONOMISTS' ROLES AND EXPERIENCE

As the previous discussion demonstrated, holistic ergonomics is a very broad area. Whole books can and have been written to detail what is required to prevent injuries and improve productivity via effective design (see, for example, McCormick, 1976; Chengalur, Rodgers, & Bernard, 2004). However, most people in the field think of ergonomics much more narrowly. Most practitioners consider macroergonomics to be the field of designers and engineers and theoreticians and not ergonomists. Ergonomists in the field tend to deal with a narrow set of conditions related to **repetitive motion,** fatigue, and back injuries. Most of the Occupational Safety and Health Administration's regulations and guidance relating to ergonomics have been concerned with repetitive motion (see, for example, OSHA, 1988; 2004a).

Here are some expert descriptions of the role of the ergonomist. The *International Encyclopedia of Ergonomics and Human Factors* (Karwowski, 2006) states: "As a professional, an ergonomist uses the skills and knowledge from the various human sciences and engineering sciences. The ergonomist matches jobs/actions, systems/products, and environments to the capabilities and limitations of people." According to the Human Factors and Ergonomics Society, "ergonomics professionals apply human-system interface technology to the design, analysis, test and evaluation, standardization, and control of systems for such purposes as improving human and system performance, health, safety, comfort, and quality of life" (p. 181).

This encyclopedia goes on to quote A. Chapanis, who states that "*ergonomic design or engineering* is the application of human factors information to the design of tools, machines, systems, tasks, jobs, and environments for productive, safe, comfortable and effective human functioning" (p. 181). And this encyclopedia also notes (p. 181) that "[e]rgonomists apply their skills in business, industry, government, and academia to:

▨ Increase human productivity, comfort, health, and safety, and to

▨ Reduce injury, illness, and the likelihood of errors."

The Board of Certification in Professional Ergonomics (BCPE) has two levels of expertise defined, the certified ergonomics associate (CEA) and the certified professional ergonomist (CPE) or certified human factors professional (CHFP). Many practitioners in the field are more in line with the CEA level of expertise and practice than with the CPE or CHFP level, and many do not have either certification. An organization may need an ergonomist at either or both of these levels, depending on the type of intervention and expertise needed. If an organization was taking on the holistic problem, it would need to look for a CPE or CHFP to help it through the process. If an organization was looking for workstation redesign or another fairly narrow set of ergonomic issues, then it would look for the CEA level of expertise. Professional certification in ergonomics is not required for solving many problems, as certified safety professionals and certified industrial hygienists have much to offer in the field of ergonomics. In fact, none of these professional certifications are absolute musts to solve either macro- or microergonomic issues, but the organization does need someone with a basic understanding of how humans actually perform work and their capabilities and limitations and someone with the ability to think differently from the way the organization currently thinks about how to organize and design work. Before the establishment of the Board of Certification in Professional Ergonomics in 1990, there were experts in the field who successfully solved ergonomic problems. These solutions were developed by people of many disciplines (sometimes licensed or certified and sometimes not) who drew on expertise in design, engineering, and the like.

FEW ABSOLUTE LIMITS

Before we move on to discuss specific types of injuries, one more thing must be understood about ergonomics, whether macro or micro. There are very few absolutes when it comes to making tasks, jobs, designs, and the like, ergonomic. In nearly all cases, some people are susceptible to injury or mistake, and some are not. The causes of this variation are beyond the scope of this chapter but fall primarily into the fields of psychology and medicine and may be psychosocial issues. Generally speaking, organizations with poor morale tend to have more ergonomic issues than organizations with high morale do. Similarly, organizations going through restructuring or downsizing may see an increase in ergonomic injuries. Once an organization gets traumatic injuries under control, ergonomic injuries can begin to surface as issues that have been there all along but were hidden by the more obvious (and usually more serious) injuries. Off-the-job activities can affect an individual's sensitivity to on-the-job exposures. People with different body structures can have different sensitivities to work exposures, and underlying disease or health factors can also affect these responses. Wilson and Corlett (2005) and Kroemer and Grandjean (1997) are among the authors who offer more complete discussions of these variations in susceptibility.

Given the variation in human sensitivity to work exposures, the field of ergonomics offers risk factors and approximations of exposures rather than the limits one sees in the OSHA permissible exposure limits (PELs), for example. PELs and the corresponding exposure limits set by the National Institute for Occupational Safety and Health (NIOSH) and the American Conference of Governmental Industrial Hygienists (ACGIH) set a *cliff point* beyond which it is expected that the overwhelming majority of any human population will start to suffer adverse effects. In fact, many of these limits are also approximations because there is variation around the point at which people start to see the effects. But in ergonomics, the limits are even less exact. For this reason it is often better to think in terms of risk factors that in some combination result in ergonomic injuries to humans.

There are four primary risk factors: force, frequency, posture, and duration. In addition, vibration (of the hand, arm, or whole body), mechanical contact stress, temperature extremes (primarily cold temperatures), lighting, noise, and static versus dynamic stress all play a part in contributing to ergonomic injuries. Scientists, physicians, practitioners, and ergonomists, among others, continue to study and conduct research to quantify the points at which injury occurs. As measurement science has progressed, we are now able to quantify to the erg the amount of force required to perform a task. What we cannot yet quantify is the impact of the other risk factors. If my hand is in a normal posture as I use a tool with a cushioned handle, I can exert lots of force without injury as long as I do not do it often or for a long time. How often is too often, and how long is too long? This is where the difficulty in quantification comes in. For each person the overlap between force, frequency, posture, and duration is different, and so each person's susceptibility to injury also varies. Add to this the psychological, medical, and psychosocial issues and one begins to see why today this field is still nearly as much art as science. How much is too much? The answer that drives everyone crazy is, it depends! Some practitioners have approached ergonomic risk factors in the same way that fire prevention experts approach fire. The *fire triangle* says that to have a fire you must have fuel, oxygen, and an ignition source. Take away any one of these, and you will not have a fire. Some ergonomics practitioners say that if you take away any of the force, frequency, posture, or duration components of a task, ergonomic injuries will not occur. In fact, the interrelationships of ergonomic risk factors are not this simple, and more than one component needs to be addressed to solve an ergonomic problem.

CUMULATIVE TRAUMA DISORDERS

This section discusses several cumulative trauma disorders, focusing primarily on the hand and wrist and on the back.

Carpal Tunnel Syndrome

The best-known CTD is carpal tunnel syndrome, which affects the hands and wrists. Carpal tunnel syndrome (CTS) involves the irritation of the median nerve as it passes through a structure known as the carpal tunnel in the wrist. To understand the cause of this irritation, one must understand the construction of the wrist. There are bones, a ligament, tendons, a nerve, and a blood vessel running through this area. The bones, the ligament, and the tendons are largely incompressible and immovable, but the nerve and the blood vessel are softer. If any swelling occurs in the area, the nerve and the blood vessel do get compressed and suffer reduced function and capacity.

If the tendons slide in their tendon sheath often enough, they can become irritated. The body's natural reaction to this type of irritation is to produce more synovial fluid in the area of the irritation. This fluid gets into the tendon sheath in the body's natural attempt to solve the problem of irritation. It now introduces a new problem, swelling in the region. The nerve or the blood vessel, or both, are compressed by the swelling. With proper rest away from the source of the activity, the body will normally fully recover. However, if this compression is repeated often enough and for a long enough time, the individual begins to suffer the effects of carpal tunnel syndrome, such as loss of feeling, pins and needles at night, and in extreme cases loss of use of the hand. CTS affects the thumb, the pointer and index fingers, and the thumb side of the ring finger, which are the parts of the fingers used in most activities, such as grasping, pointing, and operating controls. In many workers' compensations systems, loss of these fingers or loss of the use of them is considered to be loss of the hand.

Carpal tunnel syndrome cases have been declining since 1993, when the number of reported cases involving days away from work was 41,019. In 2001, 26,794 cases were reported (NIOSH, 2004), a significant reduction. Does this mean that private industry has solved the problem of CTS? This is far from the fact in the author's experience. What has occurred is that many businesses are recognizing the problem earlier and making some changes to avoid having it progress to the point that individuals must miss work. Although some changes will be complex, many can be relatively simple. Take the meatpacking industry as an example of an industry with an ongoing CTS problem. This is a deconstruction industry that starts with a whole cow, pig, or chicken and ends up with what we see in the food markets. These animals are not bioengineered to be easily disassembled by humans at a high rate. To perform the tasks required to turn a whole animal into a product for the table, workers perform high-frequency, forceful actions in potentially awkward postures in a cold environment. The meatpacking industry has aggressively tackled the CTS problem and come up with some solutions that the author has witnessed personally in a meatpacking facility. One of the first solutions is to keep the knives used by the workers very sharp to reduce the force required to slice through the meat. Every worker was observed to have two or three knives and a means of honing them to maintain sharpness right at her workstation. Every night the knives were collected and more comprehensively sharpened. Many of the knives had modified grips and angled blades that allowed the user to keep her hand in a natural posture. The knife handles had a nonslip surface and so did the cut-resistant gloves worn by all the workers. These accommodations were made to reduce the force required to use the knife, and to keep posture natural. The risk factor of frequency was dealt with by rotating job tasks within work areas so that workers did not do the exact same actions involving the same muscle and tendon groups all day. This facility, while still seeing CTS cases, had greatly reduced the incidence rate and was an industry leader in low total incidence rate for carpal tunnel syndrome.

CTS is an issue in many other walks of life, including the office. Among the people at significant risk are those who work with a computer for extended periods. This may sound on its surface to be ridiculous until some research is done into the amount of weight moved just with the hands and fingers in a single day. Also remember that with the advent of word processor programs, the typist no longer has to take a microbreak to reach up on the typewriter and return the carriage to the left. On the computer he can type uninterruptedly for the duration of the work to be done. Assuming a person spends the majority of his day typing into a computer, he will "move" up to 18.9 tons per day with just the small muscles in the forearm and the tendons in the hands and wrists. Although this sounds like a ridiculous number, here is the calculation. It takes approximately 2 to 4 ounces of force to activate the keystrokes on the average computer keyboard. For this calculation we will use 3 ounces. There are about 8 keystrokes per word, counting spaces and capitalizations. This means that typing each word requires about 1.5 pounds of force, or weight moved. Typing 60 words per minute equals 90 pounds of force per minute and 2.7 tons per hour. Allowing for breaks and lunch and time to gather material, we will assume that the typist actually types for 7 hours per day. This equates to 18.9 tons per day moved with the fingers and hands. And we haven't even attempted to account for the poor posture encountered at many typing workstations, which may not have been designed for typing (they are standard desktops with a computer and keyboard on them), may have been designed to comfortably accommodate only people of the "average" seated height, may have the mouse located in an awkward position, or may have a keyboard that made perfect sense for typewriter users but now forces computer users into awkward wrist postures. The solutions to these issues are neither costly nor difficult. Obtain a keyboard that "splits" the hands into a more normal posture, get a desk or chair that is adjustable in height (if the desk is high, provide a footrest for the shorter user so her feet do not dangle), purchase software that forces the typist to take breaks, and exercise or rotate tasks so no one is typing all day.

Other Hand and Wrist CTDs

A number of other hand and wrist CTDs are related to the force, frequency, posture, duration, and other exposures. Among these are DeQuervain's disease, which used to be called gatekeeper's thumb and is associated with repetitive movements of the thumb that cause tendon irritation and roughness; BlackBerry thumb (newly surfaced early in the twenty-first century), associated with use of the thumb to press the keys on a BlackBerry communication device; vibration white finger (Raynaud's phenomenon), which comes from holding vibrating tools; ganglionic cysts, which form in the tendon sheaths and swell up (these used to be called Bible bumps, as people would sometimes smash down on such a bump with a large family bible to break the cyst); and trigger finger, in which repetitive actions cause the tendon sheath on a finger to limit the movement of the tendon and finger movement becomes snappy or jerky. All of these are the result of overuse of the hands and fingers over time. Simple solutions range from job rotation to vibration-absorbing gloves to tool handles that allow the whole hand to be used rather than just a few fingers or the thumb. This whole-hand action allows use of the larger muscles in the forearm and upper arm and not just the small ones leading to the tendons that go via the carpal tunnel into the hand.

The elbow has one main CTD associated with it: epicondylitis, or tennis elbow. This ailment is associated with repeated or forceful rotation of the forearm and bending of the wrist at the same time, as occurs, for example, with the repeated use of a manual screwdriver to install or withdraw screws against resistance. The simple solution is to provide ratcheting or power screwdrivers. Curved screwdrivers, which allow the hand to remain in a normal posture, have also been tried, but have not been as successful because they require remaining precisely centered on the screw head. Automatic drivers are the most successful solution here, with swiveling heads being used in some applications.

The shoulder suffers two primary CTDs: rotator cuff tendinitis and thoracic outlet syndrome. Each of these is associated with tasks that require individuals to work with one or both of the elbows elevated, thus putting stress and strain on the muscles, tendons, ligaments, and possibly the bursas in the shoulder. Both involve a combination of force, frequency, awkward posture, and possibly long duration of the force or posture that causes irritation to build. Thoracic outlet syndrome is also associated with pulling the shoulders back and down or stretching to reach above shoulder height. One key difference between these CTDs is that thoracic outlet syndrome involves nerves and blood vessels in the shoulder and upper arm whereas rotator cuff tendinitis typically involves only the tendons and immediately associated nerves. Thoracic outlet syndrome is sometimes diagnostically confused with carpal tunnel syndrome, as an early symptom is numbness in the fingers. Due to the involvement of nerves and blood vessels around the shoulder, thoracic outlet syndrome is generally considered a more serious problem than carpal tunnel syndrome or rotator cuff tendinitis. Other disorders that can arise in the shoulder are degenerative arthritis and rheumatoid arthritis (Putz-Anderson, 1988).

Solutions to prevent the development of either rotator cuff tendinitis or thoracic outlet syndrome are usually a matter of relocating work to avoid the awkward postures. For example, the working height can be lowered so that people do not have to constantly raise their hands over their heads, or the work platform can be adjustable to the worker's stature. The author toured the Toyota assembly plant in Georgetown, Kentucky, years ago and saw some examples of these solutions. Each workstation had a designed and planned work content, and workers had adjustable-height platforms, workbenches, crawlers, and other devices to enable them to work both efficiently and with minimal or no discomfort. Each workstation was staffed by a team, and all team members were capable of doing each task and rotated the tasks so that they did not get excessively tired or sore and did not lose efficiency or interest due to doing the same thing over and over. This facility had recognized the issues with reaching overhead and, at least in all the instances the author directly observed, had reduced or eliminated the risk. Adjustable work platforms can be as simple as wooden blocks for people to use in various combinations to allow them to work in their comfort zone rather than bent over or reaching above their heads. Redesigning an entire facility may not be feasible or cost effective, yet much can be done without great cost.

CTDs of the Back

The human back is one of the least efficient cranes known, yet engineers (the author has a background in engineering), designers, and others continue to install workstations and design processes that require cranelike work from this inefficient crane. Figure 11.2 illustrates a typical construction crane, the kind that can be seen on any city skyline. Often called a tower crane, it has support cables and counterweights that enable it to hold up both itself and its load. The counterweight can be changed in size, depending on the expected maximum load, as can the number of support cables. In some cases these support cables will run over a support structure on top of the crane to provide even more mechanical advantage in support of the extension that is lifting the load. The actual cables that are used will depend on the weight of the object and, again, will use a pulley system to maximize the mechanical advantage. Cranes can be designed to lift up to 900 tons (Newport News Shipbuilding has one that big, used in building aircraft carriers.) If you picture the human torso as the horizontal member of the crane in Figure 11.2 and the human legs as the vertical member, you will see that it is not realistic to expect the human body to function this way.

The human back is a bit different in the way it operates. Note the key differences between the crane in Figure 11.2 and the simplified drawing of a human bending at the waist to pick up an object in Figure 11.3. The human has (1) no counterweight, (2) no exterior support cables, (3) a suspended load (the human head) at the end of the lifting beam, (4) no ability to use mechanical advantage, and (5) an unstable base that

FIGURE 11.2.   *How a crane operates.*

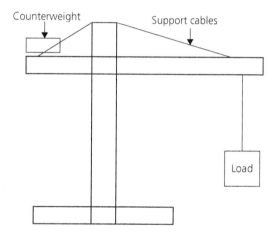

FIGURE 11.3.   *The human back in a cranelike position.*

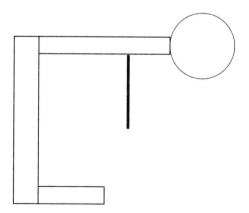

supports in only one direction rather than two. The human has internal support cables (ligaments and muscles), but these work over a very short distance and do not offer the mechanical advantage of the crane's exterior support cables. In addition, the number of these internal support cables cannot be adjusted depending on the load. An engineer who designed a crane like this would not work in the crane design business for long. Without a great deal of bioengineering the human back will not change anytime soon and in fact has taken millions of years to reach its current state of evolutionary development. Because of this inability to change the human back to make it more cranelike, we must work to reduce or eliminate lifting tasks or, at the minimum, keep all lifting in the safest range.

Arguments have raged among ergonomists, weight lifters, physicians, physical therapists, personal trainers, and members of many other groups regarding the maximum weight a person can safely lift. The actual answer to this question is that it depends. The factors governing safe lifting are many, and the most widely used model, the 1990 NIOSH lifting equation, tries to take the major factors into account. Unfortunately, many users do not read the companion manual to the equation, which clearly spells out the major assumptions made in deriving the recommendations. One of the most important is that the limits were derived from mostly young, healthy workers. Further, within that group, the limits do not apply to everyone but to 75 percent of females and 99 percent of males. When the work population doing the lifting does not match up with these assumptions, the risk is greater and different methods of calculating a maximum weight must be used (Wilson & Corlett, 2005). Another key assumption in the NIOSH equation is that the person doing the lifting does not have to carry the object(s) any distance. Lifting tasks that do involve carrying are, again, more complex and cannot use this equation.

A related tool is the handy ergonomic lifting calculator available from the National Safety Council. It functions like a slide rule and applies the guidelines and formulas of the NIOSH lifting equation. It too is accompanied by a list of reasons and assumptions that dictate against the use of the equation. Unfortunately, many users do not read this list either and have a false sense of security about their analyses of lifting tasks.

Exhibit 11.1 displays a list of tasks, from the *Applications Manual for the Revised NIOSH Lifting Equation,* for which the equation should not be used. From this list one can see the limitations of using this tool. The factors that enter into the calculations for a safe lift are many, including the worker's health, how often the worker has to lift, the posture used, the worker's underlying physical fitness, and also many nonphysical factors. The physical ones are daunting enough:

1. The distance of the center of mass of the object from the center point between the ankles

2. The distance the object has to travel when lifted or lowered

3. The object's start/stop height (below 30 inches is significantly worse)

4. The angle away from directly in front of the person

EXHIBIT 11.1. **The lifting equation should not be used for these tasks**

Lifting/lowering with one hand

Lifting/lowering for over 8 hours

Lifting/lowering while seated or kneeling

Lifting/lowering in a restricted work space

Lifting/lowering unstable objects

Lifting/lowering while carrying, pushing, or pulling

Lifting/lowering with wheelbarrows or shovels

Lifting/lowering with high-speed motion (faster than about 30 inches/second)

Lifting/lowering with unreasonable foot/floor coupling (< 0.4 coefficient of friction between the sole and the floor)

Lifting/lowering in an unfavorable environment (i.e., temperature significantly outside 66–79 degrees F (19–26 degrees C) range; relative humidity outside 35–50% range)

Source: Waters, Putz-Anderson, & Garg, 1994.

5. The frequency of lifting

6. The duration of the lifting task(s)

All lifts in the equation start with a "maximum safe lifting constant" of 51 pounds. The implication here is that for a one-time lift, under perfect conditions, 75 percent of women and 99 percent of men can safely lift 51 pounds. One problem that immediately surfaces is determining which workers are in the 25 percent of women and 1 percent of men who cannot safely do this. The sketches in Figures 11.4 and 11.5 show how to measure some physical issues associated with safe lifting.

Safe lifting and back injuries are very complex topics, as indicated in the preceding paragraphs. For further detail and analysis, please consult *Applications Manual for the Revised NIOSH Lifting Equation* as a starting point.

THE INDUSTRIAL ATHLETE

One final concept needs to be considered in this introduction to ergonomics. One often sees athletes lauded for their physical condition and activities. They bend; they jump; they run; they walk. In a professional soccer game, a good midfielder will cover over

FIGURE 11.4. *Critical dimensions for lifting.*

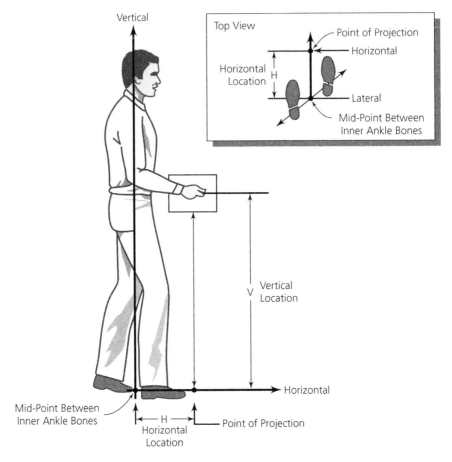

Source: Waters et al., 1994.

eight kilometers at various speeds during a ninety-minute game that has one ten-minute break in the middle. He will play at most two games in a week. A career for a top professional athlete may last up to twenty years, with the norm being less. Workers do many of the same actions during their workday, but they do them for eight hours a day, for five or more days a week, and over a thirty- or forty-year career. Professional athletes have trainers and physicians to help them condition themselves and properly warm up and loosen up prior to performing their work. Contrast that with many of the workplaces we are more familiar with: workers go directly to their workstations and start work without any warm-up. Often, depending on the time of day and off-the-job factors, they are not fully awake and alert, yet they are expected to perform at peak efficiency immediately. They will get a ten-minute break every two hours and a

FIGURE 11.5.   *Angle of asymmetry.*

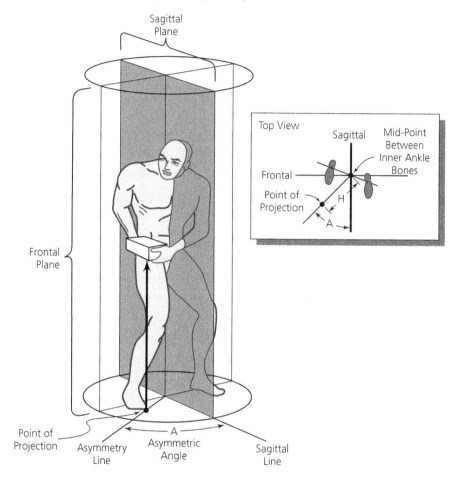

Source: Waters et al., 1994.

thirty-minute lunch. Their work might go into overtime without prior notice and might extend to twelve or more hours. They are sometimes called upon to do this seven days a week for weeks on end, due to work demands. Given all these factors, most workers are athletes just as much as or more than the sports figures who get all the attention on television and in the print media are. As the study and practice of ergonomics gains ground and more people understand what is involved in work and in preventing musculoskeletal injuries from cumulative trauma, and also understand the whole set of physical, mental, and cognitive interactions involved in workplace tasks, we will come to acknowledge the **industrial athlete** in each worker and begin to support workers in performing at their maximum effectiveness all the time.

SUMMARY

Ergonomics is neither new nor difficult to understand. In simple terms, if work hurts, it is wrong. The real challenge comes in tackling the ingrained habits of both leaders and workers to make the changes needed to solve the problem of tasks that do not fit human capabilities well. This can be a massive undertaking if organizations attempt to change whole systems. It can also be done piecemeal, attacking the problems that are hurting people right now. The best time to problem solve for a whole system is whenever a total redesign or new equipment installation occurs. The best time to problem solve for the individual issues is whenever the organization comes to a realization of the benefits of tackling ergonomic issues and challenges.

KEY TERMS

cumulative trauma disorders
holistic approach
industrial athlete
macroergonomics

musculoskeletal disorders
microergonomics
repetitive motion

QUESTIONS FOR DISCUSSION

1. How new is the field of ergonomics. and what are the key disciplines involved in a full understanding of the issues and challenges?

2. What are the differences between a macro and a micro approach to ergonomics?

3. When you think of your workplace, what ergonomics issues come to mind?

4. Of the issues you just identified, which ones have a simple solution and which might need some professional assistance to resolve?

5. How many potential back injury situations do you see frequently, and what do you suggest be done to correct them?

CHAPTER

COMMUNICABLE DISEASES

After reading this chapter, you should be able to

- Identify the major communicable disease problems that can occur in the workplace.

- Discuss the epidemiology of the most common communicable diseases.

- Understand the impact of an outbreak of communicable diseases in the workplace.

- Describe the value of a partnership between the workplace and the local health department.

An outbreak of communicable diseases has always been a serious concern for workplaces in this country. A **communicable disease**, also called a *contagious disease*, is a disease that is capable of being transmitted from one person to another. Many of these diseases have been around for thousands of years, and although their incidence has declined, they still are capable of causing not only considerable morbidity and mortality but also panic and fear in the community, school, and workplace. The occurrence of a communicable disease in the workplace can pose a tremendous risk to the health of employees and their families and to company productivity and, when compounded with lack of correct information, rumors, and fear of the unknown, may cause great panic among all employees in a short period of time. Fortunately, such occurrences have been rare, but because businesses in the United States are typically not prepared for these outbreaks, they face having to react to the problem after it happens.

The tremendous work of public health and environmental health agencies has rendered communicable diseases such as typhoid fever, cholera, and influenza, the great killers of the twentieth century and earlier, less of a concern for businesses and society. A *Morbidity and Mortality Weekly Report (MMWR)* article ("Ten Great Public Health Achievements . . . ," 1999), points out that control of infectious diseases has resulted in considerable part from clean water and improved sanitation. Public health agencies have also played a large part in reducing the threat from communicable diseases through contact tracing and treatment of those with communicable diseases or exposed to those diseases. At the same time, the success in controlling most communicable disease outbreaks has resulted in a relaxed attitude concerning the possibility that these diseases could ever return. It must be kept in mind that although most of the pathogens responsible for these diseases are under control, they have not been eliminated. In fact only one communicable disease, smallpox, has actually been eliminated, despite the best efforts of public health.

After reviewing some general information about the way communicable diseases are spread, this chapter looks at the impact on the workplace of specific diseases including hepatitis and influenza.

EPIDEMIOLOGY OF COMMUNICABLE DISEASES

The epidemiology of communicable diseases has been studied for more than two thousand years. Hippocrates, in an essay titled "On Airs, Waters and Places," actually suggested environmental and host factors as the cause of disease. Scientists have always been interested in how disease agents are spread from one person to another. Today, *communicable diseases* are defined as diseases caused by biological agents and then spread from a host to other individuals, usually in a short period of time (see, for example, McKenzie, Pinger, & Kotecki, 2005). A number of diseases that are spread from person to person can also be classified as *chronic diseases* (discussed in Chapter Two); they can be acquired from another person but last for a long period of time. Two examples of such diseases that are both communicable and chronic are acquired immune deficiency syndrome (AIDS) and tuberculosis. AIDS is caused by the human immunodeficiency virus (HIV), which is typically spread person to person by certain high-risk behaviors and is treatable but incurable. Tuberculosis, as discussed later in this chapter, is caused by a bacterium and is usually curable with appropriate medical treatment.

An infectious agent must be present for a communicable disease to occur (as discussed in Chapter Two and Figures 2.1 and 2.3). If the agent can be eliminated, the disease usually caused by the agent will not happen. For example, poultry products are often contaminated by salmonella bacteria, which can produce gastrointestinal illness in people. However, if the contaminated poultry is cooked at the right temperature for the appropriate amount of time, this agent is destroyed and no one will contract salmonella from consuming the product. Most people have heard of bacteria, viruses, and even protozoan parasites. Unfortunately, most people are unaware of how deadly these agents can be and how easily they can be spread to others under the right circumstances.

Many disease agents are well known, and public health departments have had the responsibility for controlling outbreaks of disease caused by these agents since such departments were first started. In fact, communicable disease control programs have always been a mandated function for all public health departments throughout this country. The word *control* is used with these agents because they have never been eliminated. They may be transmitted in different ways and their incidence may remain low, but they are always present and capable of causing large outbreaks of illness that can terrorize a population.

The stages in the spread of communicable diseases are known as the chain of infection (Chapter Two, Figure 2.1) and have been studied by epidemiologists and other medical personnel for hundreds of years (see, for example, McKenzie et al., 2005). The concept of the chain of infection is very useful in the study of communicable diseases and has been helpful in developing an information base for a majority of the infectious diseases that occur frequently throughout the world. Public health epidemiologists who investigate outbreaks of infectious diseases complete reports of their investigations and share them with the medical community, and the *MMWR* offers up-to-date information on outbreaks of communicable diseases. These reports and articles written by epidemiologists have helped medical personnel to better understand how infectious diseases are spread from one person to another and how the spread of disease can be halted by breaking or neutralizing any piece of the chain of infection, consisting of pathogen (or agent), reservoir, mode of transmission, and host. The identification of vaccine-preventable diseases is an example of this kind of understanding. If an individual who has been properly immunized against a disease is then exposed to the disease, there is no infection because the exposed individual is no longer susceptible to that particular disease agent.

The mode of transmission is the way an infectious agent travels from an infected person to a new person who is currently not ill. The route of transmission can be direct or indirect. Direct transmission involves immediate transmission of an infectious agent to a new host, whereas indirect transmission involves an intermediate vehicle or vector, such as an inanimate object (McKenzie et al., 2005).

FOODBORNE AND WATERBORNE DISEASES

In recent years there have been reports of *Escherichia coli* (E. coli) in spinach, *Listeria monocytogenes* in hot dogs, and salmonella in egg-based food products. The CDC reports that over 76 million Americans are infected annually with disease-causing organisms from food, with five thousand deaths every year.

McKenzie et al. (2005) define a foodborne outbreak as the occurrence of two or more cases of an illness associated with the consumption of a specific food item. Food acts as the vehicle of indirect transmission for more than two hundred known diseases. The outcomes of these diseases range from uncomfortable symptoms to death, so **foodborne and waterborne diseases** need to be taken very seriously in the community and the workplace.

Contaminated food and water are common sources of infection for humans worldwide, particularly in developing countries. They have not been as devastating in the United States, but prevention of contamination is still essential. The majority of human illnesses caused by the agents that are transmitted by consuming food or water are reportable by law to the local health department. This constant surveillance of food- and waterborne diseases allows public health officials to act rapidly if an outbreak of illness involving food or water has occurred.

Salmonellosis

Among the more common agents of foodborne illnesses are the salmonella bacteria, which have been responsible for many outbreaks of foodborne illnesses in the United States. In fact, over forty thousand cases of salmonellosis are reported to U.S. health officials every year, and many more cases go unreported because they are mild infections that do not require medical attention. Salmonellosis is caused by ingestion of food of animal origin, such as poultry and food containing eggs, that is contaminated with the salmonella bacteria and has not been cooked sufficiently to destroy the pathogen.

This disease has a short **incubation period**, ranging from three to seventy-two hours, with a median time from ingestion of a contaminated product to illness of twenty-four hours. Individuals who become infected with the salmonella bacteria usually recover from the illness in five to seven days without any medical treatment or drug therapy. The recovery from this illness is usually complete, although some infected people may develop pains in their joints, irritation of the eyes, and pain when urinating.

Impact on the Workplace

Businesses that deal in food service or food production can be implicated in outbreaks of food poisoning that can produce illness and then loss of business and lawsuits that can severely affect the business. Because there is no vaccine to prevent foodborne illnesses, the only way to eliminate such illness is to use proper food-handling techniques and to educate individuals who are responsible for producing or serving food products.

Businesses need to develop comprehensive rules for the handling of food prepared on site and served to their employees. Foods that are most commonly associated with outbreaks of salmonellosis need to be handled with particular caution, including ensuring proper cooking and cooling of these foods and not allowing ill people to prepare and serve food. Once again, workplace education programs concerning food- and waterborne outbreaks of illness can go a long way toward preventing workplace outbreaks of disease and panic.

TUBERCULOSIS

Tuberculosis (TB) is one of the world's leading infections, responsible for more than two million deaths worldwide each year. This disease is the leading killer of people infected with HIV, the virus that causes AIDS. It is caused by a bacterium, *Mycobacterium tuberculosis*, and most often infects the lungs. The initial infection usually goes unnoticed, and about 10 percent of those infected will go on to develop disease. The symptoms of this communicable disease include a productive, prolonged cough of more than three weeks duration and coughing up blood. Among the other symptoms are chills, night sweats, appetite loss, weight loss, and fatigue. This disease is spread person to person by aerosol droplets expelled by individuals with active disease of the lungs when they cough, sneeze, speak, or spit.

It is important to understand that not everyone infected with the bacteria that cause TB will become ill. Many TB infections are *latent* and unable to infect others. Moreover, individuals with active TB can be treated and cured if they seek medical care. This is one of the reasons why TB is a reportable disease in every state in this country. The major problem with TB in the workplace is not usually the risk of infection but the panic that spreads through the entire workforce when people lack information about the disease and its treatment.

The major risk factors for acquiring TB are the following ("Trends in Tuberculosis Incidence . . . ," 2007):

- HIV infection

- Low socioeconomic status

- Alcoholism

- Homelessness

- Crowded living conditions

- Diseases that weaken the immune system

- Migration from a country with a high number of cases

- Being a health care worker

Although the United States has seen thirty years of decline in TB cases, the average annual decline has slowed since 2000, and TB still remains a threat in this country, with individuals who are members of racial or ethnic minority populations and foreign-born persons representing a large number of the new cases ("Trends in Tuberculosis Incidence . . . ," 2007). In addition, drug-resistant TB has become an emerging infection in recent years and a great concern for public health officials. Employers must be prepared for the possibility that this and other emerging infections could occur in their workplaces.

Impact on the Workplace

Employers need to recognize that TB can become a real problem for their workers, especially if their company finds it has an employee with a drug-resistant infection. The most important requirement when cases of tuberculosis emerge in the workplace is having accurate information and sharing that information with the workforce.

Researchers writing in the *Morbidity and Mortality Weekly Report* ("Trends in Tuberculosis Incidence . . . ," 2007) point to a national need for improved case management, better contact investigation, testing of high-risk populations, improvements in treatment and diagnostic tools, and an improved understanding of TB transmission. These recommendations can be incorporated into a comprehensive TB preparedness plan for the workplace. This plan should include education of employees and TB prevention and control.

TB Education for Employees

The best way to prevent panic in the workplace if a case of TB is identified is to provide an education program about the epidemiology of this disease. Employees will require up-to-date and accurate information about how the disease is contracted and what the company is planning to do about the current case(s) of this disease in their workplace. This information can be disseminated through planned educational seminars, e-mails to employees, and meetings with concerned workers. The key to success with this educational strategy is to put it into action immediately after a case (or even a rumor of a case) of TB has appeared in the workplace.

TB Prevention and Control

Once a case of TB has been confirmed in the workplace, the local health department needs to be contacted immediately to conduct counseling and testing of contacts. This testing will cover family members and friends of the confirmed case as well as coworkers. Again, it is important that this component of the TB strategy occur immediately, before the company is forced into compliance due to panic in the workplace.

HEPATITIS

Hepatitis is a disease of the liver caused by a virus. There are several types of hepatitis, with different incubation periods and different modes of transmission, but the most common forms are hepatitis A, B, and C. Because the infected individual usually becomes very ill and the virus is known to damage the liver, there is usually panic surrounding the occurrence of this disease in a member of the workplace, especially among those individuals who have had contact with the infected person.

Hepatitis A

Hepatitis A is a disease of the liver caused by the *Hepatitis A virus*. It is spread person to person through ingesting the feces of an infected person, and most often involves bad personal hygiene (such as poor hand washing) or bad sanitation. Most cases involve contact with a family member or sexual partner who already has the disease. Casual contact, as in a school or workplace setting, does not usually spread the virus and cause outbreaks of illness.

The incubation period for hepatitis A is between fifteen and fifty days but usually individuals start showing symptoms of disease in twenty-eight days. If symptoms occur, they will usually include fever, fatigue, anorexia, nausea, dark urine, and jaundice (a yellowing of the skin and the whites of the eyes).

There are three ways to prevent hepatitis A;

1. Vaccination. A vaccine is available to prevent hepatitis A, but it is recommended only for those individuals traveling to areas with a high incidence of hepatitis A cases.

2. Administration of immunoglobulin. This antibody can be given before or after suspected infection; it can protect individuals from hepatitis A if given within two weeks of exposure to the virus.

3. Prevention education.

Impact on the Workplace

Hepatitis A is another example of an infectious disease that can wreak havoc on a workplace if a communicable disease plan is not available to deal with a diagnosis or even a rumor of hepatitis A in the workplace. Businesses that deal in handling food are especially susceptible to the occurrence of hepatitis A in the workplace. Another high-risk setting is day-care centers.

The best method of dealing with workplace exposure to hepatitis A is to offer educational programs to managers and staff before an outbreak occurs. This educational program needs to cover effective hand-washing techniques and proper handling of food products. Washing hands after using the bathroom, changing a diaper, or handling food needs to be stressed to all workers. The virus can also be killed by heating food to 185 degrees F for one minute.

In addition to education programs, workplaces require written procedures on the process to be followed in the event that a case of hepatitis A is reported in the workplace. These procedures should include restricting infected workers' duties so they do not perform any tasks that might expose fellow workers or consumers to the virus.

Hepatitis B

Hepatitis B is a much more serious infection than Hepatitis A. It is caused by a virus that attacks the liver and can cause cirrhosis, liver cancer, liver failure, and death. The incubation period for this type of hepatitis is very long, ranging from 45 to 180 days, with an average time from exposure to infection of 60 to 90 days.

The CDC (2007c) reports that this form of hepatitis is spread when blood from an infected person enters the body of a person who is not infected. The most common modes of hepatitis B transmission are having unprotected sex with an infected person, sharing hypodermic needles when using illicit drugs, and accidentally receiving a needle stick from a needle used by an infected person. In addition, an infected mother may pass the virus to her baby during birth. The symptoms of hepatitis B are the same as the symptoms for hepatitis A.

Impact on the Workplace

According to the CDC (2007c), one out of every twenty people in this country will become infected with hepatitis B. There is no cure for this disease at the present time, but there is a vaccine to prevent hepatitis B. The virus can survive outside the human body for at least seven days, but it can be removed from surfaces with a solution that is one part household bleach and ten parts water.

This virus should be of great concern for the health care industry and other industries that deal with human blood or blood products. These industries need to issue strict guidelines to ensure the practice of *universal precautions*, a set of practices defined by the CDC for avoiding contact with bodily fluids. For industries in which workers are not handling or being exposed to blood or blood products, education programs are usually all that are required.

Hepatitis C

Hepatitis C is also a disease of the liver; it is caused by the *Hepatitis C virus*, which is found in the blood of infected individuals. The incubation period can range from two weeks to six months but commonly runs six to nine weeks. There are blood tests for this viral infection, but no vaccine is available.

Hepatitis C is usually spread from person to person by direct contact with human blood. The mode of transmission is very similar to that for to hepatitis B. The high-risk behaviors that predispose someone to this infection include sharing needles with an infected person; receiving a blood transfusion; having frequent contact with blood or blood products, especially through needle sticks; sharing razors or toothbrushes with an infected person; and having sex with an infected person.

Impact on the Workplace

This virus should be of great concern for the health care industry and industries that deal with human blood or blood products. Workers in these industries need to practice universal precautions. For workers in industries where they are not handling or being exposed to blood or blood products, education programs are usually all that is required.

HIV AND AIDS

Acquired immunodeficiency syndrome (AIDS) is caused by infection with the human immunodeficiency virus (HIV). In just over twenty-five years, **HIV/AIDS** has become the principal viral infection affecting this country. It is predominantly an infection of the young, and thanks to better treatment, it is both an acute and a chronic disease. There is promising treatment available for those infected with HIV and AIDS, but there is no cure.

In the beginning of the HIV/AIDS **epidemic**, when the cause was still unknown, this disease was thought to be spread only by homosexual sex and was called gay-related immune disease (GRID). As time passed and information became available about this new infection, it became clear that HIV/AIDS was not a disease caused by belonging to a high-risk group but rather a disease caused by high-risk behaviors.

The human immunodeficiency virus is spread by the practice of high-risk health behaviors, and over 40,000 Americans become infected every year. There is strong evidence that prevention efforts are working, but they need to be expanded if we are ever going to gain control of this epidemic.

Impact on the Workplace

The CDC (2007b) reports that over 1 million individuals in the United States are living with HIV/AIDS. Better treatments for HIV/AIDS are allowing those infected to live long lives and many continue to work. Although HIV is communicable because it can be passed from one person to another, HIV/AIDS is also a chronic disease because people can live with it and be productive for many years before it causes or contributes to death. This makes it important for both employers and employees to understand how HIV is transmitted.

Understanding HIV Transmission

This disease has been studied by researchers for more than twenty-five years, and it has been proven that the disease is spread person to person by high-risk behaviors. These behaviors include having sexual contact with an infected person, sharing hypodermic needles with someone who is infected, and less frequently, receiving a transfusion of infected blood. The CDC (2007b) reports that there is no known risk of HIV transmission to coworkers, clients, or consumers in the workplace. The real threat posed by HIV in the workplace is the fear and panic that can arise if even a rumor of an infected coworker surfaces. This threat can be dealt with by offering workers updated information about HIV as it becomes available.

Businesses in which certain workers may come into contact with human blood or blood products need to make universal precautions mandatory to protect these workers from infection with HIV. Many health care settings fall into this business category. In the normal course of the workday in most businesses in this country, universal precautions to contain the spread of HIV are not necessary.

INFLUENZA

Influenza (or the flu) is a respiratory illness that is caused by a virus and can range from a temporary health problem to a fatal condition among certain groups of individuals. The primary symptoms of this infection are fever, headache, extreme tiredness, dry cough, sore throat, runny and stuffy nose, and muscle aches. The virus may be spread from person to person in droplets from coughs and sneezes. A droplet can travel up to three feet in the air from an infected person to a new host. The virus can also be spread to a new host by being deposited on an object (such as a cup or a door handle) that subsequently comes into contact with a susceptible individual. The CDC influenza pandemic operation plan (2006) reports that the time from exposure to illness is usually one to four days, with a median incubation period of two days. Moreover, individuals who are developing this disease are usually infectious for one to four days before the symptoms manifest themselves, and people continue to shed virus for up to one week after becoming acutely ill.

There are three major types of influenza viruses, labeled A, B, and C. Humans are susceptible to all three strains, but A is most associated with large outbreaks of illness. Wild birds are the natural reservoir for all known subtypes of influenza A, including H5N1, the subtype better known as avian influenza (or bird flu). The potential pandemic that we now face involves this H5N1 subtype. Swine flu (H1N1) could also instigate a pandemic.

A **pandemic** is a geographically widely distributed epidemic of a new or reemergent disease. Pandemic outbreaks of influenza occur every ten to forty-two years and usually result from the mutation of an avian virus to a form that can infect humans and can be easily passed between them. Once a pandemic begins it cannot be easily stopped, so the preparation for the pandemic must occur long before the advent of the initial cases of infection. So far the transmission of this new influenza A subtype among humans has been limited. Worldwide, the CDC (2006) reports that it has affected more than two hundred people, with a mortality rate of 50 percent. This lethality will be a particular concern if this virus becomes more easily transmissible among humans.

Impact on the Workplace

The peak of the influenza season occurs every year in this country between December and March and usually has a large impact on worker job attendance and productivity. Workers can be protected from contracting influenza by receiving an annual influenza immunization (or flu shot).

The CDC (2006) reports that in the United States there are approximately 36,000 influenza deaths each year. A pandemic involving a new strain of virus could result in 200,000 to 2 million deaths just in this country. If an influenza pandemic becomes reality, businesses across the United States can play a vital role by protecting their employees' health and safety and by limiting the spread of this disease to other businesses and the community at large. This pandemic will be widespread and extended, producing multiple waves or outbreaks of illness lasting six to eight weeks. It will pose multiple threats above and beyond morbidity and mortality for all workplaces in this country.

OSHA (2007) predicts that workplaces will experience major increases in absenteeism, changes in the patterns of commerce, and interruptions in the supply and delivery of items. The absenteeism rate could increase to 40 percent of the workforce, owing to personal illness, family illness, and fear of getting infected at work and bringing the virus home to family members. A pandemic of influenza will reduce shopping for nonmedical items and increase the demand for home delivery. The elderly and disabled will be affected to a greater extent than the rest of the population.

Preparing for a Pandemic

In order to reduce the impact of an influenza pandemic on the workplace, employers must engage in considerable planning well before the potential pandemic becomes reality. Without a plan for this potential health emergency, employers are likely to face challenges for which they are destined to suffer failure, placing their employees at high risk of a multitude of problems. According to CDC (2006) the influenza plan must include a well-developed surveillance system capable of early detection of the pandemic, containment of human cases of influenza, and treatment of those who have been infected and exposed to the virus. One issue this plan needs to address is the time gap that will occur between the first case of human-to-human transmission of avian influenza and the availability of a vaccine for the new easily transmissible strain. Businesses need to prepare their workplace for this gap, or suffer high morbidity and mortality until the vaccine becomes available.

OSHA (2007) recommends that each business in the United States develop a complete disaster plan that includes pandemic preparedness, and OSHA offers the guidance shown in Exhibit 12.1, "Preparing the Workplace for an Influenza Pandemic."

EMERGING INFECTIONS

Government cuts in the funding for public health programs, the resistance of some pathogens to antibiotics, and the importation of diseases into this country from around the world has produced new and emerging communicable disease threats for the workplace. David Satcher (1995) describes how infectious diseases maintain a large reservoir of agents that are always available to become epidemic under the right conditions. Recent large outbreaks of infectious diseases in this country underscore how easy it is to have an epidemic of communicable diseases if public health does not remain vigilant about the threat of disease.

As mentioned earlier, the only communicable disease that has ever been eliminated from the world is smallpox; this happened in 1977. Many other infectious diseases are currently under control but remain capable of reemerging as major health threats to many countries, including ours. One example of the serious nature of these infectious diseases occurred in Milwaukee, Wisconsin, in 1993. Contamination of the city water supply resulted in an outbreak of cryptosporidiosis that affected an estimated four hundred thousand people, over four thousand of whom required hospitalization. Another example is tuberculosis, which reemerged in the United States in the

EXHIBIT 12.1.   **Preparing the workplace for an influenza pandemic**

A disaster plan must be developed and communicated to the entire country. The responsibility for developing and implementing this rests with state and local public health departments. This plan needs to include the following components:

- Be aware of and review federal, state and local health department pandemic influenza plans. Incorporate appropriate actions from these plans into workplace disaster plans.

- Prepare and plan for operations with a reduced workforce.

- Work with your suppliers to ensure that you can continue to operate and provide services.

- Develop a sick leave policy that does not penalize sick employees, thereby encouraging employees who have influenza-related symptoms (e.g., fever, headache, cough, sore throat, runny or stuffy nose, muscle aches, or upset stomach) to stay home so that they do not infect other employees. Recognize that employees with ill family members may need to stay home to care for them.

- Identify possible exposure and health risks to your employees. Are employees potentially in contact with people with influenza such as in a hospital or clinic? Are your employees expected to have a lot of contact with the general public?

- Minimize exposure to fellow employees or the public. For example, will more of your employees work from home? This may require enhancement of technology and communications equipment.

- Identify business-essential positions and people required to sustain business-necessary functions and operations. Prepare to cross-train or develop ways to function in the absence of these positions. It is recommended that employers train three or more employees to be able to sustain business-necessary functions and operations, and communicate the expectation for available employees to perform these functions if needed during a pandemic.

- Plan for downsizing services but also anticipate any scenario which may require a surge in your services.

- Recognize that, in the course of normal daily life, all employees will have non-occupational risk factors at home and in community settings that should be reduced to the extent possible. Some employees will also have individual risk factors that should be considered by employers as they plan how the organization will respond to a potential pandemic (e.g., immuno-compromised individuals and pregnant women).

- Stockpile items such as soap, tissue, hand sanitizer, cleaning supplies and recommended personal protective equipment. When stockpiling items, be aware of each product's shelf life and storage conditions (e.g., avoid areas that are damp or have temperature extremes) and incorporate product rotation (e.g., consume oldest supplies first) into your stockpile management program.

Make sure that your disaster plan protects and supports your employees, customers and the general public. Be aware of your employees' concerns about pay, leave, safety and health. Informed employees who feel safe at work are less likely to be absent.

- Develop policies and practices that distance employees from each other, customers and the general public. Consider practices to minimize face-to-face contact between employees such as email, websites and teleconferences. Policies and practices that allow employees to work from home or to stagger their work shifts may be important as absenteeism rises.

- Organize and identify a central team of people or focal point to serve as a communication source so that your employees and customers can have accurate information during the crisis.

- Work with your employees and their union(s) to address leave, pay, transportation, travel, childcare, absence and other human resource issues.

- Provide your employees and customers in your workplace with easy access to infection control supplies, such as soap, hand sanitizers, personal protective equipment (such as gloves or surgical masks), tissues, and office cleaning supplies.

- Provide training, education and informational material about business-essential job functions and employee health and safety, including proper hygiene practices and the use of any personal protective equipment to be used in the workplace. Be sure that informational material is available in a usable format for individuals with sensory disabilities and/or limited English proficiency. Encourage employees to take care of their health by eating right, getting plenty of rest and getting a seasonal flu vaccination.

- Work with your insurance companies and state and local health agencies to provide information to employees and customers about medical care in the event of a pandemic.

(continued)

EXHIBIT 12.1.   **Preparing the workplace for an influenza pandemic** (*continued*)

- Assist employees in managing additional stressors related to the pandemic. These are likely to include distress related to personal or family illness, life disruption, grief related to loss of family, friends or coworkers, loss of routine support systems, and similar challenges. Assuring timely and accurate communication will also be important throughout the duration of the pandemic in decreasing fear or worry. Employers should provide opportunities for support, counseling, and mental health assessment and referral should these be necessary. If present, Employee Assistance Programs can offer training and provide resources and other guidance on mental health and resiliency before and during a pandemic.

Source: OSHA, 2007.

1980s as a formidable disease threat, especially in its new drug-resistant forms. In addition, a particular strain of *Escherichia coli* (0157:H7) has emerged as a major threat to the public in recent years (Turnock, 2007), pneumonia and influenza cause tremendous morbidity and mortality every year, and as discussed earlier in this chapter, mutations of the influenza virus pose the threat of a worldwide pandemic of disease capable of reaching this country and killing thousands.

Impact on the Workplace

The continuing battle with emerging infections requires a proactive response from workplaces across this country. Employers have to be prepared to respond rapidly to the needs of their workers and consumers in the event of reported cases of infectious diseases among their workers and workers' family members.

The most recent outbreak of illness caused by E. coli involved people in a number of states and was associated with consumption of bagged spinach. The California Food Emergency Response Team (2007) reported 205 confirmed illnesses and three deaths associated with this outbreak; 103 patients were hospitalized and 30 percent developed hemolytic uremic syndrome. This outbreak is one more example of how a disease can harm communities and workplaces. It offers further proof that we must never let our guard down when it comes to the possibility of communicable diseases in the workplace.

Emerging diseases and bioterrorism have become potential workplace issues that employers must plan to deal with. Preparation requires developing an information base about diseases and assigning staff to prepare a contingency plan to deal with an outbreak, including identifying a way to communicate rapidly with employees and consumers with information about the disease.

Infectious Disease Committee

Employers should also establish an infectious disease committee that meets regularly to develop workplace policies concerning communicable diseases and to develop educational programs that inform workers about these diseases.

SUMMARY

The occurrence and spread of communicable diseases is still a real problem for workplaces in this country. The biggest part of this problem is often not the ill worker or workers or the disease itself, but the fear it can cause among other workers, fear that increases dramatically as rumors about the disease expand. Workers become concerned about their own health and the possibility of bringing infections home to their family members. Employers need to quickly provide them with information about the disease and about the precautions that need to be taken by the workforce, clients, and family members. The infectious disease model called the chain of infection is a useful aid for explaining communicable diseases, evaluating their threat, and developing strategies to control the spread of disease among employees and customers.

The main prerequisite for a proactive approach to communicable, or contagious, diseases is an accurate and accessible educational program about these diseases that can spread easily from person to person. Employers need to respond immediately to the threat of disease that may affect their workforce. Honesty with employees and customers from the very beginning of the reported problem is the only way to deal with a communicable disease threat in the workplace.

Businesses in America need to realize that the cost-effective way to deal with outbreaks of infectious disease in the workplace is to have a well-developed plan. One outbreak of illness can cost a business a great deal of money in both current and future sales due to lowered productivity and the bad publicity associated with infectious diseases occurring in the workplace. For these reasons, all businesses need to become proactive in their planning for a communicable disease problem in their workplace.

KEY TERMS

communicable diseases
epidemic
foodborne and waterborne diseases
hepatitis

HIV/AIDS
incubation period
pandemic
tuberculosis

QUESTIONS FOR DISCUSSION

1. What are the advantages for a business of developing a plan to deal with an outbreak of communicable diseases in the workplace?

2. What should an employer do to prepare for an outbreak of avian influenza in the community and the workplace?

3. What are the differences between the three types of hepatitis discussed in this chapter?

4. What do employers and managers need to know about HIV and AIDS in the workplace?

CHAPTER

13

VISION AND HEARING ISSUES

After reading this chapter, you should be able to

- Recognize that vision and hearing injuries are preventable when appropriate precautions are taken.

- Identify the governmental agencies and standards concerned with protecting vision and hearing.

- Describe the variety of products that are available to protect vision and hearing.

- Understand that industries and companies have a responsibility to protect employees from vision and hearing injuries.

In the workplace, many workers think about accomplishing their job every day but do not consider vision or hearing safety. The statistics of vision and hearing injuries that occur daily make it imperative that employers and employees take the necessary precautions to prevent work-related injuries to the eyes and to the ears. Work-related injuries may be minor but they can also cause lifetime disabilities. It is for this reason that this chapter provides necessary information on the prevention of injuries and protection of people in the workplace.

PROTECTING VISION IN THE WORKPLACE

According to All About Vision (2007), "more than 1 million Americans 40 and over are blind from eye disease. An additional 2.3 million Americans are visually impaired. Seventeen percent of Americans who are 45 or older report some type of vision impairment even when wearing eyeglasses or contact lenses. This percentage rises with age, to 26 percent of people age 75 and older." A significant amount of the blindness and vision impairment among Americans is the direct result of injuries in the workplace. Data from the United States Eye Injury Registry (2000) for 1988 to 2000 indicate that 40 percent of serious eye injuries take place in the home and 13 percent occur in industrial premises. Kuhn, Master, Witherspoon, Morris, and Maisiak (1998) report that "eye trauma is the cause of 40,000–60,000 new cases of blindness each year. In the working-age population, eye trauma is the leading cause of visual morbidity and blindness."

Each business day, more than two thousand U.S. workers incur job-related eye injuries, with 10 to 20 percent of these injuries causing temporary or permanent vision loss. These injuries are most commonly caused by flying objects such as bits of metal and glass, tools, particles in the air, and exposure to chemicals or radiation. Ninety percent of these injuries could have been prevented or made less severe with protective eyewear (Prevent Blindness America, 2005).

Many safety issues related to the protection of the eyes involve using common sense. Many accidents are avoidable if proper precautions are taken. Uncorrected vision problems can cause accidents. It makes sense for workers to have their vision checked every year for prescription updates, focusing problems, and medical eye problems. Employers can also ensure that workers are wearing appropriate protective eyewear. Prevention is the key. The following discussion focuses on summarizing and explaining the standards set out by the Occupational Safety and Health Administration and the **American National Standards Institute** for protecting workers' vision and on describing the various types of protective eyewear.

Federal Safety Standards

Under the terms of its enabling legislation, the Occupational Safety and Health Administration (OSHA) has set standards, or rules, for eye and face protection. OSHA requires employers to ensure the safety of all employees in the work environment. Eye and face protection must be provided whenever necessary to protect against chemical, environmental, radiological, or mechanical irritants and hazards. Eye and face protection is addressed in specific standards for general industry, shipyard employment, longshoring, and the construction industry. All OSHA rules, proposed rules, and notices, including those related to eye and face protection, are published in the *Federal Register*, which is updated daily. General and final rules are then codified in the *Code of Federal Regulations* (*CFR*), which is updated annually. On its Web site, OSHA (2008) lists the *CFR* sections that relate to eye and face protection (see Exhibit 13.1). In addition, this Web site makes available the *standard interpretations* that clarify existing OSHA standards relating to vision safety and also provides *general consensus* materials, which are not OSHA standards but which contain guidance from organizations such as the American National Standards Institute about worker eye protection.

EXHIBIT 13.1. *CFR* sections concerning eye and face protection

General Industry (29 CFR 1910)
1910 Subpart I, Personal protective equipment

- 1910.132, General requirements [related topic page]

- 1910.133, Eye and face protection

- Appendix B, Non-mandatory compliance guidelines for hazard assessment and personal protective equipment selection

1910 Subpart Q, Welding, cutting, and brazing

- 1910.252, General requirements [related topic page]

  - 1910.252(b)(2), Eye protection

Shipyard Employment (29 CFR 1915)
1915 Subpart I, Personal protective equipment

- 1915.153, Eye and face protection

Longshoring (29 CFR 1918)
1918 Subpart J, Personal protective equipment

- 1918.101, Eye and face protection

Construction Industry (29 CFR 1926)
1926 Subpart E, Personal protective and life saving equipment [related topic page]

- 1926.95, Criteria for personal protective equipment

- 1926.102, Eye and face protection

Source: OSHA, 2008.

Twenty-four states, Puerto Rico, and the Virgin Islands have OSHA-approved state or territory plans (with standards identical to the federal OSHA standards) and have also adopted their own standards and enforcement policies. Some states have adopted somewhat different standards or may have different enforcement policies.

Section 5(a)(1) of the Occupational Safety and Health Act (which created OSHA) is referred to as the General Duty Clause. It requires the employer "to furnish to each of his employees employment and a place of employment which are free from recognized hazards that are causing or are likely to cause death or serious physical harm to his employees." Section 5(a)(2) requires employers to "comply with occupational safety and health standards promulgated under this Act."

Protective Eyewear

Wearing the correct type of eye protection is an essential element of on-the-job safety. The following recommendations compiled by the Department of Energy provide general guidance to all organizations for minimizing eye injuries in the workplace.

- Perform worksite hazard analyses to determine what eye hazards exist and what type of eye safety equipment will provide the right protection.

- Post safety procedures that clearly identify the appropriate eye protection in work areas where such protection is required.

- Provide prejob instruction for those workers whose tasks require eye protection, and schedule hands-on training in the use and selection of appropriate eye protectors on a regular basis.

- Ensure that no one, including top-level managers, public officials, or other visitors to the work site, is exempt from wearing eye protection in areas where it is required.

- Use eye protection in conjunction with, not as a replacement for, machine guards, engineering controls, etc.

- Ensure that eye protection fits properly (i.e., firmly and comfortably, without restricting vision).

- Wear eye protection even if prescription eyewear is worn. Although most plastic lenses of eyeglasses are impact-resistant (by Federal regulation), they are not meant for use in hazardous situations.

Source: U.S. Department of Energy, 1991.

The **American National Standards Institute** (ANSI) calls itself the "voice of the U.S. standards and conformity assessment system" (ANSI, 2009). A private, nonprofit organization, it represents the interests of governmental agencies, academic and international bodies, more than 125,000 companies, and 3.5 million professionals. It oversees the creation, promulgation, and use of thousands of norms and guidelines that directly affect businesses in nearly every industry sector. ANSI is also the official U.S. representative to the International Organization for Standardization (ISO). In August 2003, ANSI issued a new standard (ANSI Z87.1-2003) that establishes revised performance criteria and testing requirements for devices used to protect the eyes and face from injuries from impact, nonionizing radiation, and chemical exposure in workplaces and schools. (This standard does not address protection in certain medical settings involving bloodborne pathogens or around various types of radiation.) It covers all types of relevant protective devices, including spectacles and eyeglasses, goggles, face shields, welding helmets, hand shields, and full facepiece respirators. The standard contains descriptions and general requirements as well as criteria for testing, marking, selection, use, and care.

As optometrists and other eye-care professionals know, these standards are extremely important when prescribing glasses to patients. This ANSI standard has new designations for basic impact and high-impact protectors. These two levels of protection have distinct testing and marking requirements. Basic impact lenses are tested using a drop ball test (involving a three-eighths-inch metal ball dropped from a height of fifty inches). High-impact lenses and all frames have to meet more stringent high-mass and high-velocity impact tests. The new standard addresses the topic of which devices must be used in conjunction with safety spectacles or goggles. Also, respiratory equipment that offers eye and face protection has been added to the standard. This equipment includes both tight-fitting full facepiece respirators and loose-fitting respirators. To sum up the standard, safety spectacles and goggles, welding shields, and face shields may meet either the basic or the high-impact level. Respirators that also provide eye protection, such as tight-fitting full facepieces, loose-fitting facepieces, and helmets, must meet the high-impact level. In the new marking requirements, the mark that identifies the basic impact level is "Z87." The mark that identifies the high-impact level is "Z87+." The manufacturer's identifying mark or symbol plus the basic or high-impact level marking must appear at designated places on safety spectacles, goggles, face shields, and respirators.

Goggles and Spectacles When face shields and welding shields on respirators can be raised from the normal position, ANSI states that the respirator must be used in conjunction with spectacles or goggles. Many companies with specific hazardous jobs have additional requirements for safety glasses that protect the eyes and the face.

Cup goggles are designed for operations in which foreign particles might strike the eyes from the sides, top, or bottom, such as chipping, grinding, riveting, performing hand tool and machine operations, rail cutting, and spike driving. **Dust goggles** are recommended for use in cement plants and compressed air operations, where fine dust particles and powder create severe eye hazards. Dust goggles also protect against the impact of flying particles from any direction. Cover goggles are designed to fit over prescription glasses, providing greater protection than glasses alone would against all types of airborne foreign particles coming from any direction. Cover goggles might be used with jobs such as chipping, grinding, riveting, or machine tool work or any job where sparks or fairly small-scale explosion hazards are present. A specially designed goggle is available for acetylene welding, cutting, burning, brazing, and furnace operations. These goggles provide protection against harmful light rays, glare, and flying sparks. Flexible mask chemical goggles are specifically designed to offer protection against corrosive liquid splashes encountered in chemical process industries but not from flying particles. Face shields are designed to protect the eyes and face from the hazards of sawing, chemical work, buffing, sanding, light grinding, and hazards in the manufacturing of incandescent lamps, electronic tubes, and glass bottles. Many types of shields are available. These shields do not fully comply with ANSI Z87.1 requirements, so workers need to wear approved safety glasses with them. Welding helmets are designed to protect the eyes from injurious light rays emitted during welding operations. Safety glasses must be worn under welding helmets. Safety glasses look and feel like an ordinary pair of glasses except that the lenses are made of industrial specification safety glass or plastic. This offers increased eye protection from flying particles coming from in front of the eye. Plastic lenses, especially those made from polycarbonate, offer greater impact resistance than glass lenses and they are lighter. Although plastic lenses are less resistant to scratching than glass lenses, abrasion-resistant coatings are now available for plastic and polycarbonate lenses. Side shields are often needed and suggested for additional protection.

Just as some people are long and thin, so are some faces. Other faces are large and round. Not everyone can wear the same size glasses or goggles. Safety eyewear must be fitted properly to the individual's face.

Photochromic Lenses Photochromic lenses change their degree of tint depending on the amount of available light. ANSI standards allow photochromic lenses to be used indoors, but it is recommended that they be used with care in jobs requiring precise visual acuity or requiring fast reactions to visual stimuli. Although photochromic lenses absorb ultraviolet light, they are not adequate for protection in hazardous radiation environments, such as an area where X-rays are taken, and should not be used in these situations. The OSHA rules differ from the ANSI standards in the matter of the use of safety glasses with photochromic lenses, such as PhotoGray lenses. OSHA prohibits their use in indoor work locations because these variable tint lenses can cause temporary vision impairment when the light changes from bright to dim. For example, a forklift operator driving back and forth between indoor and outdoor locations should exercise caution in the lenses he or she chooses. PhotoGray lenses are allowed to be used inside when lighting conditions do not change substantially and when an employee stays constantly in one area, especially where glare or bright lights are a problem. PhotoGray lenses may be used by employees working outdoors as long as there are no ultraviolet or infrared hazards.

Contact Lenses Contact lenses have become a popular choice of eyewear over the past fifty years, but there are arguments against wearing contact lenses in some workplace environments. Dust or chemicals can be trapped behind a lens and cause irritation or damage, or both, to the cornea of the eye. Gases and vapors can cause irritation and excessive eye watering. Chemical splashes may be more injurious when contact lenses are worn. If lens removal is delayed, first-aid treatment may not be as effective and the eye's exposure time to the chemical may be increased. There are also arguments for wearing contact lenses in a workplace environment. Contact lenses may prevent some substances from reaching the eye, and thus may minimize or even prevent an injury. As a result a wide range of opinions about the safety of contact lenses in the workplace has formed, and helpful data are hard to find because occupational injury reporting systems do not typically include information about contact lens use. Basically, it is important to remember that contact lenses are not intended to be used as protective devices and are not a substitute for personal protective equipment (PPE). If eye and face protection is required for certain work operations, then all workers, including contact lens wearers, should wear the proper protective devices. Safe work conditions for all workers are possible only when basic occupational health and safety practices and procedures are followed.

An Example: Lasers

This section looks at a specific workplace hazard to vision (drawing on U.S. Department of Energy, 1991, and All About Eye Safety, 1996) to illustrate the variety of factors that may need to be considered in choosing appropriate eye protection. If the eyes are not protected adequately when working with laser beams, severe damage can occur. The correct choice of lens density and color for goggles is based on the wavelength and power of the specific laser being used. Plastic goggles, for example, should not be worn by workers who might be exposed to direct laser beams or reflections. To ensure adequate protection, these workers should wear filter safety-glass goggles. In general, laser eye protection should be selected on the basis of how well it will protect against the maximum exposure anticipated. At the same time, the greatest amount of light possible should be allowed to enter the eye to ensure proper sight. The unprotected human eye is extremely sensitive to laser radiation and can be permanently damaged from direct or reflected beams. The site of ocular damage for any given laser depends on its output wavelength. Laser light in the visible and near infrared spectrum can cause damage to the retina, whereas wavelengths outside this region (that is, the ultraviolet and far infrared spectrums) are absorbed by the anterior segment of the eye, causing damage to the cornea and to the lens. The extent of the damage is determined by the laser irradiance, exposure duration, and beam size. As laser retinal burns may be painless and the damaging beam sometimes invisible, maximum care should be taken to provide protection for all persons in settings where a laser is in use.

Protective eyewear in the form of goggles, glasses, and shields is the principal means of ensuring against injury, and must be worn at all times during laser operation.

Laser safety eyewear is designed to reduce the amount of incident light of specific wavelengths to safe levels, while transmitting sufficient light for good vision. In accordance with ANSI guidelines (ANSI Z136.3), each laser requires a specific type of protective eyewear, and factors that must be considered when selecting laser safety eyewear include laser wavelength and peak irradiance, optical density, visual transmittance, field of view, effects on color vision, absence of irreversible bleaching of the filter, comfort, and impact resistance. Ignorance of any of these factors may result in serious eye injury. Items of laser safety eyewear often look alike in style and color, so it is important to check both the wavelength and optical density imprinted on this eyewear prior to laser use, especially in multi-wavelength facilities where more than one laser may be located in the same room. Color coding of laser hand pieces and laser safety eyewear may help to minimize confusion. Laser safety eyewear should not be moved between laser rooms nor should it be carried in lab coat pockets between uses. The integrity of laser safety eyewear must be inspected regularly because small cracks or loose-fitting filters may transmit laser light directly to the eye.

With the enormous expansion of laser use in medicine, industry, and research, every facility must formulate and adhere to specific safety policies that appropriately address eye protection. All About Eye Safety (1996), states that "each laser facility must develop its own safety procedures to be enforced by an appropriately trained Laser Safety Officer for the facility." Employers should undertake an adequate risk assessment and seek competent advice from a specialist who is familiar with the specific business. Risk assessment and accident prevention measures should take into account the individual workers' differences and the various jobs that are specific to the business in order to prevent vision injuries. In an environment that is dusty, where the air is full of particulate matter, the type of protective eyewear and protective breathing equipment would vary for someone using dangerous power tools or electrical machinery. Other issues of concern:

- Good lighting in the workplace

- Safe workplace access and exit

- Well-maintained pedestrian and traffic routes in the workplace

- Clear communication and good signing of hazards and risks in the workplace

Eye injuries occur without any warning. One moment a person can have perfectly normal eyes, and the next moment he or she may be blind or at least in severe pain. Therefore employers and workers should be eternally vigilant and aware of situations that could lead to injury. All precautions should be taken to avoid injury. Repair of a grave injury is almost impossible, and prevention is most certainly better than a cure. One key role of health promotion programs in the workplace should be to promote awareness among employees about how to protect their eyes, and what to do in the case of injury.

PROTECTING HEARING IN THE WORKPLACE

The other sense that needs to be protected in the workplace is the sense of hearing. According to American Academy of Otolaryngology—Head and Neck Surgery (2006), "10 million Americans suffer irreversible noise-induced hearing loss, with 30 million exposed to dangerous noise levels each day." Noise can really hurt the human ear, and if it is loud enough, it can damage hearing. The damage caused by noise is called *sensory-neural hearing loss*, or nerve deafness. People who believe that they have grown accustomed to a loud noise have probably actually sustained damage to their hearing. There is no treatment, no surgery, and not even a hearing aid that can completely restore hearing that has been damaged by noise. However, the risk of this type of hearing loss can be reduced or prevented.

It is also true that as we age our hearing tends to become worse. For the average person, aging does not cause noticeably impaired hearing before the age of sixty. People who are not exposed to excessive noise and are otherwise healthy may have normal hearing for many years. People who are exposed to noise and do not protect their hearing begin to lose their hearing at an earlier age. For example, a twenty-five-year-old carpenter who has been exposed to loud machine noises may have the same hearing as someone who is fifty years old but who has worked in a quiet job. Excessive exposure to noise is one of the most common health hazards encountered at a construction site. Thousands of construction workers are already hearing impaired as a result of noise exposure, and thousands more are destroying their hearing through everyday work in the industry. Sources of excessive noise levels on a construction site range from power hand tools to diesel-powered trucks and other large pieces of equipment.

People differ in their sensitivity to noise. As a general rule, noise is probably loud enough to damage hearing if it requires individuals to shout to be heard over it. If the noise hurts people's ears, if the noise makes their ears ring, or if they have difficulty hearing for several hours after exposure, hearing damage may have already occurred. These circumstances should be avoided in the workplace. When individuals are exposed to loud noise over a long period of time, symptoms of hearing loss will increase gradually. Over time the sounds that they hear will become distorted or muffled, and it may become more and more difficult for them to understand simple spoken words. Because hearing loss is often gradual, people may not be aware of it until it is detected with a hearing test.

Most cases of occupational hearing loss develop gradually, and noise is only one of the possible reasons for this loss. Heat; harmful gases such as carbon monoxide; toxic chemicals such as arsenic, manganese, and mercury; and solvents such as toluene can also negatively affect hearing. However, as researchers writing in the *Morbidity and Mortality Weekly Report* ("Notifiable Disease Surveillance . . . ," 1996) have said, "there can be no effective prevention or control of disease without knowledge of when, where, and under what conditions cases occur." Efforts to prevent occupational noise-induced hearing loss have been hampered by a lack of surveillance data to systematically identify subpopulations at risk, evaluate the effectiveness of intervention strategies, and monitor progress in prevention. The following sections focus on what is known about devices to protect the ears from excessive noise in the workplace and on the testing and treatment of hearing loss.

Ear Anatomy

The ear has three main parts; the outer, middle, and inner ear. The outer ear is the area that can be seen externally and that opens into the ear canal. The eardrum separates the ear canal from the middle ear. Small bones (ossicles) in the middle ear, called the malleus, incus, and stapes, transfer sound to the inner ear. The inner ear contains sensitive hair cells and the auditory nerve (the eighth cranial nerve), which leads to the brain.

Any source of sound sends vibrations (sound waves) into the air. These vibrations funnel through the ear opening and go through the ear canal. They then strike the eardrum causing it to vibrate. The vibrations of the eardrum are passed to the small bones in the middle ear, which transmit them to the inner ear where hair cells with vibrating cilia stimulate the auditory nerve in the inner ear. The cilia in the inner ear vibrate at different rates in response to different sound frequencies. They vibrate more slowly for the low pitch of a baritone and vibrate faster for the higher pitch of a soprano. These vibrations are transformed into distinct electrical impulses that are sent via the auditory nerve to the medulla and then to the cortex of the brain. This neuro-anatomical pathway is what allows us to hear.

When noise is too loud, it begins to kill the hair cells in the inner ear. Just as a speaker can blow out from an electrical circuit overload, these vibrating hair cells can be overexcited by too much noise. More specifically, "when forced into metabolic overdrive, the cells spin off toxic oxidation products that make them swell and sometimes slowly die off. Toxic noise also compromises blood flow to the inner ear, causing further damage. The cells that go first are those that resonate to a higher pitch, and the resulting dropout of higher frequency sounds is what makes words seem garbled" (Healey, 2007, p. 58). As the exposure time to loud noise increases, more hair cells are destroyed. As the number of cells decreases so does the person's ability to hear. There is no way to restore these dead cells. The damage is permanent.

Decibels

Sound can be measured scientifically in two ways: by pitch and by loudness. Pitch is measured in frequency of sound vibrations per second. A low pitch, such as the pitch of a deep voice, produces fewer vibrations per second than the high pitch of a high voice. Intensity or loudness of sound is measured in **decibels** (dB). The scale for decibel measurements begins with the faintest sound that the human ear can detect, which is 0 decibels. Every 10-decibel increase is a tenfold increase in loudness. A rocket launch produces 180 decibels of noise. A whisper produces about 30 dB, moderate rainfall 50 dB, normal conversation 60 dB, a dishwasher 70 dB, a lawnmower engine 90 dB, a loud rock concert 115 dB, and an airplane jet engine 140 dB. Many experts agree that continual exposure to more than 85 decibels of noise can cause hearing damage.

According to the National Institute on Deafness and Other Communication Disorders (2007), part of the federal National Institutes of Health, "hearing loss from exposure to loud noises is 100% preventable. All individuals should understand the hazards of noise and how to practice good hearing health in everyday living. To protect your hearing, know which noises can cause damage (those at or above 85 decibels). Wear earplugs or other hearing protective devices when involved in a loud activity. . . . Be alert to hazardous noise in the environment."

Federal Safety Standards

The Occupational Safety and Health Administration has set standards that protect workers from hazardous noise exposure. Occupational noise exposure rules for general industry are published in 29 CFR 1910.95. This section of the *Code of Federal Regulations* includes Table G-16, which employers must use to determine permissible noise exposures. It displays the maximum hours per day during which employees may be exposed to particular sound levels. Section 1910.95(b)(1) states that "when employees are subjected to sound exceeding those listed in Table G-16, feasible administrative or engineering controls shall be utilized. If such controls fail to reduce sound within the levels of Table G-16, personal protective equipment shall be provided and used to reduce sound levels within the levels of the table." In addition, section 1910.95(i)(3) states that employees "shall be given the opportunity to select their hearing protectors from a variety of suitable hearing protectors provided by the employer." Section 1910.95(i)(4) states that the "employer shall provide training in the use of all hearing protectors provided to employees." And section 1910(i)(5) states that the "employer shall ensure proper initial fitting and supervise the correct use of all hearing protectors."

Protection and Products

In order to protect the hearing of people in the workplace, employers should take simple preventive measures and use common sense. There are many products on the market that can protect the ears from damage and ensure that a hearing loss does not occur, so it is important to gather information in order to make the best decision and select the protection that will be most appropriate in each particular work environment. (In discussing examples of these products, the author is not endorsing any product and has no interest in these products other than to provide comparative information and to suggest the qualities—such as comfort and weight and technical specifications—that should be investigated.)

For example, at the simplest level, expandable foam **earplugs** can be purchased in most hardware stores and drugstores. These plugs are made of a formable material designed to expand and conform to the shape of each person's ear canal. They are rolled into a thin, smooth cylinder that is placed into the ear canal. As long as a small amount of the plug remains outside the ear canal, these plugs are easily placed inside the ear and just as easily removed with a gentle tug. The Texas American Safety Company (2008), for instance, describes E-A-R Classic earplugs as made of a "unique soft PVC foam [that] provides a custom fit." They have a cylindrical shape that "allows easy insertion and provides equal pressure" throughout the ear canal. The plugs are bright yellow for high visibility and washable and reusable. They are also moisture resistant so they will not swell in the ear. The cost for 200 of this type of earplug is $25.00.

For people in occupational environments where noise is a potential hazard, there are types of earplugs that meet ANSI S3.19, a standard that requires a noise reduction rating (NRR) of at least 25. ANSI S3.19-1974 is the Standard for the Measurement of Real-Ear Hearing Protector Attenuation and Physical Attenuation of Earmuffs. This standard establishes methodology for measuring Noise Reduction Ratings (NRR) for determining the effectiveness of ear protection. The NRR indicates the decibel level that the hearing protector will reduce ambient noise. This standard provides a specific test method involving human subjects for determining the NRR ANSI S3 19-1974 EPA regulations.

E-A-R Express Pod Plugs with blue grips are earplugs that meet the NRR 25 standard and can be used in an environmental or occupational area where noise levels are loud and the ears need to be protected. These reusable earplugs provide a "fast and comfortable seal with low sound distortion." They are easy to use and the grip eliminates the need for rolling the earplug to fit into the ear canal (Texas American Safety Company, 2008). These earplugs cost $66.00 for 100. Moldex Rockets reusable earplugs are a similar product that comes with a pocket pack carrying case to store the plugs. The bright blue color is sold uncorded and 50 cost $45.00. The corded earplugs cost $60.00 for 50 earplugs.

Acoustic **earmuffs**, also referred to as ear defenders, offer another form of protection to safeguard hearing. This type of earmuff was created in Italy in 1982. They look like stereo headphones, but the cups that cover the ears are lined with a sound-deadening material, and noise reduction ratings range from 15 to 29. Acoustic earmuffs should be chosen according to their attenuation, suitable for the level and the spectrum of noise to which the worker is exposed. The selected earmuff has to reduce the noise level at the wearer's ears to below the appropriate action level as determined by national regulations. The most suitable earmuff ensures that the level of noise at the wearer's eardrum is between 5 to 10 dB lower than the action noise level. An acoustic earmuff includes a pad or cup made of rigid material that incorporates an opening for receiving one ear of the wearer, and a resilient sealing annulus intended for abutment with the head of the wearer, and also resilient pressure-exerting means connected to the shell of a protective helmet, a head strap, or like headgear. The earmuff provides good acoustic damping and a high degree of comfort, owing to the fact that the resilient pressure-exerting means is configured to produce a low pressing force substantially independently of head sizes, which vary within given limits. The pressure-exerting means includes, to this end, a spring element in the form of a combined torsion and bending spring.

These earmuffs may be clipped onto the sides of a hard hat so that workers can use them on construction sites. Some manufacturers have combined acoustic earmuffs with headphones, allowing the wearer to listen to music. Other manufacturers have added a communication source, so that the wearer can hear work instructions even though external noise is reduced.

The Elvex Corporation, for example, offers earmuffs that reduce the noise level by 25 to 29 decibels and have either plastic or stainless steel headbands. Elvex (2008) describes its SuperSonic 29 earmuff as having the "highest attenuation," the "lowest weight in its class," the "lowest headband force," "fully dielectric construction," and the "softest ear cushions." Its UltraSonic high-performance earmuff also has an NRR of 29 dB and "has been designed to provide excellent full spectrum attenuation, as well as superb low frequency attenuation." The headband is designed for "even distribution of the pressure" and the "improved balance required for extra deep ear cups." Elvex Corporation also makes a hearing protection device combined with a nylon mesh shield for facial and eye protection. The Brush Guard hearing and face protector is designed with operators of power equipment such as edgers and mowers in mind and protects against both noise and flying debris. For more risky work environments, as found on some assembly and production lines, high-performance earmuffs with impact- and heat-resistant face shields, such as the Elvex Cool Guard, may be a better alternative.

In determining the best product to use, employers need to consider that earplugs and earmuffs have both advantages and disadvantages. Earplugs may be mass produced or individually molded to fit the ear, and they may be reusable or disposable. They are simple to use and compared to earmuffs are less expensive and also more comfortable to wear in hot or damp work areas. On the negative side, earplugs offer less protection than some earmuffs do and should not be used in areas having noise levels exceeding 105 dB. Earplugs are not as visible as earmuffs, and a supervisor cannot readily check to see if workers are wearing them. They must be inserted properly to provide adequate protection. Earmuffs can vary with respect to the material and tightness of the headband. The headband must fit tightly enough to maintain a proper seal around the ears but not be too tight for comfort. On a positive note, properly fitted earmuffs can usually provide greater protection than earplugs. They are easier to fit and are generally more durable than earplugs. Also, earmuffs have replaceable parts. On the negative side, earmuffs are more expensive and are sometimes less comfortable than earplugs, especially in warm working areas.

In areas of extremely high noise levels, earplugs and earmuffs can be worn together to give better protection. Hearing protectors will lower the noise level, but cannot totally eliminate it. Some hearing protectors will reduce certain frequencies more than others, and this may be an important factor in some settings. Other protectors can make noise quieter without any other change in quality of the sound. There are also noise-activated hearing protectors that allow sounds having a safe volume to pass through the ear and become active only when the noise reaches hazardous levels.

Specialized protectors are worn by some musicians. Both professional and amateur musicians are at high risk for hearing impairments due to their continuous exposure to loud musical sounds. According to the University of Wisconsin Audiology Clinic (2003), "at classical musical concerts, in the audience, sounds have been recorded in excess of 120 dB. That is about as loud as an airplane during takeoff. The sources for sounds that are damaging to the ears come from amplifiers for rock musicians, and their own instrument or the instruments behind them for classical musicians."

It makes sense that any musician would wear earplugs to provide at least a minimum amount of protection. There are musicians' earplugs available that dampen the volume of the sound while protecting the acoustic accuracy of the sound. The accuracy, or integrity, is very important to any musician. These earplugs are custom molded to fit the individual's ear. They have filters in them to dampen the sound a certain amount. Filters for Chicago Symphony musicians, for example, are made by a Chicago-based company called Etymotic Research. According to Etymotic Research (2008), these earplugs can attenuate sound to 9, 15, or 25 dB and have "high fidelity custom hearing protection." The sound "is clear and natural, not muffled," and "noise fatigue is reduced." Moreover, "Musicians Earplugs are designed to replicate the natural response of the open ear. Sound heard with these earplugs has the same quality as the original, only quieter. The result is that speech and music are clear—you still hear the blend clearly, feel the bass, and distinguish each tone. Accurate sound reduction is achieved by combining a patented filter with specific acoustics of a custom earmold. The combination of the two produces a resonance at approximately 2700 Hz (as in the normal ear) resulting in a smooth, flat attenuation." The average cost for a pair of Musicians Earplugs ranges from $150 to $200.

People in professional sports may also need hearing protection because of noisy environments. Etymotic Research (2008), for example, offers a sports earplug in which "the plug and filter are flush with the ear to protect it from impact damage while playing. The plug's purpose is to allow the player to hear the calls on the field while protecting the ear from the high volume of stadium noise that usually accompanies these games." Professional sports car drivers are also exposed to loud noises. Wind noise and engine noise can exceed 115 dB, a level at which damage can occur after only fifteen minutes of exposure. Preventive and safety measures similar to those used in industrial workplaces need to be applied in professional sports.

Law enforcement officers, members of the military, and transportation workers also have special needs for protecting their hearing. Law enforcement officers who must practice shooting their guns periodically are exposed to loud noises during this process. People in various branches of the military can be exposed to loud noise from large guns and artillery, aircraft and boat engines, and armored personnel carriers. People who work on aircraft carriers directing flight traffic are exposed to constant loud noises from the engines of jet fighters. People such as baggage handlers and flight control workers for commercial flight carriers, who can be on the runways for most of their working day, are also exposed to the loud noises of plane engines during takeoffs and landings. Exposure to these dangerous sound environments not only has the potential to damage hearing, but can also induce fatigue and create the opportunities for errors due to miscommunication.

Arizona Ear Protection is one company that offers hearing protection for these needs. Its electronic hearing protection system known as SoundScope "is designed to enhance softer sounds while instantaneously capturing sharp impulse sounds, such as shotgun and rifle blasts" (Arizona Ear Protection, 2007). Another business, the Peltor Company, makes military hearing protection and communication systems. Peltor's ComTac and Swat Tac headsets can be used with two-way radios and incorporate "innovative surround technology." Not only do they "protect against hearing loss with a passive attenuation of 20 dB, [but] the outer cup microphones combined with the electronics inside the headset will instantaneously suppress dangerous gunshots and also amplify in stereo ambient surrounding voices" (Enviro Safety Products, 2008).

One final key point is that the user of ear protection devices must be comfortable wearing them. The subjective aspects of hearing protection are important to keep in mind. After all, "the only useful kind of protection is the protection that is actually worn. Some people do not accept particular kinds of protectors; every human being is different, and the anatomy of the ear and ear canal can vary significantly from person to person" (Canadian Centre for Occupational Health & Safety, 2007). It is a good idea for an employer to provide many different types of hearing protection devices to workers so that they can choose from among them. It is also important to keep in mind all safety, hygiene, and governmental regulations before providing a specific type of hearing protection to any worker. In any hazardous or risky environment, any ear protection must be used all the time to get the full and maximum benefits.

Tests and Treatments

Most companies who value their workers have many ways to test and to monitor their employees in order to detect a hearing loss. There are then ways that an employee can be further protected if a hearing loss is detected. The diagnosis of an occupational hearing loss begins with a medical history and a physical examination. A doctor or an audiologist can use the whispered speech test, which is a screening hearing test where words are whispered from behind a person in order to detect what he or she can hear. Tuning forks can be used to detect hearing loss at different frequencies. Pure tone audiometers are used to check how well a person hears sounds of different volumes and frequencies. This test is done by having the subject press a button each time he or she hears, through a set of headphones, a sound produced by the audiometer. An otoacoustic emissions test measures how well the hair cells are working. A standard hearing test and an X-ray of the head or a cranial CT scan can detect any underlying problems. Hearing loss can occur from vascular problems or tumors so these tests will help to rule out those causes.

Other forms of hearing tests include audiometry and tympanometry. Audiometry is the term used to describe formal measurement of hearing. The measurement is usually performed by an audiologist using an audiometer (as described in the previous paragraph). An audiologist is a health care professional specializing in the evaluation and rehabilitation of people with hearing losses. Audiologists have either a master's or a doctoral degree in audiology and have studied anatomy and physiology of the ear, psychoacoustics, and behavioral and electrophysiological testing and who can perform hearing aid training, lip reading, auditory training, and other rehabilitation technique training.

Tympanometry is a measure of the stiffness of the eardrum (or tympanic membrane) and it evaluates the functioning of the middle ear. This test is done by placing a soft probe into the ear canal and applying a small amount of pressure. The instrument then measures the movement of the tympanic membrane in response to the pressure changes. This test can be helpful in determining if there is fluid in the middle ear or negative middle ear pressure, if there are problems with the ear ossicles, if the eardrum is perforated, or if there is otosclerosis. Otosclerosis is a disease of ear bone degeneration that develops during the teen or early adult years. The consistency of the sound-conducting bones of the ears changes from hard mineralized bone to spongy tissue. This degeneration can cause a buildup of excess bone tissue around the stapes so that the stapes does not vibrate.

Treatment for temporary or reversible hearing loss depends on the cause of the hearing loss. Hearing loss caused by ototoxic medicines such as aspirin or ibuprofen usually improves after the medication is discontinued. Ear infections usually improve after a doctor prescribes medications or antibiotics. Head or ear injuries have the potential to improve without significant long-term effects, depending on the severity of the injury.

Treatments for occupational hearing loss include aural rehabilitation. This process teaches an individual how to work and cope with a hearing loss. Protective equipment, as previously described, can be used. The workplace can be redesigned to minimize or reduce further hearing loss. According to WebMD (2007), "permanent hearing losses contribute to loneliness, depression, and loss of independence. Treatment cannot bring back your hearing, but it can make communication, social interaction, and work and daily activities easier and more enjoyable." For serious hearing losses or permanent hearing losses, hearing aids can be fitted to one or both ears to help sounds sound better. These days, a hearing aid is a small electronic device that may be worn in or behind one or both ears. It has three parts: a microphone, an amplifier, and a speaker. The hearing aid receives sound through a microphone that converts the sound waves to electrical signals and sends them to an amplifier. The amplifier increases the power of the signals and then sends them to the ear through a speaker. It makes some sounds louder so that a person with a hearing loss can listen, communicate, and participate more fully in daily activities. A hearing aid can help people in both quiet and noisy situations. Only one out of five people who would benefit from a hearing aid actually use one. These devices should be fitted by a doctor, an audiologist, or a hearing professional.

Education

Any type of hearing protection must come with product information and user information, and these manufacturer's instructions must always be followed. The hearing protection should regularly be inspected for wear and tear. Ear cushions that are no longer pliable should be replaced. Units should be replaced when headbands are stretched so that they do not keep the ear cushions snugly against the head. Earmuffs must be disassembled to be cleaned. The cushions should be washed with a mild liquid detergent in warm water and rinsed in clear, warm water. The sound system in any earmuff should never get wet because that can cause an electrical malfunction. A soft brush should be used to remove oil and dirt that has hardened in the ear cushions.

Companies must have proper educational seminars to protect their workers and educate them on safety issues. OSHA has many policies and organizations that govern the education and training of the public when it comes to occupational and safety issues. The OSHA Directorate of Training and Education develops, directs, oversees, manages, and ensures implementation of OSHA's national training and education policies and procedures. The OSHA Training Institute provides training and education in occupational safety and health for federal and state compliance officers, state consultants, other federal agency personnel, and the private sector. OSHA Training Institute Education Centers offer the most frequently requested OSHA Training Institute courses for the private sector and other federal agency personnel at locations throughout the United States. Under the OSHA Outreach Training Program, individuals who complete a one-week OSHA training course are authorized to teach a ten-hour or thirty-hour course in construction or general industry safety and health standards. Under the Disaster Site Worker Outreach Training Program, individuals who complete a four-day OSHA training course are authorized to teach a sixteen-hour course in safety and health to workers who provide skilled support or site cleanup services. The OSHA Resource Center offers occupational safety and health training videos for loan to OSHA employees, grantees, consultation programs, state-plan states, and Voluntary Protection Program sites and to federal agency occupational safety and health trainers and OSHA outreach trainers. The Susan Harwood Training Grant Program awards grants to nonprofit organizations to develop training and educational programs, reaches out to appropriate workers and employers, and provides these programs to workers and employers.

SUMMARY

We live in a world where hazards and threats to our health are very common. Some of these hazards and threats to our health cannot be altered due to our genetic or hereditary makeup. But many of the injuries that occur daily are preventable, including most workplace injuries to vision and hearing. With the help of federal and state standards and information from public health agencies and other organizations dedicated to workplace safety, employers must identify the hazards to vision and hearing in their workplaces and then take appropriate precautions to reduce these hazards. They must offer the correct kinds of eye and ear protection when that protection is needed and offer workers appropriate education so that they know when and how to use eye and ear protection and what kinds of protection to use in their particular workplace environments.

KEY TERMS

American National Standards Institute
cup goggles
decibels

dust goggles
earplugs
earmuffs

QUESTIONS FOR DISCUSSION

1. What products are available to protect people's eyes in the workplace? Describe the major types.

2. What products are available to protect people's hearing in the workplace? Describe the major types.

3. What are audiometry and tympanometry?

4. What is ANSI? Whom does it represent and what does it do?

5. What government publication contains OSHA's general and final rules?

CHAPTER

OCCUPATIONAL HEALTH DISPARITIES

After reading this chapter, you should be able to

- Discuss the effect of social status on occupational health.

- Recognize variations in occupational health by social class, race and ethnicity, nativity, gender, and age.

- Describe the characteristics of populations who are most at risk for poor occupational health.

- Understand the causes and correlates (inside and outside the workplace) of occupational health disparities.

As the various chapters in this volume suggest, ensuring the occupational health and safety of workers is an extraordinarily complex task, requiring the collaborative efforts of employers, management, occupational health professionals, communities, local and national policymakers, and workers themselves. Adding yet another layer of complication to this work is that not all workers experience work in the same way. Because of the individual and group attributes they may bring to the workplace, certain populations of workers are more likely to suffer occupational health problems and to be in a worse position to either prevent or remedy them. This chapter examines the attributes of disparate populations in occupational health, the mechanisms by which occupational health disparities perpetuate, and the changing occupational health landscape with regard to disparate populations. (Note that in referring to the labor force, this chapter refers only to the paid labor force, which necessarily excludes the work that individuals, mostly women, have traditionally contributed in the unpaid labor force [housework, child care, and the like]. As of this writing, virtually no data exist on the occupational health status of unpaid workers.)

DISPARATE POPULATIONS

This section discusses occupational hazards in relation to social status, race and ethnicity, nativity, gender, and age.

Social Status

In every society it is the prerogative of higher status people to avoid work that they deem to be dirty, dangerous, physically demanding, unpleasant, or repetitive. Although occupational injuries and illnesses may arise in any type of work environment, they are more prevalent in precisely those types of occupations that are the dirtiest, the most dangerous, the most physically demanding, the most repetitive, and the most unpleasant. The inevitable result is that the pecking order of any society—whereby, for instance, non-Hispanic whites tend to have higher social status than Latinos—translates into different occupational health profiles for various groups based on their ability to avoid the most undesirable types of work.

At the very simplest level, **occupational health disparities** can be understood as a function of **socioeconomic status** (SES)—that is, position in a hierarchy of individuals and groups within a society based on *income, education,* and *occupation.* Higher SES gives individuals greater access to the following resources:

- Ability to avoid dirty, dangerous, repetitive, and demanding work

- Access to stable work hours, long-term job security, and a living wage

- Ability to balance demands of work and nonwork activities

- Ability and willingness to comply with safety protocols

- Access to quality health insurance and other health-promoting resources

▪ Preexisting good health

▪ Real and perceived legal protections for various types of workers

Educational and occupational attainment confers protection from occupational health risks in a number of ways. First, and simplest, more education gives individuals greater ability to avoid dangerous work; more highly educated workers tend to favor white-collar jobs that carry less risk of occupational injury and exposure to health hazards than blue-collar occupations do. The same mechanism (that is, better labor market position) that protects more highly educated workers from dangerous occupations may also be beneficial in terms of protecting them from occupations characterized by working conditions that tend to be more hazardous for individuals, such as part-time and temporary work and work that lacks employer-sponsored health insurance. More subtly, greater educational attainment may make individuals more savvy consumers of health information and thus more likely to engage in preventive health care practices such as eating a proper diet, exercising, and making routine visits to health care providers.

Greater educational and occupational attainment is strongly correlated with higher income, which gives workers greater resources to tend to their own health. For instance, greater income allows a worker to take a day off from work following a minor workplace injury without fear that the day's lost wages will severely harm his or her financial health, whereas a worker with fewer economic resources to begin with might be more likely to continue working through a minor injury, thus running the risk of exacerbating the original injury and developing long-term complications. Greater income also gives workers better resources to cope with the physical and mental demands of balancing work and nonwork demands, making these workers less susceptible to workplace injuries attributable to stress and fatigue.

Education, occupation, and income work in tandem to create and maintain occupational health differences among workers. It is not surprising that lower SES workers tend to report worse overall health than higher SES workers, given the potentially vast differences in access to material resources between, say, a high school dropout and an Ivy League–educated doctor (Borrell, Muntaner, Benach, & Artazcoz, 2004; Schrijvers, van de Mheen, Stronks, & Mackenbach, 1998). Even within occupational subgroups such as managers, higher SES managers tend to report better health than lower SES managers (Tomiak, Gentleman, & Jette, 1997), which suggests that psychosocial factors may also influence occupational health disparities. Material differences between various levels of management may be small in the grand scheme of things, but the perception of lower-level managers that they are disadvantaged relative to their coworkers may lead to greater experience of anxiety, feelings of lack of control, and other psychosocial stressors that prefigure many workplace injuries and illnesses, and may undermine workers' sense of empowerment when dealing with health issues. Moreover, the psychosocial stress of lower status translates into poorer health overall due to its correlation with depression, violence, and poor social support (Wilkinson, 1999).

Recent health research emphasizes the association of stress and health. In one study, low social status was found to be positively associated with chronic stress through individuals' increased exposure to crime, overcrowding, noise pollution, discrimination, and the like, all of which have a negative impact on health (Baum, Garofalo, & Yali, 1999). Low-status work is associated with elevated stress among workers, which in turn is associated with greater likelihood of musculoskeletal disorders (Lundberg, 1999) as well as with greater incidence of depression among workers; interestingly, the latter relationship is found to be stronger among men than women, suggesting that women are less protected from depression by their occupational status, perhaps because they may rely on their jobs less as a source of social validation (Zimmerman, Christakis, & Vander Stoep, 2004).

Worker health outcomes are always an interplay between individual workers— who come in with certain psychosocial characteristics, who interact with other workers of varying statuses, and whose behaviors are responsive to the occupational environments in which they find themselves—and the occupational environment itself, which offers a specific array of both hazards and opportunities. A fruitful example of this relationship and its effect on worker health can be found in the association between smoking behavior and occupational status. Tobacco use is an occupational hazard that is more likely to be confronted by low-status workers, both because of the environments in which they work and their responses to that environment, making the establishment of causation (and the design of interventions) quite complex.

Lower SES is associated with a higher level of health risk behaviors and attributes, including physical inactivity, failure to use seat belts, obesity, and tobacco use. Moreover, because smoking rates are declining more rapidly among the highly educated, the association between smoking and education has become stronger since 1990: whereas in 1990 a person with less than a high school degree was twice as likely to smoke as someone who had completed college (28.9 percent prevalence versus 14.3 percent, respectively), in 2004 a high school dropout was approximately three times as likely to smoke as a college graduate was (29.4 percent versus 10.6 percent) (Harper & Lynch, 2007). Smoking prevalence is greater among blue-collar, farm, and service workers than among white-collar workers, and the prevalence increases as income declines (Barbeau, McLellan, et al., 2004). The strong association of smoking with socioeconomic status is attributable to individual factors (the greater stress of day-to-day economic insecurity), interpersonal factors (relationships with friends and family that abet smoking behaviors), organizational factors (whereby blue-collar workers face greater hazards, greater income insecurity, and less autonomy than white-collar workers), and neighborhood and community factors (the greater prevalence of smoking advertisements and tobacco vendors in lower-income communities) (Sorensen, Barbeau, Hunt, & Emmons, 2004). Workers in very hazardous jobs, such as chemical workers, are also more likely to smoke than are workers in less hazardous jobs, which is to some extent associated with the job-related stress; by the same token these workers are also more likely than workers in nonhazardous jobs to report that they want to improve their health through behaviors such as quitting smoking and lowering fat intake (Sorensen et al., 1996). However, other studies have found that although there seem to be no SES patterns in actual quit attempts, higher SES workers are more likely to be successful in their attempts to quit, due partly to their better access to cessation resources (Barbeau, McLellan, et al., 2004).

Smoking is an occupational hazard only insofar as workplaces are organized in ways that make it easier and more acceptable for workers to smoke on the premises. Although great strides have been made in the past two decades to diminish tobacco smoke as a workplace hazard, these efforts have not reached all workers equally: individuals employed in blue-collar occupations, such as manufacturing and the construction trades, as well as in service occupations such as restaurant work, housekeeping, and maintenance, are much more likely than white-collar workers to work at sites that lack no-smoking policies (Barbeau, Krieger, & Soobader, 2004; Bourne, Shopland, Anderson, & Burns, 2004). Whereas 75 percent of white-collar workers enjoy smoke-free workplaces, only 43 percent of food service workers work in smoke-free facilities (Shopland, Anderson, Burns, & Gerlach, 2004). In other words, although tobacco smoke has largely vanished from offices and boardrooms, it persists in factories and workshops and restaurants, meaning that due to a lack of regulation, the workers in the latter sites face greater exposure to secondhand smoke during their work hours as well as less external pressure to quit smoking themselves.

Race and Ethnicity

In our society some individual attributes carry more weight at work than others, so that, for example, in a typical workplace one's musical preferences are not very important with regard to one's status but one's educational attainment is an important characteristic that shapes one's opportunities, rewards, and occupational trajectory. Certain attributes are so heavily weighted according to the perception of their importance in determining an individual's abilities, temperament, and other relevant job characteristics, that they become **master statuses**, meaning the individual is judged on one of these attributes above and beyond all the rest—as happens, for instance, when a woman is not hired for a manual labor job based solely on the assumption that she will be weaker because of her sex, in spite of any other qualifications she may possess (such as a strong physique, an exemplary work history, and years of experience). Although gender, age, nativity, and disability are all common master statuses in our society, by far the most prominent master status—that is to say, the one attribute most likely to be viewed by others as an overriding factor and thus to profoundly influence an individual's life experiences and opportunities—is race and ethnicity; accordingly, we see a great deal of variation in occupational health along these lines. Figure 14.1 illustrates the pattern for nonfatal work injuries and illnesses by race and ethnicity; in this graphic from the National Institute for Occupational Safety and Health (NIOSH) we see that for both Hispanic and non-Hispanic black workers, the injury rate exceeds the employment rate, whereas for whites and Asians, a greater percentage of workers are employed than suffer work-related illness or injury. Figure 14.2, which focuses on the forestry, agriculture, and fishing industries, illustrates that although whites make up the majority

FIGURE 14.1. *Distribution of employed U.S. workers in 2000 and nonfatal occupational injury and illness cases with days away from work in private industry in 2001 by race and ethnicity.*

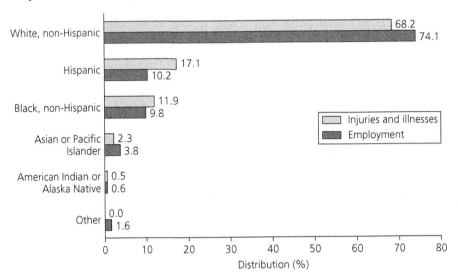

Source: NIOSH, 2004, fig. 1-30.

FIGURE 14.2. *Number and rate of fatal occupational injuries by race in the agriculture, forestry, and fishing industries, 1992–2001.*

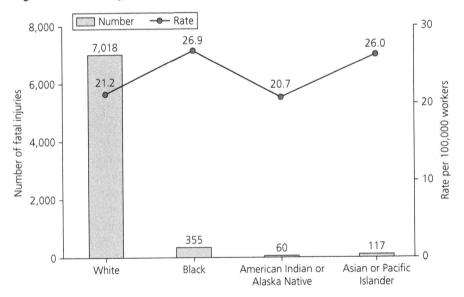

Note: Fatality data exclude New York City.
Source: NIOSH, 2004, fig. 3-4.

of work-related fatality cases, the *rate* of workplace fatalities is actually higher among both black workers and Asian or Pacific Islander workers.

Race and Ethnicity and SES For many of the racial and ethnic occupational health disparities, the mechanisms by which non-Hispanic whites tend to have better occupational health outcomes than racial and ethnic minorities do are the same as the mechanisms operating in socioeconomic status health disparities; because blacks and Latinos tend to have lower educational attainment, lower income, and are less likely to be represented in white-collar occupations compared to whites and Asians (Table 14.1), they are also more likely to suffer from worse occupational health outcomes.

For instance, although smoking poses an occupational health hazard to many workers and disproportionately to racial and ethnic minorities, this is entirely attributable to socioeconomic disparities: after controlling for income, education, and occupation, there is no difference between smoking rates of whites and minorities (Shavers, Lawrence, Fagan, & Gibson, 2005). Similarly, Oh and Shin (2003) find no association between race and nonfatal work injuries after controlling also for education, work experience, and other human capital (skill) differences (although these authors then go on to point out that disparities of education, work experience, and human capital might themselves be attributable to race—for instance, minority workers may have shorter job tenures than comparably skilled whites due to discrimination, which would also contribute to having less human capital). In a study of teenage workers, Zierold and Anderson (2006) find that minority teens are much more likely to sustain serious occupational injuries compared to white teens, which cannot be explained by minority teens working more dangerous jobs compared to white teens' jobs; however, minority teen workers were likely to work more hours per week, work shifts later at night, and

TABLE 14.1. **Median income, education, and occupation for selected racial and ethnic groups, 2006**

	Percentage with high school diploma or higher	Median household income	Percentage of workers in management and professional occupations
Non-Hispanic White	91%	$50,784	34.7%
Asian	87	61,094	47.7
Black	81	30,858	26.2
Hispanic (any race)	59	35,967	16.1

Source: Data are from Bureau of Labor Statistics and U.S. Census Bureau, 2006.

work under less supervision, all of which might contribute to higher injury rates. Although this disparity is reported as an effect of race and ethnicity, the mechanism for the longer work hours and later shifts of minority workers can likely be traced to their greater economic burden, which would make this an SES effect rather than an effect of race and ethnicity.

However, not all racial and ethnic occupational health disparities can be traced to socioeconomic status. Although the effects of race and ethnicity can be difficult to disentangle from the effects of socioeconomic status, recent research suggests many of the more subtle mechanisms by which minorities suffer disproportionately. **Occupational segregation** emerges as a primary mechanism for health disparities, and such segregation can be attributed to both SES factors such as education as well as racial and ethnic factors such as selective hiring and task assignment bias, relegating minority workers to more dangerous occupations, jobs, and tasks (Murray, 2003; McGwin, Enochs, & Roseman, 2000; Richardson & Loomis, 1997); the intra-occupational assignment of different groups of workers to different jobs and tasks may also explain a small but persistent difference in occupational mortality (Loomis & Richardson, 1998) and injury (Simpson & Severson, 2000). Residential and environmental exposure differences may also play a role in occupational health disparities, as they are found to do for health disparities more generally. Because there is a high degree of residential segregation in the United States, especially between whites and blacks (Massey & Denton, 1989), it is likely that disparate exposure to neighborhood and environmental hazards may exacerbate occupational illness and injury (Frumkin, Walker, & Friedman-Jimenez, 1999). Members of various racial and ethnic groups appear to experience some degree of increased susceptibility to certain occupational illnesses through mechanisms that are not always understood; for instance, death from occupationally linked leukemia and lung cancers are higher than expected among blacks and Latinos in industries such as textile, chemical, and rubber production (Loomis & Schulz, 2000). Susceptibility to mental illness also appears to be heightened among racial and ethnic minorities; for instance, black workers tend to score higher on depression indexes than white workers do, an outcome that has been linked to various attributes of jobs such as job security, job status, and physical demands (Zimmerman et al., 2004). Likewise, as indicated in Figure 14.3, Hispanics bear a disproportionate burden of anxiety, stress, and neurotic disorder cases relative to their representation in the U.S. workforce (currently at 13.3 percent of workers). Increased susceptibility may also interact with residential patterns; for instance, because blacks are more likely than whites to be urban dwellers, they may be more susceptible to diseases that are exacerbated by poor air quality (asthma and lung diseases) and population density (infectious diseases) (Frumkin et al., 1999).

In addition to facing greater risk of injury and illness to begin with, in most cases minority workers also face differences in their post-injury experiences. One study, which established few differences between whites, blacks, and Hispanics with regard to reporting occupational injury and illness, nevertheless found that blacks and Hispanics are likely to miss more days of work from occupational health problems

FIGURE 14.3. *Distribution and number of anxiety, stress, and neurotic disorder cases involving days away from work in private industry by race and ethnicity, 2001.*

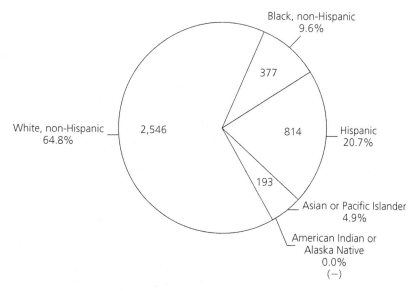

Source: NIOSH, 2004, fig. 2-5.

(Strong & Zimmerman, 2005). Another study found that African Americans and low-SES workers are more likely to report more pain, poorer mental health, and greater financial burden following a lower-back injury, which may be attributable to lower standards of care due to discriminatory health care worker attitudes, extra-occupational environmental hazards such as poor living conditions and other neighborhood effects, and poorer working conditions including lower pay, less autonomy, and more repetition (Chibnall, Tait, Andresen, & Hadler, 2005). Minorities are also more likely than whites to be forced into early withdrawal from the labor market and retirement for occupational health reasons (Flippen & Tienda, 2000), which suggests that the cumulative, decades-long effects of small but persistent disparities can have significant costs for minority workers at the end of their working years.

One of the specific occupational hazards faced by racial and ethnic minorities, and conceptually distinct from the synchronic effects of socioeconomic status and racial and ethnic identity, is the persistence of racism and discrimination. Racism is itself an occupational hazard, reported by approximately 37 percent of all racial and ethnic minority workers (Krieger et al., 2006). Among other effects, perceived racial discrimination at work is associated with higher rates of hypertension among African Americans (Din-Dzietham, Nembhard, Collins, & Davis, 2004). Visible minorities are often at greater risk of discriminatory physical and mental abuse at the hands of coworkers, superiors, and clients (Facey, 2003). Moreover, workplace discrimination is associated with poorer mental health, including lower job satisfaction, greater job burnout, greater stress, and more frequently reported instances of poor overall mental health (Roberts, Swanson, & Murphy, 2004).

Trends and Implications   Trends in racial and ethnic occupational health disparities present a mixed picture. Data from the 1980s indicate that the gap between whites, blacks, and other minorities in occupational death rates closed somewhat during that decade (Stout, Jenkins, & Pizatella, 1996); more recent data show that fatality rates have declined among all groups and that the gap between whites and blacks has been largely eliminated, although the gap between Hispanics and non-Hispanic whites has grown (National Center for Health Statistics, 2006) (see Figure 14.4). Black men, who previously had the highest rate of occupational fatalities, have been overtaken by Hispanic men as the group with the highest occupational fatality rate (Richardson, Loomis, Bena, & Bailer, 2004). The vulnerability of Latino workers is particularly troubling given their increasing representation in the labor force, which is projected to continue well into the foreseeable future (U.S. Census Bureau, 2004).

Because minority workers tend to have poorer overall health due to both occupational and extra-occupational factors, employee wellness programs targeted toward minority workers are particularly beneficial. For instance, black men have higher incidence of and mortality from prostate cancer but are less likely to participate in routine

FIGURE 14.4.   *Fatal occupational injury rates among Hispanic and non-Hispanic workers in the construction industry, 1992–2001.*

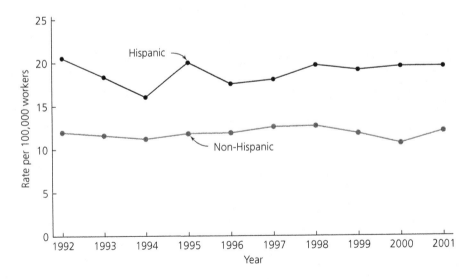

Source: NIOSH, 2004, fig. 4.22.

screenings; worksite-based screening initiatives have been shown to increase screen-ing rates substantially, which can improve an employer's health cost exposure (Weinrich, Greiner, Reis-Starr, Yoon, & Weinrich, 1998; see also Fowler & Risner, 1994). Greater attention to the diversity of workplaces in both hiring and job and task assignment can mitigate some disparities by equalizing exposure to workplace haz-ards; however, a fair amount of the occupational health disparities by race and ethnic-ity might best be addressed through social policies that equalize educational access, health care access, and environmental quality across racial and ethnic categories.

Nativity

Anyone who has glanced at a high school civics textbook in the past five or six decades is no doubt familiar with the idea of the United States as a "melting pot" of immigrants from all over the world. Never has that been more true than at the present time: both the absolute number and the rate of immigration to the United States are at an all-time high, surpassing even the number and rate during the Great Migration of a century ago, in the early years of the twentieth century (U.S. Department of Homeland Security, 2006). The most recent wave of immigration presents new challenges in the U.S. workplace in that many of the new immigrants—as with immigrants of a century ago—are coming into the United States with little education or material resources, and additionally (unlike older waves of immigrants) are increasingly people of color. Whereas Great Migration immigrants were overwhelmingly of European origin, Latin America and Asia are the primary regions of origin in today's Second Great Migration (Mosisa, 2002). Therefore current immigrants typically face the same disadvantages in occupational health faced by native-born workers who are of low socioeconomic status or who belong to racial and ethnic minorities. Additionally, however, new immi-grants often face another level of disadvantage by virtue of having little familiarity with the legal protections afforded to them as workers and residents; the health care resources available to them and the various means for gaining access to those resources; and often even the fundamental language, customs, and cultures of U.S. society. All of these factors make recent immigrants some of the most vulnerable workers in the labor force today (see Figure 14.5).

Lacking familiarity with the English language and possessing few marketable skills, new immigrants are disproportionately concentrated in low-wage jobs such as construction, agriculture, day labor, and sweatshop work, occupations that increase their exposure to a variety of occupational hazards (McCauley, 2005). Immigrants may be particularly vulnerable to injury even among workers in more hazardous occu-pations because a large proportion of them are temporary workers and therefore less likely to receive training in safety procedures (Azaroff, Levenstein, & Wegman, 2004). Poor language skills often consign people to more dangerous jobs simply because these may be the only jobs that can be performed without a command of the English language (Facey, 2003). Some industries are de facto new immigrant ghettos; for instance, the West Coast garment industry employs a disproportionate number of

FIGURE 14.5. *Distribution of foreign-born and native-born workers by occupational group, 2000 (percentage).*

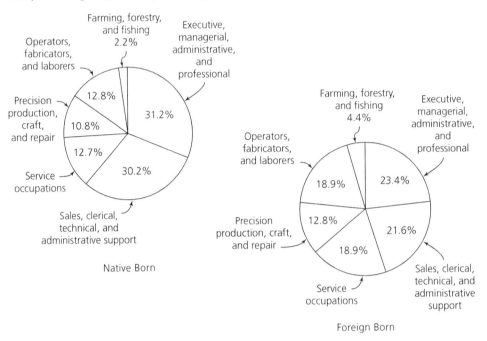

Source: Data from Mosisa, 2002.

recent Asian immigrants, who consequently suffer disproportionately from the repetitive stress disorders that typify garment production (Burgel, Lashuay, Israel, & Harrison, 2004). As noted earlier, employers often seek particular types of workers based on stereotypes about the attributes of particular subpopulations, especially racial and ethnic populations, and this can also be seen in the hiring of immigrant Asian women in garment production and computer chip assembly owing to employers' belief that Asian women are especially docile and nimble (Hossfeld, 1994). To the extent that immigrant workers are often constrained in their ability to be competitive in the job marker due to language and cultural barriers, lack of skills, and lack of familiarity with their rights, the perceived docility of immigrant workers may be a euphemism for "easily exploitable." With respect to occupational health, injuries and illnesses to immigrant workers are widely understood to be underreported (Burgel et al., 2004; Azaroff et al., 2004); among other reasons, new immigrants are not familiar with worker's compensation, and so do not perceive any benefit to reporting hazardous workplace conditions (Azaroff et al., 2004). Moreover, because workers are not familiar with their labor protections and rights and often fear losing their hard-won jobs, otherwise preventable injuries are not prevented, even when prevention might involve something as simple as raising the height of a worktable to improve ergonomics (Burgel et al., 2004).

Protecting the occupational safety of immigrants is a complex task, due both to language and cultural barriers and to typically low levels of health literacy among new immigrant populations. Not only are new immigrants less likely to receive health and safety training on the job, due to the types of occupations and jobs they are offered, but additionally they may have trouble comprehending the health and safety information that they do receive (Bouchard, 2007). Language and cultural differences can also interact with the effective communication of occupational health information in unforeseen ways, resulting in bad **cultural ergonomics**; one study of hazard symbol interpretation demonstrated that workers in Ghana assigned meanings and connotations to commonly used U.S. and international hazard symbols that deviated substantially from their intended meanings, even though English is the official language of Ghana (Smith-Jackson & Essuman-Johnson, 2002). As with disparities faced by racial and ethnic minorities, measured and assumed disparities in the occupational health of immigrants merit special attention. Protecting the occupational safety of immigrants is difficult; in addition to workplace interventions, community-based worker centers and clinics have shown some measure of success in educating and assisting new immigrant worker populations (Burgel et al., 2004; Cho et al., 2007).

Gender

The occupational health disparities faced by the groups already mentioned—low SES individuals, racial and ethnic minorities, and immigrant workers—all occur along similar lines. The mechanisms of worse health all fall from having lower occupational status and therefore an inability to avoid dangerous work. When we look at women and men separately, however, the mechanisms by which their occupational health profiles differ are not nearly so straightforward, due to women's unique history in American culture and in the U.S. labor market. Nor do women constitute a special population by virtue of nearly always having worse occupational health prospects and outcomes—on the contrary, because women have traditionally been excluded from some (though by no means all) of the most dangerous forms of labor, on some measures they fare much better than male workers. However, as the sex composition of occupations, industries, and the labor force as a whole continues to change, we can expect to see an ever-shifting pattern of occupational risk for both men and women.

To fully understand the complexity of occupational health disparities by gender, we must first look to the vast changes in the status of women in the labor force that occurred in the latter half of the twentieth century. First, women constitute a greater proportion of the paid labor force at this point in U.S. history than at any previous time. From 1950 to 1998, the proportion of women in the paid labor force rose from 34 percent to 60 percent (Fullerton, 1999), a trend spurred largely by the entry of married and middle-class women into the paid labor force due to the escalation of living costs and the stagnation of male wages (Padavic & Reskin, 2002). Second, although there is still a high degree of occupational sex segregation, women are increasingly making inroads into traditionally male occupations, which increases the exposure of women to particularly hazardous, traditionally male professions such as construction and manufacturing (although this is not to say that several traditionally female occupations are not also quite hazardous, as can be the case in domestic work and health care).

As shown in Figure 14.6, men suffer disproportionately from occupational fatalities: men are victims of 92 percent of occupational fatalities even though they represent only 54 percent of the paid labor force. As with occupational fatality rates, overall nonfatal occupational injury rates are also lower among women (see Figure 14.7). Women's occupational health, particularly with regard to occupational fatality, is commonly held to be enhanced by their greater attention to safety protocols and concern for personal safety, as well as their limited representation in the most hazardous occupations. In general, women have been shown to have greater aversion to risk than men do (Hesch, 1996); men's greater willingness to face risk is generally attributed to both the **gender socialization** of men to prove their masculinity through risk-taking behaviors and the reinforcing effects of the highly masculinized "shop floor cultures" existing in traditionally male blue-collar occupations (see Halle, 1987; Willis, 1981). However, occupational subculture may in some cases trump gender socialization, meaning that women in certain hazardous and highly localized occupations, such as agriculture, may enjoy no substantial gender socialization protection, and their injury and fatality rates are therefore equivalent to those of their male coworkers (Cole, Westneat, Browning, Piercy, & Struttmann, 2000). As women continue to make inroads into male occupations and come to integrate traditionally male occupational preserves, it is likely that the impact of gendered socialization and culture on the

FIGURE 14.6.   *Employment and fatality profiles by sex, 2002.*

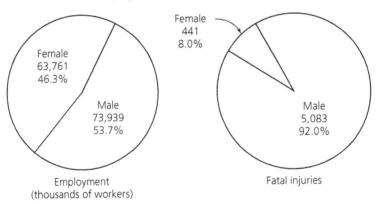

Source: NIOSH, 2004, fig. 2-20.

occupational health of men and women will diminish; although occupational fatalities declined overall in the latter part of the twentieth century, they dropped more slowly for women than for men (Loomis, Bena, & Bailer, 2003).

Women's occupational health may be enhanced by occupational segregation and sociocultural factors, but it may also be undermined by similar mechanisms. Moreover, complex disparities may be obscured by looking at overall, or crude, rates, which are not adjusted for factors such as occupation, seniority, hours worked, and other factors, all of which may be confounding factors: for instance, because women work fewer hours on average compared to men, their rate of injury per hour worked will be higher than the crude rate. Smith and Mustard's (2004) study of occupational injury rates in Ontario illustrates one way in which crude figures may be misleading. They found that women have lower rates of injury in manual occupations but higher rates in nonmanual occupations. Nonmanual occupations are ones that do not require the handling of light or heavy loads; however, they might require a great deal of repetitive motion, as, for example, clerical work and garment finishing do. Moreover, as Smith and Mustard concede, it is likely that women within either of these divisions of manual and nonmanual may be relegated to jobs with greater risk of repetitive stress, thereby conferring an advantage relative to male manual laborers but a disadvantage relative to male white-collar workers. In a similar vein, women working in construction have lower mortality rates overall than men, but only because they are more likely to work desk jobs—mortality rates among male and female laborers are virtually identical (Welch, Goldenhar, & Hunting, 2000). In yet another example of the measurement complexities in assessing occupational health disparities, Kelsh and Sahl (1996) found in their study of the electrical industry that after adjusting for age, job tenure, and occupation, women's rate of injury in this industry was higher in nine out of ten occupational groups, ranging from one and a half to three times higher than men's occupational injury rate. This study indicates that another source of occupational health disparities is the way in which jobs are designed. Because many of the more hazardous occupations have traditionally been performed by men, workplaces and equipment have evolved to accommodate men's biological advantages of size and musculature, with the result that women's advantage from their greater risk aversion may be partly offset by their greater ergonomic risk in manual labor occupations. (Figure 14.7, for example, illustrates the finding that women experience somewhat more musculoskeletal disorders (MSDs) than other nonfatal problems and men experience the reverse.)

Occupational Sex Segregation Because women and men are still concentrated in different industries, in different occupations within industries, in different jobs within occupations, and even assigned to different tasks within jobs, they also display divergent occupational health patterns, and these patterns do not uniformly favor one sex over the other. It is widely documented, for instance, that women are at far greater risk of carpal tunnel syndrome, due to their concentration in higher-risk jobs for this injury, such as clerical work and light assembly; however, when both men and women perform clerical work, their risk is roughly equal (McDiarmid, Oliver, Ruser, & Gucer,

FIGURE 14.7. *Distribution of MSD cases and all nonfatal injury and illness cases involving days away from work in private industry by sex, 2001.*

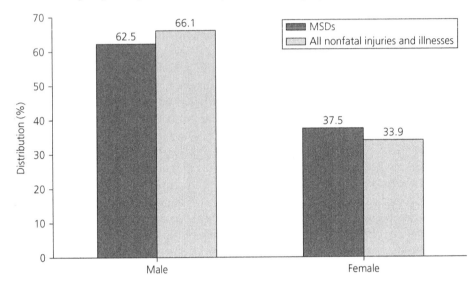

Source: NIOSH, 2004, fig.2-40.

2000; Tanaka, Wild, Cameron, & Freund, 1997). Women's concentration in health care, domestic services such as cleaning, and child care translates into higher exposure to both infectious diseases and cleaning agents intended to prevent disease; the latter are often themselves quite toxic (Stellman, 2000). Service sector employment, particularly in types of work that require some degree of **emotional management** as well as mental or physical labor, also poses a greater risk to the mental health of women given their disproportionate representation in service occupation (de Castro, Agnew, & Fitzgerald, 2004). In general, occupational stress is more prevalent among women than among men, and stress is not only an occupational health problem in and of itself but also a precursor to other occupational health problems (Swanson, 2000; Zeytinoglu, Seaton, Lillevik, & Moruz, 2005) (see Figure 14.8).

Same Job, Different Patterns Although occupational sex segregation explains some disparities, it by no means fully explains them; even within the same jobs, men and women may have different health outcomes. Research among manufacturing workers suggests that the mechanisms for men's occupational injuries tend to be job-related factors such as high ambiguity over a job's future and high variance in workload; for women, occupational injuries show a high degree of correspondence to social mechanisms such as high intragroup conflict and low job control (Nakata et al., 2006). Men and women also frequently suffer disparate injury patterns in the same jobs; for

FIGURE 14.8.   *Distribution of anxiety, stress, and neurotic disorder cases involving days away from work in private industry by sex, 1992–2001.*

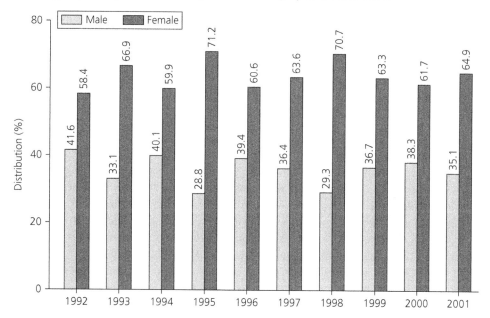

Source: NIOSH, 2004, fig. 2-4.

instance, the leading precursor of injury for male truck drivers is overexertion from lifting, whereas injuries for female truck drivers are most commonly attributed to vehicular collision (Biddle & Blanciforti, 1999). A similar pattern is found in construction: male workers are more likely to die from falls, whereas female construction workers are more likely to die in motor vehicle accidents (Welch et al., 2000). Smith, Lincoln, et al. (2005) find that even controlling for occupation, men suffer more occupational eye injuries than women, a finding they attribute to women's greater attention to safety protocols.

Consequences of Women's Occupational Health Problems   Because the sexual division of labor does not begin and end in the workplace, issues of women's occupational health also extend beyond the formal work environment. Even as women have joined the paid labor force in vast numbers, they continue to shoulder the greater share of nonmarket labor, including housework, child care, and elder care (Padavic & Reskin, 2002). In earlier times, men's ability to face their occupational demands was subsidized by women who took care of cooking and cleaning, raised children, administered to elderly relatives, and nursed the occasionally sick or injured breadwinner back to health. The economic realities of today have placed this type of arrangement out of reach of most American families, who find that they need more than one paycheck to make ends meet. And as women's increased paid workforce participation exposes them to a broader array of occupational health hazards, their ability to balance the demands of paid and unpaid labor becomes increasingly precarious, even with the help of men who have picked up some of the unpaid labor burden themselves. Not only does this pose a hazard to female workers, by increasing their overall fatigue and stress and thus rendering them more vulnerable to injury themselves, but it also poses a threat to the occupational health of all workers, fewer and fewer of whom have the support of unpaid labor in the home.

Age

Young Workers   As it is among male relative to female workers, one of the causal mechanisms for injury rates among teenaged workers is an increased propensity for risk taking that leads to injury (Acosta, Sanderson, Cooper, Perez, & Roberts, 2007). And like economically insecure workers, younger workers are more likely than older workers to be seasonal or part-time and also inexperienced, which further exposes them to acute occupational injury risks. Because worker fatalities are not adjusted for hours worked, some statistics may underestimate the likelihood that part-time workers will suffer occupational injuries and also underestimate the likelihood that workers in subgroups more likely to work part-time—including younger workers—will suffer occupational fatalities (Herbert & Landrigan, 2000). More recent data from the Bureau of Labor Statistics lend partial support to this contention, albeit not for the youngest worker cohort: compared to their representation in the labor force, workers aged sixteen to nineteen have fewer injuries per work hour, but workers aged twenty to forty-four have a greater rate of injury per work hour (see Figure 14.9).

Older Workers   Although workers aged twenty to forty-four sustain the most injuries relative to the number of hours worked, older workers have a higher incidence of severe workplace injuries (Grandjean et al., 2006). Moreover, the number of workdays lost per injury increases with the age of the worker; workers aged fifty-five to sixty-four lose ten days of work on average per injury, well over the median of six days for all workers (NIOSH, 2004). Fatality rates per work hour also climb with age. Workers just under retirement age, aged fifty-five to sixty-four, work 9.3 percent of all hours worked but suffer 14.2 percent of all workplace fatalities; workers past retirement age, sixty-five and older, work 2.0 percent of total work hours but suffer 9.0 percent of workplace fatalities (NIOSH, 2004). Occupational fatality rates are declining overall, but increasing among older workers, especially those over the age of sixty-five (Bailer, Stayner, Stout, Reed, & Gilbert, 1998). Among other reasons, the rise in fatality rates among older workers may be linked to better health care, whereby workers who might have died at earlier ages in previous decades now survive long enough to work up to and past retirement age. Also, older workers in the past might have been limited to those in better health; now, as the retirement age climbs and economic pressure on all age groups increases, workers may postpone retirement even when their health is precarious.

FIGURE 14.9. *Distribution of hours worked and occupational injury and illness cases with days away from work in private industry by age of worker, 2001.*

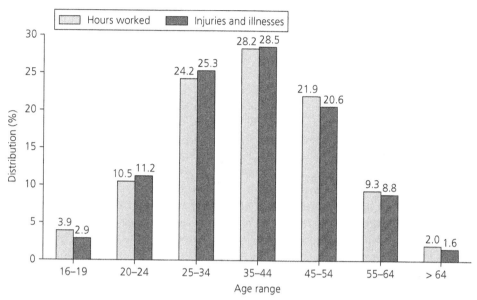

Source: NIOSH, 2004, fig. 1-27.

HOW DO HEALTH DISPARITIES PERSIST?

Many of the social and economic mechanisms that create and perpetuate occupational health disparities have been discussed in previous sections as they pertain to specific populations. In an effort to convey both the interdependence of the major occupational health disparities and the far-reaching scope of these issues, this section will examine a few of the primary factors that are implicated in the current major disparities and that are likely to continue shaping the occupational health landscape in the years to come.

Occupational Segregation

Jobs are often unofficially earmarked for certain groups, thus ensuring that different types of workers will have different levels of exposure to specific occupational hazards. Occupational segregation persists for several reasons. First, different groups of workers tend to come to the labor market with different credentials and skills and this influences their occupational opportunities and thus their exposure to hazards. Because Latinos, on average, complete fewer years of schooling than other minority groups do, they are also likely to have fewer labor market options and to be offered the most dirty, dangerous, or unpleasant types of employment, thus also increasing their exposure to occupational hazards. Because women and men are likely to be socially rewarded for learning different skills, cultivating different proficiencies, and pursuing different tasks, jobs, and occupations, they are likely to have exposure to different hazards and have different occupational health profiles. Age opens up some job opportunities while effectively closing others and may simultaneously enhance some skills and erode others, with the result that we will continue to see different health outcomes for younger and older workers overall and different outcomes in the occupations that selectively employ them.

Second, employers may enact discriminatory preferences for certain types of workers, based on their real or perceived labor market characteristics; this is equally true for high-status and low-status jobs. For instance, computer chip assembly employers in the U.S. Northwest show some preference for immigrant women for their perceived docility and fine motor dexterity, as well as their propensity to accept somewhat lower wages than native-born and male workers (Hossfeld, 1994).

Third, occupational segregation is maintained through informal hiring mechanisms, whereby employers preferentially hire workers who are friends or relatives of current workers, thus increasing the likelihood that the new workers will be similar in social status to the established workforce. Poultry processing, like many other types of labor-intensive assembly and processing, is heavily reliant on low wage costs; in the South, black women have traditionally been given the lowest wages because of their perceived dual disadvantages of gender and race, thus making them preferred employees in poultry-processing plants. Now that this work is typically associated with women, men are less likely to apply for poultry-processing jobs, less likely to be alerted to job opportunities in poultry-processing plants by current workers, and less likely to be seen as a "good fit" for the job by prospective employers. Black women in this region therefore have an elevated risk of neck and upper-back complaints compared to other workers (Lipscomb, Epling, Pompeii, & Dement, 2007).

Job Tenure, Hours, and Security

Just as race, ethnicity, gender, age, nativity, and other social status attributes may influence the types of work (and workplace hazards) that individuals experience, so too do these same attributes influence individuals' degree of attachment to work. As a general rule, workers with lower status face greater uncertainty in their job conditions, meaning that they are more likely to be subject to long and irregular hours; more likely to work in a temporary, seasonal, or part-time capacity; and less likely to experience long-term income or job security. Each of these variables has important health consequences for workers and differentially affects workers based on their gender, race, ethnicity, nativity, and age.

All other things being equal, temporary workers have more frequent occupational injuries than permanent workers do; one study pegs the injury rate for temporary workers at nearly four times the rate for permanent workers (Saha, Kulkarni, Chaudhuri, & Saiyed, 2005). The association between job tenure and workplace injury is likely due to less knowledge of workplace protocols and hazards, as length of employment tends to reduce injury incidence (Benavides et al., 2006). The association of job tenure with injury rates is more pronounced among men, older workers, and those in manual labor occupations (Breslin & Smith, 2006).

Working overtime schedules and working long hours (meaning shifts of twelve hours or longer) are both associated with greater risk of occupational injury. In one study, overtime schedules raised the injury rate by 61 percent over standard schedules, while working consecutive shifts of twelve or more hours was associated with a 37 percent increase in occupational injuries, even after controlling for industry; moreover, long work-hour and work-week schedules tend to proliferate in inherently hazardous occupations, thus exacerbating the hazard to workers (Dembe, Erickson, Delbos, & Banks, 2005). Similarly, nonstandard shifts—rotating, evening, night, and irregular—are also associated with greater injury rates (Dembe, Erickson, Delbos, & Banks, 2006).

On a broader scale, economic uncertainty often subjects workers—in many instances voluntarily—to work situations and schedules that increase their risk of occupational injuries (Facey, 2003; Dembe et al., 2005, 2006). The result is frequently that workers must choose between their economic health and their physical health; one study of taxi drivers chronicles how the economic pressure to keep up with their living costs and taxi leases causes drivers to subject themselves to such health-compromising conditions as working extremely long hours, skipping meals and bathroom breaks, and picking up abusive, violent, and other risky customers (Facey, 2003).

Unions have traditionally done much to safeguard the health of unionized workers, including but not limited to ensuring access to health resources; offering protection from excessive hours, irregular shifts, low wages, and job insecurity; lobbying for worker protection legislation; and promoting the consistent application of safety equipment and protocols in the workplace (Johansson & Partanen, 2002). However, union membership has been in decline for decades. From 1984 to 2004, union membership dropped from 20.1 percent to 12.5 percent of all workers (Bureau of Labor Statistics, 2005b). Although black men are more likely than white men to be union members, due to black men's higher concentration in blue-collar jobs, union membership has declined most precipitously among black men (Uchitelle, 2005), a trend that is likely to further exacerbate black-white occupational health disparities.

Preexisting Disparities and Neighborhood Effects

A major confounding factor in assessing the extent to which occupations contribute to health disparities is the fact that many of the populations discussed here have poorer health to begin with, due to social inequities in health care access and the quality of communities of residence. Although not absolving employers, managers, and health officers from responsibility for worker health, preexisting disparities may account for some portion of the persistent occupational health disparities among workers, if for no other reason than that an unhealthy worker may be more vulnerable to additional injury or illness than a healthy worker. Accordingly, the overall health disparities for each population discussed here run more or less parallel to the occupational health disparities by population discussed previously; with regard to health care access and outcomes, some of these groups (workers of low socioeconomic status, racial and ethnic minorities, and immigrant workers) fare worse almost uniformly, whereas for other groups (women and the elderly), the overall picture is mixed, reflecting the more complicated sources of these types of inequality, with the comparison groups (men and the young, respectively) faring better on some measures and worse on others.

For instance, health insurance is a basic feature of health care access; those without it are consigned to seek care within the tattered "safety net" of free clinics and emergency rooms, which essentially guarantees that the uninsured will have little access to routine and preventive health care. Those with annual incomes below the poverty line, currently $20,000 for a family of four, are disproportionately likely to be without health insurance (being 13 percent of the overall population, but 25 percent of the population without insurance); for that matter, those below 300 percent of the federal poverty line, or $60,000, are also somewhat more likely to be without medical insurance (17 percent of the population; 19 percent of the population without insurance). Immigrants, who constitute 7 percent of the population, are 21 percent of the uninsured. Lack of insurance is also prevalent among young adults, but diminishes with age; childless adults under the age of sixty-five are most likely to be without insurance in that, unless disabled, they are categorically ineligible for any form of government health insurance program (that is, Medicare or Medicaid). As seen in Figure 14.10, Hispanics, blacks, and American Indians are disproportionately represented among the uninsured.

Another facet of preexisting health disparities, which again is particularly relevant to the health status of minority, immigrant, and low-SES workers, is the effect of community of residence on health. Lower income and minority communities are disproportionately susceptible to a wide array of social and environmental conditions

FIGURE 14.10.   *Distribution of the uninsured and total U.S. population by race and ethnicity in 2004.*

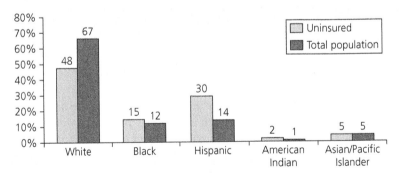

Source: U.S. Department of Health and Human Services, Office of the Assistant Secretary for Planning and Evaluation, 2005, fig. 6.

that expose residents to greater health risk in the places where they live, including but not limited to proximity to hazardous waste sites, poor quality housing, and poor air quality. One study finds that both minority race and low social class SES increase the likelihood of living near hazardous waste sites and decrease the regulatory activity and expenditure applied to clean up such sites (Brown, 1995). Substandard housing stock, a common feature of lower income areas, is associated with higher rates of both infectious and chronic disease, due to problems with consistency of potable water supply, insect and rat infestations, and inadequate food storage resources. Poor housing also increases the incidence of acute injuries, especially those associated with exposed heating sources and structural defects of windows and stairs. Disadvantaged neighborhoods are often characterized by factors such as close proximity to noisy and air-polluting bus and subway lines, lack of safe parks and playgrounds, and few or no grocery stores and pharmacies, all of which undermine healthy lifestyles (Krieger & Higgins, 2002). Neighborhoods may also affect individual health behaviors in more subtle ways through social network effects, which are just beginning to be comprehensively documented (Christakis & Fowler, 2007; Diehr et al., 1993). For instance, individuals living in neighborhoods with high unemployment are more likely to smoke and to consume a high-fat diet, even after controlling for factors such as income and race, suggesting that workers' social relationships within their neighborhoods can influence their personal health behaviors and thus their overall health (Diehr et al., 1993).

Globalization

Globalization is an important occupational health issue not only because it changes the landscape of occupational hazards but also because it disproportionately lays these hazards at the feet of workers who are disadvantaged in the labor force to begin with. As discussed earlier, because of changes in the economy, lower income workers are increasingly pressed; because they face greater economic uncertainty, they are also more likely to be exposed to occupational hazards and the correlates of these hazards, such as long and unstable work hours, shorter job tenure, and the like. These workers are more likely to be minorities or recent immigrants, or both (Guidotti, 2003). But even beyond this immediate reality, globalization is potentially problematic for occupational health because of the way it changes the organization of work domestically and because of the impact that cross-national economic activity has on workers in developing countries, exacerbating global inequalities and creating new occupational health challenges.

Many trends in workplace organization—such as organizational restructuring, a renewed emphasis on lean production, and an increased use of contingent workers—are likely to have a negative impact on worker health (Landsbergis, 2003). In the auto industry, for example, technological changes in the production process do not deliver the promised benefit of empowering workers but do seem to increase the risk of musculoskeletal injuries (Landsbergis, Cahill, & Schnall, 1999). The overall risk to workers in the United States is on the decline, both overall as well as within industries (Stout et al., 1996). However, these declines have less to do with changes in the production process than with changes in the overall labor market structure; in other words, work is not necessarily any less intrinsically dangerous, rather the most dangerous types of work employ fewer workers than previously, and the less dangerous industries have added jobs (Loomis, Richardson, Bena, & Bailer, 2004; Richardson & Loomis, 1997).

Where have the more dangerous jobs gone? Particularly in manufacturing and production work, the decrease in U.S. occupational injury and fatality rates can be attributed to the export of many dangerous jobs to the developing world. In short, we have outsourced some of our occupational hazards along with the labor-intensive manufacturing jobs that occasion them (Subramanian, Desai, Prakash, Mital, & Mital, 2006). Developing countries bear an increasing burden of occupational health problems as, in an era of rapidly increasing global economic interconnectedness, they scramble to enter and compete in the global economy, which often translates into overlooking some aspects of worker welfare and well-being in an attempt to lure international investors with low wage rates and a "business-friendly environment." And as workplaces reorganize work to maintain global competitiveness, often at the hands (or at least the behest) of investors and owners from the United States and other developed nations, workers suffer from increased variability as well as from physical changes in the work environment that make it more dangerous to workers and surrounding communities. For instance, when the adoption of the North American Free Trade Agreement (NAFTA) prompted the privatization of Mexico's sugar companies (most of which were snapped up by U.S. soft-drink manufacturers), rapid restructuring and modernization of the industry ensued; the consequences of this process included fewer worker protections as new owners abandoned old union-negotiated contracts, increased injury rates due to the introduction of new sugar-processing machinery and the faster speed of production, and increased worker stress stemming from both of the preceding factors (Lemus-Ruiz, 1999).

Although the trend of worsening occupational health may not currently be a top priority in developing countries, it can have a huge impact on economic development insofar as an unhealthy labor force will in the long run be more costly to both businesses and governments (Loewenson, 2001). Potential countervailing tendencies in developing countries include increased pressure to reduce health costs, which may bring a greater emphasis on both worker safety protocols and preventive health measures; an increased respect for individuals, which may prompt better and more stringent regulations; and the increasing consumer value of fair labor practices, which can be seen in the premium placed on such goods as fair-trade coffee and sweatshop-free apparel (Leamon, 2001).

FUTURE TRENDS IN HEALTH DISPARITIES

Occupational health disparities have received considerably more attention from health researchers in the past decade, due in no small part to the 1996 National Occupational Research Agenda issued by NIOSH, which contained an explicit call for research addressing the diversity of the American workforce. Other recent social, political, and economic developments may also bode well for the future reduction and eventual elimination of occupational health disparities. First, although great educational and occupational inequalities between worker subgroups persist, disadvantaged worker populations continue to make gains, which bodes well for the occupational health of future generations of workers. Women's college attendance rate now surpasses that of men, and the income gap between men and women has slowly but consistently narrowed; blacks have also made substantial income, educational, and occupational gains in the past few decades (Padavic & Reskin, 2002). Second, as Americans become increasingly aware of the changing demographics of the United States due to an ongoing wave of immigration from Latin America and Asia, and as national concern grows over the rapidly escalating cost of health care, the political will to address occupational health disparities of racial and ethnic minorities and foreign-born workers may be increasing, particularly as Hispanics gain political clout due to their swelling numbers and their new status as the largest U.S. minority group (U.S. Census Bureau, 2004).

SUMMARY

Various populations in society have widely different occupational health profiles; the major disparities are associated with social class, race and ethnicity, gender, and nativity. Because of the societal division of labor, some groups face greater exposure to specific occupational hazards and are more likely to do intrinsically dangerous, dirty, or repetitive work. Additionally, some groups face greater stress and burden in their daily lives because of their status in society, the effects of which spill over into their workplace experiences.

Several factors affect the direction of occupational health disparity trends. Occupational health disparities often reflect and track broader status disparities in society; preexisting health disparities and neighborhood conditions may further exacerbate disparities caused by occupational organization and practices. Because of recent globalization trends affecting the nature of work overall as well as advances in worker protections, U.S. workers are somewhat less likely than they were to face hazards. However, as old hazards fade, new hazards emerge; the dangerous work escaped by some individuals and groups is often merely displaced onto other individuals and groups, without changing the overall incidence and prevalence of occupational injury and illness. The globalization of labor markets has, if anything, exacerbated this trend. Further, the reorganization of work processes in the United States has compromised worker health to some degree, as workers are increasingly subjected to various forms of contingent work arrangements.

The future direction of occupational health disparity trends is uncertain; although some disparities have diminished, and will likely continue to diminish due to improving social conditions, other disparities are exacerbated by population flows of low-skilled workers to the United States. However, as disadvantaged populations gain economic and political clout, they may be in a better position to press for positive policy changes to eliminate occupational health disparities.

KEY TERMS

cultural ergonomics
emotional management
gender socialization
master statuses

occupational health disparities
occupational segregation
socioeconomic status

QUESTIONS FOR DISCUSSION

1. What are the characteristics of the populations that are most at risk for occupational health disparities?

2. In what ways are occupational health disparities linked to social status? To race or ethnicity? To gender?

3. Looking at your current or most recent job, determine whether it presents any occupational health disparities. If so, what are these disparities, and why do they persist?

4. Given that many variations in occupational health are accounted for or influenced by factors outside the workplace, how might our society best think about employers' level of liability for these disparities and responsibility for mitigating them?

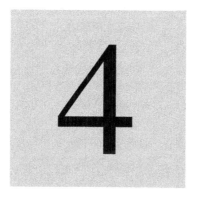

4

EVALUATION AND LEADERSHIP ISSUES IN PREVENTION

CHAPTER

ECONOMIC IMPACTS
OF PREVENTION

After reading this chapter, you should be able to

- Understand the value of conducting an economic evaluation of workplace prevention efforts.

- Discuss the concept of years of potential life lost.

- Describe the value of a cost-benefit analysis.

- Discuss the burden of workplace injury and illness.

It seems that the creation of the Occupational Safety and Health Administration (OSHA) and the National Institute for Occupational Safety and Health (NIOSH) by the federal government in 1970 was never viewed as a positive development by employers in this country. It was thought of as a punishment for bad working conditions that caused great morbidity and mortality among American workers. The business sector has historically been resistant to NIOSH and OSHA because they were perceived to lack value and their standards and recommendations were assumed to have profit-cutting consequences. These federal agencies compounded their credibility problem by having difficulty proving value for their research, regulation, and compliance programs. Therefore their budgets continued to be cut by Congress, and there was discussion in recent administrations of disbanding the entire agency assigned to workplace safety and health.

A company goes into business to make a profit. Without profits it is virtually impossible to stay in business for a long period of time. OSHA fines for violating workplace safety mandates have never really offered an incentive for businesses to significantly change they way they address safety and health for their employees. So employers have generally complied at the most minimal levels that would avoid OSHA penalties. Only when employee safety and health programs can be proven to increase profits through healthy employees will they be embraced by business and industry leaders. This chapter examines some concepts and methods that can help public health professionals and others determine the value of workplace prevention programs.

PREMATURE MORTALITY

Before we can evaluate the remedy for a public health problem, we need to accurately evaluate the seriousness of that problem. One way to do this is to measure both some causes of premature death and the extent of premature death. One popular measure for premature mortality is **years of potential life lost** (YPLL). It can be defined as "a public health measure that reflects the impact of deaths occurring in years preceding a conventional cut-off year of age" ("Years of Potential Life Lost . . . ," 1992). Often the cut-off year of age is seventy-five, because that is about the present average life expectancy in this country. YPLL is typically determined for specific causes of death. When this calculation is compared over dynamic populations, it is helpful to calculate the rate per one thousand people in each age group. YPLL has been often used by public health officials over the last several years in intense evaluation of prevention programs.

EMPLOYER HEALTH INSURANCE COSTS

To attract competent workers after wage and price controls were implemented in the 1950s, employers started offering fringe benefits to workers instead of increases in wages. These benefits were exempted from taxes and were very effective in attracting and retaining much-needed workers.

According to an article found on Medscape Today (2004), employers spend more on health insurance for their employees than they spend on any other single benefit, and the cost of providing health insurance to employees is one of the largest costs of doing business in the United States. An analysis of Bureau of Labor Statistics data found that health insurance benefits accounted for 23 percent of nonwage employee compensation in the first quarter of 2004. These costs are projected to continue increasing every year well into the future. This report also discovered that employers spent an estimated $330.9 billion to fund employee health insurance benefits in 2003, representing an increase of 12.1 percent over 2002 and a 51.4 percent increase since 1998. Once used to attract and retain employees for a business, the health insurance benefit has become extremely costly for employers to continue to offer to all their employees, and at times it affects their ability to remain competitive. Indeed, the health insurance coverage issue has become a nightmare, not only for employers but also for employees.

According to a study by economists Kenneth Thorpe and David Howard (Health Affairs, 2006), health care spending will constitute 18.7 percent of gross domestic product (GDP) by the year 2014. Over the last twenty years, two major trends have been developing in the delivery of health insurance to employees: a significant decrease in the number of workers receiving health insurance from their employers and a sharp increase in the insurance premiums paid by workers as companies pass increased costs along. U.S. census figures released in August 2006 (Bureau of Labor Statistics & U.S. Census Bureau, 2006) revealed that the number of people having health insurance provided by their employer dropped from 62.6 percent in 2001 to 59.5 percent in 2005. As health care costs continue to rise above the inflation rate, many groups, from state and federal legislators to business owners, are struggling to reduce the costs associated with delivering health care to their respective constituents. This decline in health insurance coverage has been most profound in the small employer segment of American business, but all companies are feeling the pressure. The *Wall Street Journal* reported in 2006 that 11 percent of the small business owners who offer their employees health benefits were considering dropping these benefits in 2007 (Breeden, 2006). Overall, the percentage of small firms offering health benefits dropped by 9 percentage points from 2000 to 2005, according to a survey published by the Kaiser Family Foundation in 2005. The firms not offering employees health insurance cited high premiums as the most important reason for not doing so. If the costs of health insurance could be controlled or reduced, businesses seem interested in continuing the insurance coverage.

Robert W. Fogel, a professor at the Graduate School of Business, University of Chicago and a Nobel Laureate, predicts that by the year 2030 about 25 percent of the GDP will be spent on health care. Victor Fuchs, an economist at Stanford, agrees with that projection but argues that the issue is not how much is being spent on health care but whether the extra dollars are buying marked improvements in health (Kolata, 2006). We know, for example, that Medicare beneficiaries treated for five or more chronic conditions account for virtually all program spending growth in recent years (Health Affairs, 2006). The American workforce is growing older and sicker, and workers are bringing their medical health issues, developed in their working years, into retirement with them. A major health factor behind the Medicare spending increase was overweight and obesity.

According to Robert W. Woodruff, professor and chair of the Department of Health Policy Management at Emory University's Rollins School of Public Health,

"We need interventions that go beyond what current Medicare policy does, to reach the 'near elderly' and work with people before they approach the age of Medicare eligibility to fight obesity and chronic disease" (Health Affairs, 2006). These near elderly can be found in the workplace, and for many years have been practicing the high-risk health behaviors that have predisposed them to multiple chronic conditions.

A recent survey conducted by Hewitt Associates (2008) points out that businesses in this country are seeing health and productivity as a business issue. This survey also revealed that the majority of employers plan to invest in long-term solutions designed to improve the health and productivity of their workers over the next few years. To make these changes, the possible interventions by businesses need to be thoroughly evaluated. Part of this evaluation will include an economic evaluation of prevention programs in the workplace.

THE PURPOSES OF ECONOMIC EVALUATION

Employers are in need of government help as they deal with their growing problem of keeping their employees healthy and productive at a reasonable cost. This is a role that could be easily assumed by OSHA and NIOSH as American business comes to rely on lowering costs, particularly labor costs, to remain internationally competitive.

Gorsky and Teutsch (1995) state that decision makers in public health need to consider costs and effectiveness when it comes to offering preventive services to Americans. They need not only to identify those preventive programs that work but also to consider the additional costs associated with the use of these interventions. Businesses are charged with finding affordable ways of keeping their workforces healthy and productive. The expense of providing health insurance to their workers is a good investment only if the workers remain healthy and productive. OSHA and NIOSH have the resources and tools to help the business community select programs that contribute to a healthy and productive workforce. Fielding and Briss (2006) argue that improvements in the health of the population can be achieved through better use of evidence-based decisions, so that our finite resources will be used to do the right thing at the right time. What is needed is faster and better use of scientific information that increases the return on the investment in prevention and treatment by having the desired effect on the health of the public.

THE BURDEN OF INJURY AND ILLNESS

According to the CDC ("Workers' Memorial Day . . . ," 2009), a total of 5,488 U.S. workers died from occupational injuries in 2007. In addition, 49,000 workers died from work-related diseases. An estimated four million workers were involved in a nonfatal occupational injury or illness, resulting in half of this total being transferred, restricted, or forced to take time off from work. Injuries and illnesses represent one of the most serious public health problems facing our country and especially our workplaces. These numbers do not include the very large numbers of workers incubating chronic diseases in the workplace.

The CDC ("Workers' Memorial Day . . . ," 2009) also reports that an estimated 3.4 million workers visited emergency departments in 2004 because of occupational injuries, and eighty thousand of these visits resulted in hospitalizations. Work-related injuries and illnesses are very expensive for employers. In 2006, employers spent $87.6 billion on workers' compensation and lost a tremendous amount of productivity because of time away from work.

These work-related injuries are for the most part preventable, but the effort will require an investment in time and money by the employer. Fielding and Briss (2006) explain the fact that many improvements in health result from evidence-informed programs that affect the likelihood of acquiring a disease, the severity of the disease, and the receipt of appropriate and timely medical care. Prevention programs should improve the quality of life, reduce the incidence or severity of a disease or injury, and reduce premature death through early detection or interventions to reduce risks or exposures associated with incidence.

The CDC (Gorsky & Teutsch, 1995) has developed an approach to preventive health program evaluation called the Basic Assessment Scheme for Intervention Costs and Consequences (**BASICC**). (Exhibit 15.1 contains an outline of the six data elements the assessment requires.) This is a very rational approach to developing an evaluation strategy that looks at both what a program or other intervention uses in resources and how it performs. Although other evaluation methods will be discussed in this chapter, they all revert back to many of the components found in the BASICC approach.

EXHIBIT 15.1.   **BASICC: six required data elements**

- A complete description of the program, the units in which the service(s) are provided, and the time frame of the program.

- Health outcome(s) averted by the prevention program and the estimated time between its implementation and when the health outcome is averted.

- The rates and societal burden of the health outcome.

- The preventable fraction for the health outcome, with the program in place and used in a realistic manner (i.e., the proportion of the health outcome averted through the program).

- Intervention costs per unit of intervention, including the cost of any intervention side effects.

- Direct medical treatment cost of the health outcome prevented.

Source: Gorsky & Teutsch, 1995.

The success of prevention activities is be defined by their effectiveness in delaying or averting morbidity and mortality from illness or injury. According to Gorsky and Teutsch (1995) prevention effectiveness integrates the best available information into evaluating the choices made for averting illness and injury in the workplace.

The BASICC model offers an excellent approach to the evaluation of preventive health initiatives for use in the workplace. Consider, for example, needing to evaluate a smoking cessation program. According to "Annual Smoking-Attributable Mortality . . . ," 2005), tobacco use is one of the leading causes of preventable mortality in the United States. In determining the effectiveness of a smoking cessation program, it would make sense to include averted poor health outcomes as an important part of the evaluation process.

TYPES OF ECONOMIC ANALYSIS

"Efficacy refers to the scientific basis for 'what works' in reducing adverse health outcomes. It is the improvement in health outcome that a prevention strategy can produce" (Gorsky & Teutsch, 1995). Evaluations of efficacy attempt to discover the value of interventions, to show whether or not they are succeeding in their efforts to keep individuals healthy at a reasonable cost. Evaluating efficacy allows us to see whether there is evidence of improvement in health as a result of resources being allocated to a prevention strategy or intervention. There are several economic tools available to measure these improvements and rank them in some logical order of success. The major methods used in **economic evaluation** are cost analysis, cost-effectiveness analysis, cost-utility analysis, and cost-benefit analysis.

Cost Analysis

Cost analysis (CA) looks at all the costs of an illness including both direct and indirect costs. As an economic evaluation technique it involves the systematic collection, categorization, and analysis of program costs. The results are a measure of the burden of disease for a defined period of time.

Cost-Effectiveness Analysis

Cost-effectiveness analysis (CEA) compares the costs of intervention with the resulting improvement in health. It can be used to compare the costs of alternative interventions that produce a common health effect. For example, Exhibit 15.2 shows various health interventions that analysis has proven to be cost effective to offer to the population. According to the Partnership for Prevention study that discusses these findings, the three most cost-effective preventive health services that can be offered in medical practice are smoking cessation, aspirin therapy, and childhood immunizations. This study is a good example of using economics to assist in making decisions about the utilization of scarce health resources.

EXHIBIT 15.2. Cost-effective preventive health services

1. Aspirin therapy
2. Childhood immunizations
3. Tobacco use, screening and intervention
4. Colorectal cancer screening
5. Measuring blood pressure in adults
6. Influenza immunizations
7. Pneumococcal immunization
8. Alcohol screening and counseling
9. Vision screening for adults
10. Cervical cancer screening
11. Cholesterol screening
12. Breast cancer screening
13. Chlamydia screening
14. Calcium supplement counseling
15. Vision screening in children
16. Folic acid
17. Obesity screening
18. Depression screening
19. Hearing screening
20. Injury prevention counseling
21. Osteoporosis screening
22. Cholesterol screening for high-risk patients
23. Diabetes screening
24. Diet counseling
25. Tetanus-diphtheria boosters

Source: Johnson, 2006.

Cost-Utility Analysis

Cost-utility analysis (CUA) is a special type of cost-effectiveness analysis that uses years of life saved combined with quality of life during those years as a health outcome measure. These measures allow direct comparisons of interventions.

Nas (1996) points out that because of the difficulty in identifying and quantifying outcomes, research on health care services usually uses CEA or CUA when determining value in the use of health resources. CEA provides a good measurement tool for determining the efficiency of a particular procedure or program in meeting its goal. The outcome in CEA is usually represented by a single health outcome such as years of life saved or improvement in health status.

Cost-Benefit Analysis

Cost-benefit analysis (CBA) is a type of economic analysis that compares both costs and benefits in dollar terms. They are adjusted to their present value through a process called discounting. If a program demonstrates a net benefit after the computations, the program is considered to provide good economic value and should be continued or perhaps expanded.

Gorsky & Teutsch (1995) point out that prevention-effectiveness analysis, a form of CBA, could be used to measure the effects of public health programs. In order to compare different prevention strategies and document which programs and activities provide the greatest benefit for the funds expended, an organization needs reliable and consistent cost and effectiveness data. Table 15.1 shows how each of these analysis methods can be applied to document the economic effectiveness of programs.

TARGET AREAS FOR EVALUATION

Employers are not capable of dealing with every health problem that may affect their workers. They do not have the ability or the desire to evaluate the effects of wellness initiatives that may or may not work in reducing their health insurance premiums. Nonetheless, businesses have started to realize that injury and disease prevention programs are an investment in the future of the health of their employees. They need to be able to choose the injury and disease prevention programs that have the best chance of success while consuming the smallest amount of finite business resources.

Some interventions lend themselves to pure economic evaluation using cost-benefit analysis or cost-effectiveness analysis criteria. Other programs use qualitative analysis at first, until true costs and benefits can be determined. Much more research is necessary in this case because evaluators are dealing with issues like quality of life measurements, which are very subjective and on which it is difficult to place a monetary value. Workplace illness and injury prevention is, in the long run, economically beneficial to both workers and business. Program areas in which this has already been demonstrated include smoking cessation, diabetes prevention, and injury prevention, as discussed in the following sections.

TABLE 15.1. Overview of economic evaluation methods

Economic evaluation method	Comparison	Measurement of health effects	Economic summary
Cost analysis	Used to compare net costs of different programs for planning and assessment	Dollars	Net cost Cost of illness
Cost-effectiveness analysis	Used to compare interventions that produce a common health effect	Health effects, measured in natural units	Cost-effectiveness ratio Cost per case averted Cost per life-year saved
Cost-utility analysis	Used to compare interventions that have morbidity and mortality outcomes	Health effects, measured as years of life, adjusted for quality of life	Cost per quality-adjusted life year (QALY)
Cost-benefit analysis	Used to compare different programs with different units of outcomes (health and nonhealth)	Dollars	Net benefit or cost Benefit-to-cost ratio

Source: CDC Evaluation Working Group (1999).

Smoking Cessation Programs

Tobacco use by workers is clearly one of the most important triggers for worker illness, disability, and death in this country. It is also linked with a tremendous loss of productivity in the workforce. There is no doubt that this dangerous product is responsible for a dramatic reduction in the profits of many companies in America, yet many companies are not even aware of the loss. Tobacco use by workers results in poor health, lost wages, and lost productivity. The CDC ("Annual Smoking-Attributable Mortality . . . ," 2005) reports that smoking cost the nation about $92 billion in the form of lost productivity in the years 1997 to 2001, up from $10 billion from the annual mortality-related productivity losses for the years 1995 to 1999. The lost-productivity estimate combined with smoking-related health care costs, which were reported at $75.5 billion in 1998, now exceeds $167 billion per year in the United States. This represents an enormous loss in profits for American businesses. According to the CDC (2004), reducing adult smoking rates by 1 percent could result in more than 30,000 fewer heart attacks, 16,000 fewer strokes, and savings of over $1.5 billion over five years.

There are only two ways to reduce consumption of this deadly and costly product in the workplace. They are regulation of tobacco use in the workplace and smoking cessation programs that include education and therapy. The outcomes of tremendous savings in medical costs, an increase in productivity, and a reduction in mortality make the reduction of tobacco use in the workplace a very important future goal.

Injury Prevention Programs

The CDC ("Achievements in Public Health, 1900–1999 . . . ," 1999) reports that over the last sixty years deaths from unintentional work-related injuries in the United States have decreased nearly 90 percent, from thirty-seven deaths per one hundred thousand workers in 1933 to four deaths per one hundred thousand workers in 1997. Simon and Fielding (2006) argue that worker productivity has improved because of the reduction in injuries. This higher productivity has reduced business costs and is due in large part to public health interventions that are low cost compared with the medical care that would have been needed if the injuries had not been prevented. Despite these facts, injuries still remain a tremendous source of morbidity, mortality, and economic cost to American businesses, and they are still the leading cause of death in individuals between the ages of one and forty-four.

For example, since OSHA's inception, work-related health problems such as coal workers' pneumoconiosis (black lung), and silicosis—common at the beginning of the century—have come under better control; severe injuries and deaths related to mining, manufacturing, construction, and transportation also have decreased; and since 1980, safer workplaces have resulted in a reduction of approximately 40 percent in the rate of fatal occupational injuries.

Smith, Wellman, et al. (2005) found that injuries on the job constitute about 30 percent of all medically treated injuries to adults aged eighteen to sixty-four years. This fact alone makes it important that workplace conditions be examined in an effort to reduce the impact of injuries on society. Christoffel and Gallagher (2006) believe

FIGURE 15.1.   *A six-step framework for program evaluation.*

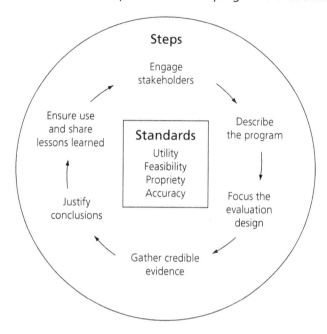

Source: CDC Evaluation Working Group, 1999.

that evaluation of the effectiveness of injury prevention programs should be done on a routine basis. Unfortunately, employers and public health agencies do not always have the luxury of engaging in carefully designed and controlled studies, and it is not always easy to offer quantitative data to prove the worth of injury control programs.

The CDC Evaluation Working Group (1999) has developed a six-step framework for conducting program evaluations (see Figure 15.1), and it also offers supporting materials (of various more recent dates) that include a workbook, an evaluation primer specific to injury prevention programs, and an evaluation Web site (http://www.cdc.gov/eval/index .htm) from which these and other materials can be downloaded. Another interesting model of injury prevention program evaluation has been prepared by Christoffel and Gallagher (2006). This model evaluates injury prevention programs in qualitative stages, using formative evaluation, process evaluation, and **impact and outcome evaluation**.

Prevention of Ergonomic Injuries

An evaluation of the prevention of ergonomic injuries must always start with a look at the potential costs of ergonomic injuries compared to the costs incurred to prevent them. If one looks at the broad nature of ergonomics including the fundamental design of the operation, the costs of doing it right can appear excessive. However, in the personal experience of the author, when engineers and designers are educated on the impacts of design choices, often a simpler, less expensive, and more productive design can and will be chosen. While involved with design reviews for a $500 million new machine installation, the author met with the designers and engineers. As part of the review, ergonomic issues and concepts were discussed to ensure the engineers understood our concerns. After the initial discussion, the author noticed an engineer busily drawing and writing on a notepad. When this engineer took a break from writing, the author asked what he was thinking. The engineer replied, "I have redesigned this operation based on your education work, and this new design will be simpler to build, operate, and maintain than what we had before, which was the 'industry standard.' I wish I had known this information before to prevent problems elsewhere." The author was floored that some simple design concerns and concepts being shared led to such improvements that quickly.

On the issue of soft tissue injuries associated with ergonomics, the costs of preventing or treating injuries often fail the "common sense" test. Solutions to soft tissue injuries can be as simple as requiring job rotation among the workforce to keep exposures below approximate threshold limits as discussed in Chapter Eleven. This does not cost anything except some additional training to ensure the workers are all equally competent at the rotated work unless there is contractual language that does not allow job rotation. In the event of contractual language precluding job rotation, other options should be pursued or negotiations begun to enable job rotation. If job rotation is not feasible, then the costs of changing the job must be examined in light of the cost of injuries. As discussed in Chapter Eleven, sometimes small solutions such as modifying the height or access to machines can improve the operation to the point that it is no longer a major concern. Compare these costs to the average cost of one carpal tunnel injury that requires surgery, rehabilitation, and potentially job placement, and the prevention costs start to look good, especially in light of the fact that one carpal tunnel injury is most likely the warning sign of more to come.

Safety Inspections

Another area where prevention more than pays for itself in any cost-benefit calculation is the area of safety inspections. Depending on the level of safety inspection and the material used to conduct this inspection, costs of conducting this can range from a minimal part of normal operations up to several thousand dollars if specialized equipment and techniques are used. In some cases the specialized techniques include X-ray examination of equipment, which requires all other work in the area to be shut down while the equipment is set up and calibrated. This can cost thousands of dollars to conduct. What is it being used to examine? Often this is used in pressure vessels or pressurized pipes to ensure structural integrity of the metal and or welds done on the same. The cost of not doing this? An explosion (See Exhibit 15.3).

One can only imagine the total cost to Marcus Oil and Chemical Company from this incident. There would have been OSHA fines as well as lawsuits due to damage and injuries to individuals affected by the explosion. In 2005 BP America paid a fine of over $21 million to OSHA for issues related to a fatal explosion at its Texas City,

EXHIBIT 15.3. Final report from U.S. Chemical Safety Board on 2004 explosion calls on Houston to enact stricter pressure vessel regulations

Houston, Texas, June 6, 2006—In its final investigation report on a December 2004 chemical plant explosion in southwest Houston, the U.S. Chemical Safety Board (CSB) today called on the city to adopt new safety regulations governing the construction and modification of pressure vessels—industrial process and storage containers that hold pressurized gases or liquids. The case study report issued at a news conference this morning describes the violent explosion of a 50,000-pound steel pressure vessel on the evening of December 3, 2004, at the Marcus Oil and Chemical facility on Minetta Street in southwest Houston. The explosion was felt over a wide area in Houston and ignited a fire that burned for seven hours. Three Houston firefighters were slightly injured during the response to the blaze. Several residents sustained cuts from flying glass, and steel fragments from the explosion were thrown up to a quarter-mile from the plant. Building and car windows were shattered, and nearby buildings experienced significant structural and interior damage.

The Marcus Oil facility, which was established in 1987, refines polyethylene waxes for industrial use. The crude waxes, which are obtained as a by-product from the petrochemical industry, contain flammable hydrocarbons such as hexane. At Marcus Oil, the waxes are processed and purified inside a variety of steel process vessels. The vessel that exploded was a horizontal tank 12 feet in diameter, 50 feet long, and operated at a pressure of approximately 67 pounds per square inch.

CSB investigators determined that the failed vessel, known as Tank No. 7, had been modified by Marcus Oil to install internal heating coils, as were several other pressure vessels at the facility. Following installation of the coils, each vessel was resealed by welding a steel plate over the two-foot diameter temporary opening. The repair welds did not meet accepted industry quality standards for pressure vessels. Marcus Oil did not use a qualified welder or proper welding procedure to reseal the vessels and did not pressure-test the vessels after the welding was completed.

Source: U.S. Chemical Safety Board, 2006.

Texas, plant (OSHA, 2005). This incident, which caused fifteen fatalities in addition to extensive damage to the facility, was not specifically a failure of safety inspection processes but shows the scale of costs that can result from not properly installing, maintaining, and inspecting a facility.

Older Workers

Still another issue pertains to the growth of the percentage of older workers in the workforce. Over the last few years, a new trend has started to emerge in many U.S.

workplaces: individuals over the age of 65 are continuing to work rather than retire. In addition, due to demographic changes, the workforce continues to age in most fields. According to studies by the National Research Council of the National Academies (Wegman & McGee, 2004, p. 1), in 2003, 44 percent of the civilian population was age forty-five and over, and projections are that by 2050 that figure will be 55 percent. Projections for the workforce show similar changes and percentages across the United States. In fact, data from Europe and Japan (Taylor, 2002, p. 4) indicate that an older workforce with physical, medical, and mental issues related to age will be an issue for the entire developed world. This will bring a changed and different dynamic to many aspects of running an operation. This will be driven by older workers who tend to have different needs, desires, mental and physical abilities, and medical issues than a younger workforce. This section will discuss some of the problems and opportunities associated with the aging workforce and some solutions that can be implemented immediately to avoid the negative aspects of an older workforce as well as recommend some long-term interventions that must be considered. Of significant note is that few detailed studies of the impacts of an older workforce on productivity, safety, medical costs, and related issues have been completed. The National Research Council publication *Health and Safety Needs of Older Workers* (Wegman & McGee, 2004, pp. 10–12) specifically calls for more and more detailed studies to understand all aspects of the changes and impacts of a workforce with many more older workers than today's workforce.

The following issues related just to the physical changes an older workforce faces show the reader that working to redesign the workplace to accommodate these changes can clearly offset the costs likely to be incurred once these problems surface in performance and operations. For the purposes of this section we will ignore the medical and mental changes and issues an older workforce faces even though these will, in many cases, be more costly than accommodating the physical changes.

There are many possible issues and problems associated with older workers and their participation in the workforce. These range from mild physical impairments limiting their ability to perform the physical work to significant mental and psychological issues and impairments that limit their ability to process information and make decisions related to work tasks. The data show that not all older workers will suffer all or even most of the possible impairments, but in very few cases are they predictable. Thus prudent employers will need to start immediately to analyze their workplace to determine whether or not they are capable of fully and appropriately utilizing workers in their fifties, sixties, and older. This analysis will look at the physical demands of the work, the decision making requirements, visual aids, and other solutions to be addressed later in this chapter.

The physical issues for older workers start with some effects that simply occur with aging such as reduced stamina, weaker eyesight (Haight, 2003), reduced physical flexibility, and reduced hearing ability (Haight, 2003). Each of these manifests itself as a person gets older although very unevenly and usually quite slowly, at such a rate that the individual hardly realizes the losses.

Vision manifests itself as a loss of visual acuity with such issues as loss of light transmittance (an individual requires more light to see objects, especially small print or parts), reduced ability to track moving objects, and reduced ability to make out images due to cataracts and macular degeneration. These all show themselves to advance with advancing age, but individual variations increase with age such that generalizations for the population of older workers are fine but for any specific worker or even a small workforce may not be valid. Many of the research studies done to date to assess age-related performance have utilized driving a motor vehicle (Haight, 2003). The data show that older drivers have more difficulty reading highway signs, especially at night, a reduced ability to track and predict the path of moving objects and—as part of a mental decrement–to decipher what all the complexity might mean to them potentially leading to an accident. In the workplace this could imply that insufficient lighting (for energy conservation or lack of understanding of the needs of older workers for increased illumination) will lead to an increased opportunity for older workers to be unable to see their work and can consequently lead to errors and accidents.

Hearing loss is another malady that all older adults suffer (presbycusis) in varying degrees. Of particular note is the fact that the first sound frequency an older worker loses is the high frequency (Wegman, 2004, p. 179): sounds that coincide with the generalized female voice as well as many alarms, sirens, and so on. This loss is very gradual unless an individual is exposed to a significant noise that causes immediate loss. Individuals may not even realize that they have lost a significant percentage of their hearing ability and therefore cannot look for help. For a workplace, this can mean that workers are unable to hear alarms, are unable to hear coworkers and may be unable to sort out multiple sounds that require action by the individual. This is a particular issue when the workplace is one with multiple sound sources such as a manufacturing facility, a control room for a complex process and/or a motor vehicle. The reduced hearing ability can lead, as with reduced visual ability, to errors and/or accidents.

Physical stamina and flexibility, similar to hearing and vision decrement, normally present themselves slowly and with great variation between individuals. Persons who keep physically fit and utilize strength and flexibility exercises will be better able to adapt to physical demands than do those whose only exercises are conducted at work (Wegman & McGee, 2004, p. 197). Limitations gradually increase in the absence of exercises and subject individuals to an increasing risk of injury if their job duties require any significant degree of physical exertion. In addition, back injuries are increasingly likely with an older workforce due to the age-related deterioration of the disks in the back (data from the BLS, 2006, show an approximately 2:1 back pain and hurt back ratio based on percentage of workforce for older workers compared to younger workers). The age-related deterioration of the disks starts in the mid-twenties and gradually saps the integrity of the back. Data shared in a training session attended by the author indicate that a fifty-five-year-old male, bending over at the waist with straight legs, will exert enough force on the disks in the lower back to rupture a disk without lifting anything. When excess weight, especially around the middle, is added to the equation, the reduced flexibility and strength are even more of an issue and make individuals more at risk for injury. This is due to the added weight placed forward of the fulcrum (low back) when lifting.

Formative Evaluation   Formative evaluation occurs while the program or intervention is being designed. It involves developing a base of knowledge from stakeholders and other relevant parties through personal interviews or focus groups. The information gathered is used as feedback for the program developers to help with the final design of the program. It is nothing more than an early test of the appropriateness of the program.

Process Evaluation   Process evaluation is concerned with program implementation as designed and whether or not the program is reaching the target population. It is an ongoing evaluation process that continues through the life of the program. Organizations that concentrate on outcomes only will find it easy to ignore this part of the evaluation process, but it is an essential step in building an accurate picture of the program.

Impact and Outcome Evaluation   Impact and outcome evaluation is concerned with achievement of the objectives and goals of the program or intervention, that is, it determines whether the injury prevention program is a success or a failure. If it is a success, data from this evaluation will serve as documentation of that effectiveness. These data may be quantitative or qualitative or both, and they will answer such questions as this: Has there been a reduction in injuries or in the severity of the injuries that have occurred?

SUMMARY

Economic evaluation of workplace illness and injury reduction programs makes good sense in order to prove their worth and thus attract new interest and resources for their expansion. These health promotion efforts also need to prove their worth in order to continue and expand current funding and resource allocation. Public health departments have a great deal of experience in the development of prevention programs that can easily be adapted to the workplace. Best practices in workplace prevention programs need to be applied in order to improve workers' health at a reasonable cost in order to provide a positive return on investment for employers.

The cost of supplying health insurance to workers in this country is increasing at such a rapid rate that many businesses are passing more and more of the costs of health insurance on to the employee. At the same time, workers' productivity is decreasing because of poor health due to the effects of chronic diseases developed and manifested during the working years. Employers are looking for help in confronting these workplace issues, retaining their employees, and keeping their workers healthy and productive. To meet the goal of reducing the incidence of injuries and diseases in the workplace, employers need to form partnerships with public health departments and other relevant federal and state departments. Public health departments have the requisite tools to help employers develop workplace wellness initiatives, implement these initiatives, and prove their worth through qualitative and quantitative evaluation techniques.

The purpose of economic evaluation is to make value judgments about intervention strategies. In other words, if a company is attempting to improve the health of its workers, it needs to know the value of the intervention and the costs associated with the intervention in order to determine whether it is a good investment for the company. This approach can be called evidence-based health care, population-based medicine, and cost-effectiveness analysis.

KEY TERMS

BASICC
cost-benefit analysis
cost-effectiveness analysis

economic evaluation
impact and outcome evaluation
years of potential life lost

QUESTIONS FOR DISCUSSION

1. How would you explain the concept and the purpose of the measure called years of potential life lost?

2. Why are employers decreasing their contribution to employees' health insurance costs?

3. What are the six components of the Basic Assessment Scheme for Intervention Costs and Consequences?

4. What are the similarities and differences between cost-benefit analysis and cost-effectiveness analysis?

IMPACTS OF LEADERSHIP AND CULTURE

After reading this chapter, you should be able to

- Understand how to use leadership skills to improve workplace safety and health.

- Describe how the empowerment of workers affects workplace wellness issues.

- Understand how team development can reduce workplace injuries.

- Discuss the advantages of having a proactive approach to occupational health and safety in place.

- Explain the actions management needs to take to have a safety and health focus in the workplace.

If we are to improve the health and safety of American workers, a great deal of change must occur in the way the workplace treats all of its workers. This change will require not only laws but also a leader's vision of a safe and healthy place to work. Occupational safety and health problems are a result of management failures, worker failures, process failures, or a combination of all three of these types of failures. The benefit to everyone from correcting these failures is a safe and healthy working environment for all employees, an outcome that is too great to ignore. In fact, improving worker health and safety needs to become one of the most important tasks for every business in America. The cost of illness and injury in the workplace goes way beyond any fine levied by the Occupational Safety and Health Administration (OSHA) or losses arising from bad publicity for the business. It involves subjecting human beings to preventable injury and illness that may result in death.

Making progress on health and safety issues requires establishing workplace systems and processes that accomplish business goals and production concerns while maintaining a health and safety focus for those who are accomplishing the work. This is a change in the way business is usually conducted, because it elevates the concern for people to the same level as the concern for production. According to Nahavandi (2009), providing a vision is by far the greatest function that can be carried out by a leader during the process of change. The leader who understands the value of making the workplace safer and healthier must be able to convince everyone, including the workers, of the value of this change to everyone involved in the work process. In other words, he or she must produce a mutually acceptable vision of a safe and healthy workplace.

To improve health and safety, a business needs to put a greater emphasis on the entire process of work. McKenzie, Pinger, and Kotecki (2005) argue that workplace illnesses and injuries are usually the result of process errors that could be prevented with leadership, employee empowerment, and the development of a culture of preventing work-related problems within the business. We will discuss all three of these areas in this chapter. The process of work needs to be redesigned to produce a better product or service while at the same time not compromising worker safety and health. No one benefits from sick or injured workers; therefore this seems like a natural area for management and labor to work together in, for the common good of the business and its employees.

This change can achieve success only with commitment from management and employees. It is at this point that leadership has to emerge from management and empowerment has to become the norm for company employees. Zero defects, continuous improvement, committed workers, and good citizenship behavior in the workplace are just words unless they are given meaning by a leader who shares power with workers to make the best product or service in the safest working environment.

Hammer (2007) explains that process-based change is difficult to accomplish and requires changing jobs and increasing training if the new or redesigned process is to have a chance of success. It requires the entire organization to recognize and accept the need for the change in the process. This type of change will require strong leadership from the top to the bottom of the organizational chart. Everyone in the organization needs to become part of the change process and work together to make the new or redesigned process successful.

It is also extremely important that both formal and informal leaders play a role in the prevention of illness and injury in the workplace. The formal leader has power that has been granted by the organization, whereas the informal leader has the power generated by his or her own expertise and charisma. In order to accomplish the objectives of the organization, the formal leader needs to obtain the support of the informal leaders. Both these leaders are required to forge and nurture the culture necessary to keep workers safe in the workplace.

Leaders can create a culture in an organization where they are the key motivators for undertaking new tasks and accepting change as the opportunity for growth. Smircich and Morgan (2006) argue that leadership consists of the leader exercising an obligation and a right to structure the real world, which includes developing a vision for others to follow. In other words, the leader must gain the ability to control the behavior of followers through allowing them to see and believe in the vision of the formal leader. Kouzes and Posner (2006) point out that the very best leaders have the ability to inspire followers to believe that the vision being discussed belongs to everyone, not just the leader. This is probably what has been lacking in the ongoing effort to achieve safer and healthier workplaces. Those responsible for accomplishing this vision have never taken or been given any type of ownership in the attainment of the vision. Safety and health in the workplace has to become one of the most important values of a business rather than just something that must be done because of a new management directive. It must be seen by all employees as something that is as important as the marketing, production, and quality control of products or services. Until employee safety and health is taken to this level, it will never receive the attention by everyone that is required to make it everyone's everyday focus.

It must be looked at as a never-ending process. The vision has to include the protection of workers from injury and illness when they come to work and it has to inspire a team effort or it is destined to fail. Strong, consistent, visible worksite leadership is essential for sending a message of support to the workers that everything will be done to protect them from injury and illness in their particular business. It is the same concept that drives continuous quality improvement, only in this case it is applied to safety and health rather than producing products or services. A company can never achieve complete success because the environment is constantly changing. The best that it can hope for is that it has improved since yesterday and is now prepared to improve some more tomorrow.

Exhibit 16.1 shows the major categories of injuries and illnesses that are associated with specific agents and work settings. These injuries and illnesses are all preventable if management and labor work together. The prevention effort has to be a continuous process involving every employee.

Sull and Spinosa (2007) argue that employees engage in change activities or disengage from those activities according to whether they do or do not buy into company

EXHIBIT 16.1. Categories of occupational illnesses and injuries

- Hearing loss

- Lung disease

- Cancer and lead poisoning

- Carbon monoxide poisoning

- Allergic and irritant dermatitis

- Fertility and pregnancy abnormalities

- Infectious diseases

- Low-back disorders

- Musculoskeletal disorders of the upper extremities

- Traumatic injuries

- Adverse mental health outcomes

Source: Adapted from Friis, 2006, table 13-3.

priorities. Managers are not able to make changes in the way work is done unless they rethink the process of work. Sull and Spinosa also discuss the fact that businesses need to practice **promise-based management,** that is, they need to make a promise of safe work and safe products to fellow workers and customers. The culture of the business needs to become adaptive to continuous change in the improvement of the process of work.

USING VISION AND MANAGEMENT SKILLS

The leader must have a **vision** of wellness for the organization's workers. This vision has to be articulated to workers so often that it becomes an accepted norm of the culture of the business. To assist workplaces in improving safety and health leadership, OSHA has developed the Safety and Health Program Management module, which addresses the following management actions required to achieve this goal (OSHA, 2009b):

- Establishing a safety and health policy

- Establishing goals and objectives

- Providing visible top management leadership and involvement

- Ensuring employee involvement

- Ensuring assignment of responsibility

- Providing adequate authority and responsibility

- Ensuring accountability for management, supervisors, and rank-and-file employees

- Providing a program evaluation

If these actions are carried out, the chances of producing an excellent workplace safety and health program increase dramatically. The two key components of the process are assigning ownership and developing an evaluation process. Both of these components involve managers and workers. The way the program is evaluated is especially critical. The organization must develop an evaluation process that includes the measurement of goals, objectives, and the various program elements.

Completing this list of actions will go a long way toward improving the health and safety of employees, which in turn will reduce health and disability costs while also improving worker productivity. Many of these components can be catalysts for a long healthy life and the prevention of premature death. The leader has to be aware of how the workplace can influence workers' health and the quality of life for workers and their families. Because of these high stakes the leader needs to pay a great deal of attention to possible injuries and illnesses among his or her followers during and even after their working years. The diseases or injuries produced in the workplace are taken with the worker into retirement.

The health of workers is definitely affected in many ways during their time in the workplace. Although the workplace can be dangerous, it can also be a source of opportunity for wellness if visionary leadership is present. A workplace focused on wellness can move people from potential poor health to high-level wellness through positive actions that reduce and prevent injuries and chronic diseases and their complications during the working years. The improvement of the process of work to reduce or eliminate workplace injuries and illnesses requires the emergence of leadership committed to protecting the workplace.

OSHA has instituted the **Voluntary Protection Program** (VPP) to increase worker protection, cut business costs, and improve employee productivity and morale. According to OSHA (2004b), this program was developed to benefit workers and management by offering each side incentives to keep workers safe and healthy. OSHA points out that this program has had tremendous success, reporting that for every $1 saved on medical or insurance costs (direct costs), an additional $5 to $50 more is saved on indirect costs, such as repair to equipment or materials, training of new workers, or losses due to production delays. This is why innovative safety and health programs have to be developed, implemented, and evaluated. Then a set of best practices for workplace health and safety can be shared with all businesses in America, allowing all employees and employers to share in the successful ventures. Once real value, in terms of cost savings, can be proven, it will become much easier to sell the prevention concept to all employers. This is why leadership in occupational safety and health is such an important topic for all businesses.

USING POWER EFFECTIVELY

There are so many descriptions and definitions of leadership that it is virtually impossible to discover one definition that is accepted by everyone. However, leadership is often described in terms of some type of power relationship between the leader and followers. By using the concept of power development and power sharing, we can gain a better understanding of what the leader can and cannot do for the organization. It comes down to realizing that a leader's potential for success diminishes when his or her power is not validated by the followers in the workplace.

Dubrin (2007) believes that leadership involves the ability to acquire from the employees the respect and support that is necessary to accomplish the goals of the organization. Leaders may possess several types of power. Legitimate, reward, and coercive power are usually found in the leadership of a bureaucratic organization, and charisma and expertise are usually found in the leadership of newer, organic organizations. Charisma and expertise are highly valued in organizations experiencing rapid change, which probably includes the majority of businesses in modern America. These two types of power are usually found in the individual; they are not given to people along with a supervisory title. They are what make exceptional leaders.

The leader is responsible for creating a vision that the organization will embrace and that will encourage people to move toward accomplishing many goals, including a safe and protective place to work. If a leader has charisma supplemented by expertise, it becomes much easier to persuade employees to accept a new vision and the change it brings. Hammer (2007) argues that leaders are responsible for developing the culture of the company to emphasize accountability and for helping managers to develop an understanding of the need to be responsible for processes rather than activities. In order to do this, leaders must foster the development of a bond between management and workers. Rice (2007), for example, argues that leaders need to be able to go beyond competence and be able to build bonds with employees and customers. These qualities are necessary to build the trust required to make great things happen.

For the business to succeed at accomplishing its major goals, leadership must involve the sharing of power with every worker in the company. There is no goal more important than keeping the employees of the company safe and healthy at work. Every worker in the company also shares in this responsibility for the safety and wellness of himself or herself and of coworkers while producing goods and services for the business. Leadership for occupational safety and health involves forming partnerships with all employees to reduce the incidence of threats to the workers' safety and health while at work. According to Dubrin (2007), the leader who is gifted with charisma has the ability to communicate a vision of a workplace that is capable of inspiring workers to accomplish the goals present in the vision. The vision articulated by the leader is capable of attracting others to want to be part of the vision. It brings workers together in wanting to be part of the successful completion of the vision.

Kouzes and Posner (1995) also discuss the leader's role in enabling others to act. In the case of occupational safety and health this role is paramount because followers are the key ingredient necessary to make and keep the workplace free of hazards. Collaboration among managers and workers can build the spirited team that is so necessary to produce the extraordinary effort that will keep the workplace safe and free of disease. Manning and Curtis (2007) point out that clarity of purpose can result in decisions that inspire others to follow the vision put forth by the leader. This clarity of purpose allows everyone to understand the reasons for the decisions made by the business.

The Institute of Medicine (2003) reports that small businesses employ more than half the workers in this country. One-third of all worker mortality occurs in workplaces employing ten or fewer workers. The National Institute for Occupational Safety and Health believes that this epidemic of mortality in small workplaces is a result of a lack of onsite occupational safety and health professionals and an inability to recognize and control workplace hazards. Compounding this problem is the fact that OSHA in recent years has gotten away from an emphasis on regulation and now favors a "voluntary compliance strategy," defined as reaching agreement with industry associations to, basically, regulate themselves. This new strategy is fine for a large business with resources available to employ occupational safety and health personnel. The small business does not have the resources to police the workforce for hazards and therefore needs to provide its own leadership for hazard identification and abatement.

According to OSHA (2009b), a safety and health management system is "an established arrangement of components that work together to attain a certain objective, in this case to prevent injuries and illnesses in the workplace." The elements of this system are all interrelated and require the involvement of management and employees because a problem in one part of the system will probably affect other parts of the system. The manager must supply the workers with the required resources and authority to discover the hazards in the worksite. Once the hazards are uncovered, the appropriate training must be given to all employees to prevent these workplace hazards from becoming catalysts for workplace health and safety problems. Measurement of leadership effectiveness in this area is difficult. How do you measure that which didn't happen?

OSHA (2009a) points out that without strong leadership where top executives have not only up-to-date knowledge concerning safety issues but also the willingness to correct problems, these issues will never be resolved. A leader must show the resolve to accept nothing less than zero defects when it comes to health and safety. This requires a leader who has developed the appropriate leadership style to make the health and safety vision into reality.

EXERCISING TRANSFORMATIONAL LEADERSHIP

The style of the leader is very important in the development of successful health and safety workplace programs. Any serious attempt to keep workers safe and healthy is going to require the development of trust between employees and employers. This trust becomes even more important when attempting to develop workplace wellness programs where a great deal of personal data will be gathered from employees. The recent literature is strongly supportive of a **transformational leadership** style that uses the personal power of the leader to inspire people to adopt new ways. This style involves an understanding and compassion for the followers that is real.

Northouse (2007) argues that a transformational leadership style is a necessity for getting workers more motivated and involved in supporting the betterment of the company and the entire workforce rather than seeking only their own self-interest. The transformational leader works very hard to develop a supportive environment for listening to workers in an attempt to get them to self-actualize and become the best at what they do at work. The transformational leader also has a very clear vision of where he or she wants the organization to be in future years. It is certainly possible to include as part of this vision a workplace that is free of injuries and illness without the need of burdensome government regulation and fines for noncompliance.

André (2008) points out that transformational leadership pushes followers to move beyond their personal self-interest to the good of the group or the organization. This trait is helpful in getting employees to work together to produce a safer and healthier workplace. The leader needs to realize that the improvement of health and safety is going to require continuous effort by every worker, not just the leader.

Modern organizations require inspiration from leaders in order to accomplish revolutionary change (Nahavandi, 2009). It is certainly going to require revolutionary efforts to change our injury- and illness-prone workplaces into sources of wellness for all. The charismatic leader will need to form a bond with workers in order to improve the health and safety of all employees in the workplace. All employees of the company will have to buy into the vision of improvement espoused by the leader.

Northouse (2007) points out that transformational leadership uses the leader's vision to give the followers a sense of identity with the organization. The followers are then capable of working together as a team to ensure the successful completion of the vision. Positive results achieved by this team are most often associated with strong team leadership, in which the leader constantly helps the team members to keep their focus on goal achievement. In other words, the leader requests each follower to form a partnership with other team members and to collaborate in realizing the vision of a safe and healthy workplace.

Safety and health issues in the workplace are so important that we need to have a way of uniting management and employees in the pursuit of this common goal. The style of the leader can be extremely important in bringing all the key players together in reaching the common goal of a safe and healthy workplace. These players include managers, employees, public health experts, and OSHA personnel. A transformational leadership style can help in bringing such a diverse group of individuals together to work on a common problem.

CHANGING THE PROCESS OF WORK

The process of producing a good or service usually involves an input, management of the input, and a resultant output, or outcome. Unfortunately, this process of work also involves the possibility of workers becoming ill or injured while completing their tasks or their input into the work process. There are incentives present for management and workers to prevent injuries and illnesses in the workplace, but these injuries and illnesses still occur.

The majority of the quality problems in the workplace are caused by management. McLaughlin and Kaluzny (2007) point out that management is typically responsible for the design of the work process and employees produce the output of the work process. Therefore responsibility for both the good and the bad results (including injuries) produced by the work process is the ultimate responsibility of the leadership of the business. It is ironic that even though the leader designs this process, the only ones who can make the process safe for the workers are the workers themselves, who often are not included in the design process. Total quality management programs as they relate to workplace injury and illness programs have to be a top-down process. Although the expertise necessary for a quality work process free of worker injury and illness resides largely in the workers, the change in the work process needs to be ignited by the workplace leader, because he or she controls the resources and training necessary to reduce workplace injuries and illnesses.

MOTIVATING EMPLOYEES

The leadership of the business needs to put forth the goal of a healthy and safe workplace, but then the problem becomes getting employees to buy into this goal and become motivated to accomplish it. Ponder (2005) points out that an understanding of motivational theory can be very useful in getting workers to become serious about safety in the workplace. The leader has to motivate each employee to want to be part of the workplace changes that are necessary to improve the safety and health of all employees in the business.

Rewards are usually very effective motivators and will usually work much better than punishments in helping the workforce to improve the process of work. Workers' interest tends to increase in areas where management has increased its focus. In other words, if a leader is concerned about potential dangers from the work process, the workers become more interested in keeping the process safe. The process also has to offer incentives for goal accomplishment.

Northouse (2007) discusses the concept of inspirational motivation. In this case the leader communicates high expectations to followers, inspiring them to become part of the vision for a safe and healthy working environment. This vision put forth by the leader should attract the commitment of the employees to act on making the vision reality. This change produced by the leader and the workers can certainly become a positive force in the development of a workplace free of illness and injuries.

Dubrin (2007) discusses how coaching can be an effective leadership skill when attempting to motivate employees to attain the vision espoused by the leader. Dubrin also points out that expectancy theory can be an excellent starting point in understanding how to motivate employees. The three major parts of expectancy theory are valence, instrumentality, and expectancy. Valence is the value of the outcome to the employee. Instrumentality refers to the probability that the performance by the employee will lead to certain outcomes. Expectancy then becomes the individual's assessment of the probability that his or her effort will lead to correct performance. Applying this motivational theory to achieving occupational safety and health tells us that there needs to be a strong belief among employees that a safe and healthy workplace is desired by all and that if they use their skills they can make this vision a reality. The leader must also ensure that workers have the requisite skills and empowerment they will need to use once they are motivated.

One of the more intriguing theories of motivation was put forth by Abraham Maslow in the 1940s and posits that individuals are motivated by a hierarchy of needs that range from lower-level physiological and safety needs to higher-level social, esteem, and self-actualization needs (Lussier & Achua, 2004). Only unmet needs can be a source of true motivation, and the lower-level needs must be met before the individual is able to move on and attempt to satisfy higher-level needs. Workers may or may not be aware of all of the potential safety needs not being met by their current place of employment and particular occupation. The leader has the ability to educate them about all the needs that can affect them as they continue their employment with the business.

BUILDING A CULTURE

The leader is most effective when he or she has the ability to make a task for a follower meaningful. The task of building a culture of continuous quality improvement in the workplace is likely the most important responsibility of a leader in today's work environment. A central part of quality improvement is a culture of workplace safety and health.

Culture is a combination of the learned beliefs, values, rules, and symbols that are common to a group of people. Kotter and Heskett (1992) describe how strong cultures can have powerful consequences because they enable groups to become proactive in the way they deal with problems confronting the group. Strong cultures also result in most of the managers in a business sharing a set of relatively consistent values and methods of completing work. Hickman (1998) argues that a corporate culture that pushes positive change understands the value of the individuals and the processes that create change. These companies truly believe in their workers and respect their customers, and it shows every day in the way top management acts in the workplace. They demonstrate a performance-enhancing culture that takes pride in its workers and customers and would never do anything to hurt either group. These companies take the extra step necessary to produce goods and services with zero defects and zero negative consequences for their workers in the production process.

OSHA (2009c) states that the creation of a strong safety culture has the greatest impact on accident reduction of any intervention in any type of workplace. In this type of culture, all employees feel an obligation to immediately report unsafe working conditions and behaviors to their immediate supervisor. Workplace leaders have convinced these employees that reporting potentially unsafe behavior is not only appropriate but will be respected and rewarded.

According to OSHA (2009c), the safety culture can be nurtured by a number of factors:

- Management and employee norms, assumptions, and beliefs
- Management and employee attitudes
- Values
- Policies and procedures
- Supervisor priorities, responsibilities, and accountability
- Production and bottom-line pressures versus quality issues
- Actions or lack of actions to correct unsafe behaviors
- Employee training and motivation
- Employee involvement or buy-in

When these factors are present they can develop and nurture a **thick culture**, that is, a culture that is widespread and found throughout most of the organization, and that supports the goals of a safe and healthy workplace. A company that encourages the practice of these factors in the workplace creates a culture of excellence that will not tolerate workers' suffering injury or illness while at work.

OSHA (2009c) has also identified three basic elements of a safety and health culture:

1. All individuals within the organization believe they have a right to a safe and healthy workplace.

2. Each person accepts personal responsibility for ensuring his or her own safety and health.

3. Everyone believes he or she has a duty to protect the safety and health of others.

The interesting thing about companies with this type of culture is that as they continue to grow and prosper because of their culture, they inspire other companies to do the same. The culture is capable of determining the values that the company holds. The company that is successful in embedding the concept of workplace safety in its culture will see fewer risk-taking behaviors in its place of work. This proactive development of a safety culture will usually result in low accident rates, low turnover, low absenteeism, and high productivity. It will also result in higher profits. A portion of the higher profits can be returned to the proactive employees as a bonus, which will motivate other employees to value safety in the workplace.

According to OSHA (2009c), workplace leaders can further the expansion of the safety culture by naming a safety director, investigating accidents immediately, and providing constant training in the relevant areas of safety for all employees, including managers. There is no reason why this type of thick culture cannot be expanded to address all sources of workplace injuries and illnesses including workplace violence, impaired employees, and workers with communicable and chronic diseases. The catalyst for the development and expansion of workplace wellness programs may very well be the inclusion of these programs in the new culture of the workplace.

Keyton (2005) points out that problem solving may be the starting point for the formation of a thick culture. Formal or informal leaders can help worker groups become active in solving workplace problems. Positive experiences with using their expertise to reduce or eliminate workplace injuries will allow the workers in these groups to begin to accept these solutions as normative. New workers then become accepting of these solutions when they are expressed as norms by more senior workers during new worker orientation programs.

Keyton (2005) also suggests that the culture of an organization forms through a process of successful interaction during which the culture is assimilated by everyone in the workplace. This interaction is a learning and teaching experience for workers on how the process of work is accomplished. The leader of the interaction needs to obtain commitment from the workers to a shared set of values. This attempt at culture formation will work only if all workplace members are part of the process. Participation must be voluntary and be a result of the workers buying into the leader's vision of a safe workplace for all workers. It is a continuous process that will never end because there will always be room for improvement in the work process.

EMPOWERING WORKERS

In order to achieve this thick culture the leader must work very hard at empowering workers to build it. Successful leaders spend a great deal of their time and energy attempting to empower all employees to embrace the goals of the organization and actively work with leaders to accomplish those goals. **Empowerment** involves the complete sharing of power with lower-level employees who are critical to the successful attainment of goals. These goals include maintaining a safe place for all employees to work and grow.

Earlier we discussed the five types of power that leaders may hold: legitimate, reward, coercive, charisma, and expertise. The sharing of any of these forms of power with others generally improves their commitment to the task at hand. Dubrin (2007) argues that the power held by a leader can only increase when he or she shares that power with others in the workplace. Dubrin also defines true employee empowerment as the sharing of decision-making authority and responsibility for production between manager or leader and the members of the workgroup. In order for this sharing of power to work for the employee it must be wanted by the employee and be real. Many leaders talk about empowerment of employees but are reluctant to release real power to them.

One of the most important forms of power is expertise concerning the work process. This is an especially important form of power when it comes to identification of potential workplace hazards and the development of a strategy to prevent these hazards from affecting the workers. This power is usually already present in the workers and just needs to be activated by the leader. There are several ways in which the workplace leader can empower the workers in an attempt to make their employment setting a safe and healthy place to work. According to Dubrin (2007), the easiest way to accomplish this task is by requesting greater initiative and responsibility for safety and health issues at work from all employees. Another method of empowerment of employees is to make workplace safety and health issues part of the strategic goals of the organization. In other words, evaluate employees on their success or failure in contributing to the health and safety of the place where they work.

Finally, Bossidy and Charan (2002) state that for the leader's vision to materialize, the leader must build and sustain employees' momentum. The leader needs to consistently search for people who want to win and who are empowered to translate short-term wins into long-term successes. This is very important when trying to improve health and safety in the workplace.

IMPROVING TEAM EFFECTIVENESS

Although leadership is critical in the improvement of employee safety and health, the use of teams to point out what needs to be done is of equal importance. The leader can only accomplish so much in moving toward this very large goal. He or she needs help from all employees in order to achieve success. According to McKenzie et al. (2005), employees need to be involved because they are in contact with potential safety and health problems, they are more likely to support safety if they are involved in the process, and as a group they can offer a wide range of experiences. Employees need to be separated into teams with specific responsibilities in order to make this assignment successful. André (2008) notes that one of the most important components of developing a team is choosing individuals who can develop cohesion to keep the process going.

The formal leader also needs to recognize that each group will also host at least one or more informal leaders. It is very important to use the expertise and the other powers of this informal leader in order to achieve health and safety objectives. If the team is to be effective, its members and leader need to be given the respect they deserve. They are the ones who can be the real catalyst in the process of change.

SUMMARY

Occupational safety and health has to be the most important duty of the top management of every business in this country. This enormous task can be started by one person but requires everyone in the workplace to support the process. It is going to require not just leadership but a special style of leadership. A transformational leadership style that convinces workers to move above self-interest and consider the interests of all employees

The workplace leader needs to learn how to use his or her interpersonal skills to attract each employee's interest in the development of a workplace that is obsessed with preventing illness and injury. It will take a united effort to achieve this lofty goal; management and workers need to join together in supporting the safety and wellness of everyone in the workplace. Leaders need to be able to use appropriate leadership skills to develop and fine-tune motivated workers who are truly empowered to accomplish the goal of a workplace free of injury and illness.

The major ingredient required to prevent occupational safety and health problems in the workplace is a supportive thick culture that envelops both labor and management and that has zero tolerance for workers getting hurt in the workplace. A thick culture that supports the worker as the most important part of the process of work has a deep understanding and appreciation of the value of a safe and healthy place in which the workers can produce their goods and services. Leaders have the unique ability to develop and fine-tune these workplace cultures that are capable of increasing productivity for the company and at the same time protecting workers from disease and injury.

KEY TERMS

empowerment
promise-based management
thick culture

transformational leadership
vision
Voluntary Protection Program

QUESTIONS FOR DISCUSSION

1. Why has the development of leadership skills become such an important component in the improvement of health and safety in the workplace?

2. What role should workplace teams play in discovering how to correct work processes that are likely to result in employee injuries?

3. How can we motivate employers and employees to develop a health and safety improvement program in their workplace?

4. What are the characteristics of the transformational leadership style, and how does it relate to the development of worksite health and safety programs?

REFERENCES

Achievements in Public Health, 1900–1999: Improvements in Workplace Safety—United States, 1900–1999. (1999). *Morbidity and Mortality Weekly Report, 48,* 461–469.

Acosta, V., Sanderson, M., Cooper, S. P., Perez, A., & Roberts, R. E. (2007). Health risk behaviors and work injury among Hispanic adolescents and farmworkers. *Journal of Agricultural Safety and Health, 13*(2), 117–136.

Adams, P. F., & Schoenborn, C. A. (2006). Health behaviors of adults—United States, 2002–2004. *Vital and Health Statistics, 10*(230).

Adult participation in recommended levels of physical activity—United States, 2001 and 2003. (2005). *Morbidity and Mortality Weekly Report, 54,* 1208–1211.

Agency for Toxic Substances and Disease Registry. (2006). *A toxicology curriculum for communities: Trainer's manual.* Retrieved August 10, 2006, from http://www.atsdr.cdc .gov/training/toxmanual/modules/lecturenotes.html.

Akinci, F., Healey, B., & Coyne, J. (2003). Improving the health status of US working adults with type 2 diabetes mellitus. *Disease Management & Health Outcomes, 11,* 489–498.

All About Eye Safety. (1996). *Laser safety.* Retrieved April 15, 2009, from http://www .eyesafety.4ursafety.com/laser-eye-safety.html.

All About Vision. (2007). *Statistics on eye problems, injuries and eye diseases.* Retrieved April 15, 2009, from http://www.allaboutvision.com/resources/statistics-eye-diseases .htm.

American Academy of Otolaryngology—Head and Neck Surgery. (2006). *Noise-induced hearing loss in children.* Retrieved April 15, 2009, from http://www.entnet.org/About Us/upload/NoiseInduced_small-2.pdf.

American Diabetes Association. (2002). Standards of medical care for patients with diabetes mellitus. *Diabetes Care, 25*(1), 213–229.

American Legacy Foundation. *Employer-sponsored tobacco cessation programs are inexpensive and effective* (News Release). Retrieved May 4, 2009, from http://www .americanlegacy.org/407.aspx.

American National Standards Institute. (2009). *About ANSI overview.* Retrieved April 10, 2009, from http://www.ansi.org/about_ansi/overview/overview.aspx?menuid=1.

American Psychological Association. (2004). *Stress: When and how to get help.* Retrieved March 28, 2009, from http://www.apahelpcenter.org/articles/article.php?id=27.

André, R. (2008). *Organizational behavior: An introduction to your life in organizations.* Upper Saddle River, NJ: Pearson Education.

Annual smoking-attributable mortality, years of potential life lost, and productivity losses—United States, 1997–2001. (2005). *Morbidity and Mortality Weekly Report, 54,* 625–628.

Azaroff, L. S., Levenstein, C., & Wegman, D. H. (2004). The occupational health of Southeast Asians in Lowell: A descriptive study. *International Journal of Occupational Medicine and Environmental Health, 10*(1), 47–54.

Arizona Ear Protection. (2007). *Electronic SoundScope.* Retrieved April 15, 2009, from http://www.azearprotection.com/electronic.htm.

Awofeso, N. (2004). What's new about the "new public health"? *American Journal of Public Health, 94,* 705–709.

Bailer, A. J., Stayner, L. T., Stout, N. A., Reed, L. D., & Gilbert, S. J. (1998). Trends in rates of occupational fatal injuries in the United States (1983–92). *Occupational and Environmental Medicine, 55,* 485–489.

Barbeau, E. M., Krieger, N., & Soobader, M. J. (2004). Working class matters: Socioeconomic disadvantage, race/ethnicity, gender, and smoking in NHIS 2000. *American Journal of Public Health, 94,* 269–278.

Barbeau, E. M., McLellan, D., Levenstein, C., DeLaurier, G. F., Kelder, G., & Sorensen, G. (2004). Reducing occupation-based disparities related to tobacco: Roles for occupational health and organized labor. *American Journal of Industrial Medicine, 46,* 170–179.

Barnett, D. J., Balicer, R. D., Blodgett, D., Fews, A. L., Parker, C. L., & Links, J. M. (2005). The application of the Haddon matrix to public health readiness and response planning. *Environmental Health Perspectives, 113,* 561–566, doi: 10.1289/ehp.7491.

Baum, A., Garofalo, J. P., & Yali, A. M. (1999). Socioeconomic status and chronic stress: Does stress account for SES effects on health? *Annals of the New York Academy of Sciences, 896,* 131–144.

Bayer, R. (2000). Editor's note: Whither occupational health and safety? *American Journal of Public Health, 90,* 513.

Benavides, F. G., Benach, J., Muntaner, C., Delclos, G. L., Catot, N., & Amable, M. (2006). Associations between temporary employment and occupational injury: What are the mechanisms? *Occupational and Environmental Medicine, 63,* 416–421.

Benjamin, G. C. (2006). Putting the public in public health: New approaches. *Health Affairs, 25,* 1040–1043.

Biddle, E. A., & Blanciforti, L. A. (1999, September). Impact of a changing U.S. workforce on the occupational injury and illness experience. *American Journal of Industrial Medicine,* (Suppl. 1), 7–10.

Blascovitch, J., Brennan, K., Tomaka, J., Kelsey, R. M., Hughes, P., Coad, M. L., et al. (1992). Affect intensity and cardiac arousal. *Journal of Personality and Social Psychology, 63,* 164–174.

Borrell, C., Muntaner, C., Benach, J., & Artazcoz, L. (2004). Social class and self-reported health status among men and women: What is the role of work organisation, household material standards and household labour? *Social Science & Medicine, 58,* 1869–1887.

Bossidy, L., & Charan, R. (2002). *Execution: The discipline of getting things done.* New York: Crown Business.

Bouchard, C. (2007). Literacy and hazard communication: Ensuring workers understand the information they receive. *AAOHN Journal, 55,* 18–25.

Bourne, D. M., Shopland, D. R., Anderson, C. M., & Burns, D. M. (2004). Occupational disparities in smoke-free workplace policies in Arkansas. *Journal of the Arkansas Medical Society, 101*(5), 148–154.

Brauer, R. L. (1994). *Safety and health for engineers*. Hoboken, NJ: Wiley.

Breeden, R. (2006, August 15). *Firms consider end to employee health insurance*. Retrieved August 22, 2006, from http://www.wallstreetjournal.com.

Breslin, F. C., & Smith, P. (2006). Trial by fire: A multivariate examination of the relation between job tenure and work injuries. *Occupational and Environmental Medicine, 63*, 27–32.

Brown, P. (1995). Race, class, and environmental health: A review and systematization of the literature. *Environmental Research, 69*, 15–30.

Brown, S., & Peterson, R. (1993). Antecedents and consequences of salesperson job satisfaction: Meta-analysis and assessment of causal effects. *Journal of Marketing Research, 30*, 63–77.

Brownlee, S. (2007). *Overtreated: Why too much medicine is making us sicker and poorer*. New York: Bloomsbury.

Brownson, R., Remington, P., & Davis, J. (Eds.). (1998). *Chronic disease epidemiology and control* (2nd ed.). Washington, DC: American Public Health Association.

Bureau of Labor Statistics. (2005a, August). *National census of fatal occupational injuries in 2004* (USDL05–1598). Washington, DC: U.S. Department of Labor.

Bureau of Labor Statistics. (2005b). *Women in the labor force: A databook*. Washington, DC: U.S. Department of Labor.

Bureau of Labor Statistics. (2005c, September). *Workplace homicides declined in 2004*. Retrieved April 15, 2009, from http://www.bls.gov/opub/ted/2005/aug/wk5/art04.htm.

Bureau of Labor Statistics (2006). *National Census of Fatal Occupational Injuries in 2006*. Retrieved April 3, 2009, from http://www.bls.gov/news.release/archives/cfoi_08092007.pdf.

Bureau of Labor Statistics. (2007). *Workplace injuries and illnesses in 2006*. Retrieved April 15, 2009, from http://www.bls.gov/news.release/pdf/osh.pdf.

Bureau of Labor Statistics. (2009). *Census of fatal occupational injuries (CFOI)—Current and revised data*. Retrieved April 15, 2009, from http://www.bls.gov/iif/oshcfoi1.htm.

Bureau of Labor Statistics & U.S. Census Bureau. (2006). *Current Population Survey*. Washington, DC: U.S. Census Bureau.

Burgel, B. J., Lashuay, N., Israel, L., & Harrison, R. (2004). Garment workers in California: Health outcomes of the Asian Immigrant Women Workers Clinic. *AAOHN Journal, 52*, 465–475.

California Food Emergency Response Team. (2007). *Investigation of an Escherichia coli 0157:H7 outbreak associated with Dole pre-packaged spinach*. Alameda, CA: U.S. Food and Drug Administration; Sacramento: California Department of Health Services.

California Task Force on Youth and Workplace Wellness. (2005). *Fit businesses: Fit business award winners*. Retrieved June 2006 from http://www.wellnesstaskforce.org/fitbusiness-0405winners.html.

Canadian Centre for Occupational Health & Safety. (2007). *Hearing protectors*. Retrieved April 15, 2009, from http://www.ccohs.ca/oshanswers/prevention/ppe/ear_prot.html.

Casey, S. N. (1998). *"Set phasers on stun": And other true tales of design, technology, and human error*. Santa Barbara, CA: Aegean.

CDC Evaluation Working Group. (1999). Framework for program evaluation. *Morbidity and Mortality Weekly Report: Recommendations and Reports, 48(RR-11)*. Retrieved August 28, 2006, from http://www.cdc.gov/eval/index.htm.

Centers for Disease Control and Prevention. (2002). *Emergency preparedness and response.* Retrieved April 3, 2009, from http://emergency.cdc.gov/radiation/emergen cyfaq.asp.

Centers for Disease Control and Prevention. (2004). *The health consequences of smoking: What it means to you.* Washington, DC: Office of Smoking and Health, National Center for Chronic Disease Prevention and Health Promotion, Centers for Disease Control and Prevention.

Centers for Disease Control and Prevention. (2005). *The burden of chronic diseases and their risk factors: National and state perspectives 2004.* Retrieved August 29, 2008, from http://www.cdc.gov/NCCDPHP/burdenbook2004/Section01/tables_access.htm.

Centers for Disease Control and Prevention. (2006). *CDC influenza pandemic operation plan (OPLAN).* Retrieved April 10, 2007, from http://www.cdc.gov/flu/pandemic/cdcp lan.htm.

Centers for Disease Control and Prevention. (2007a). *Emergency preparedness and response: Bioterrorism overview.* Retrieved May 4, 2009, from http://www.bt.cdc.gov/ bioterrorism/overview.asp.

Centers for Disease Control and Prevention. (2007b). *HIV and its transmission.* Retrieved August 10, 2008, from http://www.cdc.gov/hiv/resources/factsheets/transmission.htm.

Centers for Disease Control and Prevention. (2007c). *Viral hepatitis.* Retrieved April 7, 2007, from http://www.cdc.gov/ncidod/diseases/hepatitis/b/fagb.htm.

Centers for Disease Control and Prevention. (2008a). *New report estimates more than 2 million cases of tobacco-related cancers diagnosed in the United States during 1999–2004* (Press Release). Retrieved April 2, 2009, from http://www.cdc.gov/media/pressrel/ 2008/r080904a.htm.

Centers for Disease Control and Prevention. (2008b). *Preventing tobacco use.* Retrieved May 5, 2009, from http://www.cdc.gov/NCCdphp/publications/factsheets/Prevention/ tobacco.htm.

Centers for Disease Control and Prevention. (2009a). *Chronic diseases: The power to prevent, at a glance.* Retrieved April 15, 2009, from http://www.cdc.gov/nccdphp/ publications/AAG/chronic.htm.

Centers for Disease Control and Prevention. (2009b). *Framework for evaluating public health surveillance systems for early detection of outbreaks.* Retrieved April 15, 2009, from http://www.cdc.gov/mmwr/preview/mmwrhtml/rr5305a1.htm.

Centers for Disease Control and Prevention. (2009c). *Overview: Surveillance for selected public health indicators affecting older adults—United States.* Retrieved April 15, 2009, from http://www.cdc.gov/mmwr/preview/mmwrhtml/ss4808a1.htm.

Centers for Disease Control and Prevention. (2009d). *Preventing obesity and chronic diseases through good nutrition and physical activity.* Retrieved May 5, 2009, from http://www.cdc.gov/nccdphp/publications/factsheets/prevention/obesity.htm.

Centers for Disease Control and Prevention, National Center for Chronic Disease Prevention and Health Promotion. (2005). *General alcohol information.* Retrieved September 15, 2006, from http://www.cdc.gov/alcohol/factsheets/general_information.htm.

Centers for Disease Control and Prevention, National Center for Injury Prevention and Control. (2002). *Impaired driving.* Retrieved September 22, 2006, from http://www .cdc.gov/Motorvehiclesafety/index.html.

Chengalur, S. N., Rodgers, S. H., & Bernard, T. E. (Eds.). (2004). *Kodak's ergonomic design for people at work* (2nd ed.). Hoboken, NJ: Wiley.

Chibnall, J. T., Tait, R. C., Andresen, E. M., & Hadler, N. M. (2005). Race and socioeconomic differences in post-settlement outcomes for African American and Caucasian workers' compensation claimants with low back injuries. *Pain, 114,* 462–472.

Chiras, D. (2006). *Environmental science.* Sudbury, MA: Jones and Bartlett.

Cho, C. C., Oliva, J., Sweitzer, E., Nevarez, J., Zanoni, J., & Sokas, R. K. (2007). An interfaith workers' center approach to workplace rights: Implications for workplace safety and health. *Journal of Occupational and Environmental Medicine, 49,* 275–281.

Christakis, N. A., & Fowler, J. H. (2007). The spread of obesity in a large social network over 32 years. *New England Journal of Medicine, 357,* 370–379.

Christoffel, T., & Gallagher, S. (2006). *Injury prevention and public health. Practical knowledge, skills, and strategies* (2nd ed.). Sudbury, MA: Jones and Bartlett.

Clapp, R., Howe, G., & Jacobs. M. (2006). Environmental cancer and occupational causes of cancer revisited. *Journal of Public Health Policy, 27,* 61–76.

Cohen, J. T., Neumann, P. J., & Weinstein, M. C. (2008). Does preventive medicine save money? Health economics and the presidential candidates. *New England Journal of Medicine, 358,* 661–663.

Cole, H. P., Westneat, S. C., Browning, S. R., Piercy, L. R., & Struttmann, T. (2000). Sex differences in principal farm operators' tractor driving safety beliefs and behaviors. *Journal of the American Medical Women's Association, 55*(2), 93–95.

Cooper, C. L., Dewe, P. J., & O'Driscoll, M. P. (2001). *Organizational stress: A review and critique of theory, research and applications.* Thousand Oaks, CA: Sage.

Cooper, K. T. (2003). Introduction: Occupational stress and its management. *International Journal of Stress Management. 10*(4), 275–279.

Critical Incident Response Group, National Center for the Analysis of Violent Crime. (2002). *Workplace violence: Issues in response.* Quantico, VA: Federal Bureau of Investigation.

Daschle, T. (2008). *Critical: What we can do about the health-care crisis.* New York: Thomas Dunne Books.

de Castro, A. B., Agnew, J., & Fitzgerald, S. T. (2004). Emotional labor: Relevant theory for occupational health practice in post-industrial America. *AAOHN Journal, 52*(3), 109–115.

Dembe, A. E., Erickson, J. B., Delbos, R. G., & Banks, S. M. (2005). The impact of overtime and long work hours on occupational injuries and illnesses: New evidence from the United States. *Occupational and Environmental Medicine, 62,* 588–597.

Dembe, A. E., Erickson, J. B., Delbos, R. G., & Banks, S. M. (2006). Nonstandard shift schedules and the risk of job-related injuries. *Scandinavian Journal of Work, Environment & Health, 32,* 232–240.

Dever, G.E.A. (2006). *Managerial epidemiology: Practice, methods, and concepts.* Sudbury, MA: Jones and Bartlett.

Diehr, P., Koepsell, T., Cheadle, A., Psaty, B., Wagner, E., & Curry, S. (1993). Do communities differ in health behaviors? *Journal of Clinical Epidemiology, 46,* 1141–1149.

Din-Dzietham, R., Nembhard, W. N., Collins, R., & Davis, S. K. (2004). Perceived stress following race-based discrimination at work is associated with hypertension in

African-Americans: The metro Atlanta heart disease study, 1999–2001. *Social Science & Medicine, 58*, 449–461.

Dishman, R. K., Oldenburg, B., O'Neal, H., & Shephard, R. J. (1998). Worksite physical activity interventions. *American Journal of Preventive Medicine, 15*, 344–361.

Doll, R., & Hill, A. B. (1950). Smoking and carcinoma of the lungs: Preliminary report. *British Medical Journal, 2*, 739.

Dubrin, A. J. (2007). *Leadership: Research findings, practice, and skills* (5th ed.). New York: Houghton Mifflin.

Eldin, G., & Golanty, E. (2006). *Health and wellness.* Sudbury, MA: Jones and Bartlett.

Elvex Corporation. (2006). *Ear muffs—hearing protection.* Retrieved April 15, 2009, from http://www.elvex.com/ear-muffs.htm#ElvexMaxiMuff.

Enviro Safety Products. (2008). *Peltor military and tactical headsets.* Retrieved April 11, 2009, fromhttp://www.envirosafetyproducts.com/category/peltor-tactical-headsets-peltor-comtac.html.

Etymotic Research. (2008). *High fidelity hearing protection.* Retrieved April 15, 2009, from http://www.etymotic.com/ephp/erme.aspx.

Facey, M. E. (2003). The health effects of taxi driving: The case of visible minority drivers in Toronto. *Canadian Journal of Public Health, 94*, 254–257.

Federal Emergency Management Administration. (1993). *Emergency management guide for business and industry: A step-by-step approach to emergency planning, response and recovery for companies of all sizes* (FEMA 141). Retrieved April 3, 2009, from http://www.fema.gov/pdf/business/guide/bizindst.pdf.

Fielding, J., & Briss, P. (2006). Promoting evidence-based public health policy: Can we have better evidence and more action? *Health Affairs, 25*, 969–978.

Finkelstein, E. A., Corso, P. S., & Miller, T. R. (2006). *Incidence and economic burden of injuries in the United States.* New York: Oxford University Press.

Fit City, San Antonio, Texas. (2002). *Healthy vending guidelines.* Retrieved March 31, 2009, from http://www.healthcollaborative.net/assets/pdf/vendingcriteria.pdf.

Flavorings-related lung disease. (2000). *Morbidity and Mortality Weekly Report, 56*(16), 389–393.

Fleming, S. T. (2008). *Managerial epidemiology: Concepts and cases* (2nd ed.). Chicago: Health Administration Press.

Flippen, C., & Tienda, M. (2000). Pathways to retirement: Patterns of labor force participation and labor market exit among the pre-retirement population by race, Hispanic origin, and sex. *Journals of Gerontology: Series B, Psychological Sciences and Social Sciences, 55*(1), S14–S27.

Fowler, B. A., & Risner, P. B. (1994). A health promotion program evaluation in a minority industry. *ABNF Journal, 5*(3), 72–76.

Friis, R. H. (2006). *Essentials of environmental health* (2nd ed.). Sudbury, MA: Jones and Bartlett.

Friis, R. H., & Sellers, T. A. (2009). Epidemiology for public health practice (4th ed.). Sudbury, MA: Jones and Bartlett.

Frumkin, H., Walker, E. D., & Friedman-Jimenez, G. (1999). Minority workers and communities. *Occupational Medicine, 14*, 495–517.

Fuchs, V. (1998). *Who shall live? Health, economics and social choice.* Hackensack, NJ: World Scientific.

Fullerton, H. N. (1999, December). Labor force participation: 75 years of change, 1950–98 and 1998–2025. *Monthly Labor Review,* pp. 3–12.

Garrett, L. (2000). *Betrayal of trust: The collapse of global public health.* New York: Hyperion.

Giga, S., Cooper, C., & Faragher, B. (2003). The development of a framework for a comprehensive approach to stress management interventions at work. *International Journal of Stress Management, 10*(4), 280–296.

Goetzel, R. Z. (2004, October 26). *Examining the value of integrating occupational health and safety and health promotion programs in the workplace.* Presentation at the *CDC-NIOSH Steps to a Healthier Workforce Symposium.* Washington, DC: National Institute for Occupational Safety and Health.

Goodspeed, R. B., & DeLucia, A. G. (1990). Stress reduction at the worksite: An evaluation of two methods. *American Journal of Health Promotion, 4,* 333–337.

Gorsky, R. D., & Teutsch, S. M. (1995). Assessing the effectiveness of disease and injury prevention programs: Costs and consequences. *Morbidity and Mortality Weekly Report: Recommendations and Reports, 44*(RR-10).

Grandjean, C. K., McMullen, P. C., Miller, K. P., Howie, W. O., Ryan, K., Myers, A., et al. (2006). Severe occupational injuries among older workers: Demographic factors, time of injury, place and mechanism of injury, length of stay, and cost data. *Nursing & Health Sciences, 8*(2), 103–107.

Greenberg, P. E., Stiglin, L. E., Finkelstein, S. N., & Berndt, E. R. (1993). Depression: A neglected major illness. *Journal of Clinical Psychiatry, 54,* 419–424.

Gruen, R. J., Folkman, S., & Lazarus, R. S. (1988). Centrality and individual differences in the meaning of daily hassles. *Journal of Personality, 56,* 743–762.

Guidotti, T. L. (2003). Occupational health and safety in the real "new economy." *New Solutions, 13,* 331–340.

Haight, M. J. (2003). Human error and the challenges of an aging workforce: Considerations for improving workplace safety. *Professional Safety, 43,* 18–24.

Halle, D. (1987). *America's working man: Work, home, and politics among blue collar property owners.* Chicago: University of Chicago Press.

Hamburg, M. A. (2001). *Bioterrorism: A challenge to public health and medicine.* Gaithersburg, MD: Aspen.

Hammer, M. (2007, April). The process audit. *Harvard Business Review,* pp. 111–123.

Harper, S., & Lynch, J. (2007). Trends in socioeconomic inequalities in adult health behaviors among U.S. states, 1990–2004. *Public Health Reports, 122,* 177–189.

Harris, J. R., Cross, J., Hannon, P. A., Mahoney, E., & Ross-Viles, S. (2008). Employer adoption of evidence-based chronic disease prevention practices: A pilot study. *Preventing Chronic Disease, 5*(3). Retrieved June 20, 2008, from http://www.cdc.gov/pcd/issues/2008/ju/07 0070.htm.

Harrison, R. V. (1978). Person-environment fit and job stress. In C. L. Cooper & R. Payne (Eds.), *Stress at work* (pp. 175–205). Hoboken, NJ: Wiley.

Hastings, M. (1998). The brain, circadian rhythms, and clock genes. *British Medical Journal, 317*, 1704–1707.

Healey, B. (2007, July 16). Stop the decibel damage. *U.S. News and World Report*, p. 58.

Health Affairs. (2006, August 22). *Medicare beneficiaries treated for five or more chronic conditions account for virtually all program spending growth* (Press Release). Retrieved August 22, 2006, from http://www.healthaffairs.org/press/julaug0607.htm.

Hearne, S., Segal, L., Earls, M., Juliano, C., & Stephens. T. (2005). *Ready or not? Protecting the public's health from diseases, disasters, and bioterrorism 2005*. Washington, DC: Trust for America's Health.

Heffler, S., Smith, S., Keehan, S., Borger, C., Clemens, M. K., & Truffer, C. (2005, February 23). *U.S. health spending projections for 2004–2014*. Retrieved May 5, 2009, from http://content.healthaffairs.org/cgi/content/full/hlthaff.w5.74/DC1.

Herbert, R., & Landrigan, P. J. (2000). Work-related death: A continuing epidemic. *American Journal of Public Health, 90*, 541–545.

Hesch, J. (1996). Smoking, seat belts, and other risky consumer decisions: Differences by gender and race. *Managerial and Decision Economics, 17*, 471–481.

Hewitt Associates. (2008). *Two roads diverged: Hewitt's annual health care survey 2008*. Lincolnshire, IL: Author.

Hickman, G. R. (1998). *Leading organizations: Perspectives for a new era*. Thousand Oaks, CA: Sage.

Hilgenkamp, K. (2006). *Environmental health: Ecological perspectives*. Sudbury, MA: Jones and Bartlett.

Holland, J. (1997). *Making vocational choices: A theory of vocational personalities and work environments* (3rd ed.). Odessa, FL: Psychological Assessment Resources.

Hossfeld, K. J. (1994). Hiring immigrant women: Silicon Valley's "simple formula." In B. T. Dill & M. B. Zinn (Eds.), *Women of color in U.S. society* (pp. 65–93). Philadelphia: Temple University Press.

Huckabee, M. (2006). A vision for a healthier America: What the states can do. *Health Affairs, 25*, 1005–1008.

Institute of Medicine. (2003). *The future of the public's health in the 21st century*. Washington, DC: National Academies Press.

International Labour Office. (2005). *Poor workplace nutrition hits workers' health and productivity, says new ILO report* (Press Release). Retrieved May 5, 2009, from http://www.ilo.org/global/About_the_ILO/Media_and_public_information/Press_releases/lang-en/WCMS_005175/index.htm.

Johansson, M., & Partanen, T. (2002). Role of trade unions in workplace health promotion. *International Journal of Health Services, 32*(1), 179–193.

Johnson, T. D. (2006, August 1). Preventive services a good investment for health. *Nation's Health*.

Jones, T., & Eaton, C. B. (1994). Cost-effectiveness of walking in the prevention of coronary heart disease. *Archives of Family Medicine, 3*, 703–710.

Kaiser Family Foundation. (2005). *Employer health benefits 2005 annual survey*. Retrieved August 5, 2006, from http://www.kff.org/insurance/7315.cfm.

Kaplan, S. P. (1990). Social support, emotional distress, and vocational outcomes among persons with brain injuries. *Rehabilitation Counseling Bulletin, 34*, 16–23.

Karwowski, W. (Ed.). (2006). *International encyclopedia of ergonomics and human factors* (2nd ed.). Boca Raton, FL: CRC Press.

Kelsh, M. A., & Sahl, J. D. (1996). Sex differences in work-related injury rates among electric utility workers. *American Journal of Epidemiology, 143,* 1050–1058.

Kessler, R. C., DuPont, R. L., & Berglund, P. (1999). Impairment in pure and comorbid generalized anxiety disorder and major depression at 12 months in two national surveys. *American Journal of Psychiatry, 156,* 1915–1923.

Keyton, J. (2005). *Communication and organizational culture.* Thousand Oaks, CA: Sage.

Khan, A. S., & Sage, M. J. (2000, April 21). Biological and chemical terrorism: Strategic plan for preparedness and response. Recommendations of the CDC Strategic Planning Workgroup. *Morbidity and Mortality Weekly Report: Recommendations and Reports, 49*(RR-4).

Kolata, G. (2006, August 22). Making health care the engine that drives the economy. *New York Times.* Retrieved August 22, 2006, from http://www.nytimes.com/2006/08/22/health/policy/22pros.html.

Kolavic, S., Kimura, A., Simons, S. L., Slutsker, L., Barth, S., & Haley, C. E. (1997). An outbreak of *Shigella dysenteriae* type 2 among laboratory workers due to intentional food contamination. *JAMA, 278,* 396–398.

Koob, G. F. (1991). Arousal, stress, and inverted U-shaped curves: Implications for cognitive function. In R. G. Lister & H. J. Weingartner (Eds.), *Perspectives on cognitive neuroscience* (pp. 300–313). New York: Oxford University Press.

Kotler, P., Shalowitz, J., & Stevens, R. (2008). *Strategic marketing for health care organizations: Building a customer-driven health system.* San Francisco: Jossey-Bass.

Kotter, J. P., & Heskett, J. L. (1992). *Corporate culture and performance.* New York: Free Press.

Kouzes, J. M., & Posner, B. Z. (1995). *The leadership challenge.* San Francisco: Jossey-Bass.

Kouzes, J., & Posner, B. (2006). It's not just the leader's vision. In F. Hesselbein & M. Goldsmith (Eds.), *The leader of the future 2: Visions, strategies, and practices for the new era.* San Francisco: Jossey-Bass.

Krieger, J., & Higgins, D. L. (2002). Housing and health: Time again for public health action. *American Journal of Public Health, 92,* 758–768.

Krieger, N., Waterman, P. D., Hartman, C., Bates, L. M., Stoddard, A. M., Quinn, M. M., et al. (2006). Social hazards on the job: Workplace abuse, sexual harassment, and racial discrimination—A study of black, Latino, and white low-income women and men workers in the United States. *International Journal of Health Services, 36*(1), 51–85.

Kroemer, K.H.E., & Grandjean, E. (1997). *Fitting the task to the human* (5th ed.). New York: Taylor & Francis.

Kuhn, F., Master, V., Witherspoon, C., Morris, R., & Maisiak, R. (1998). Epidemiology and socioeconomic impact of ocular trauma. In D. V. Alfaro and P. E. Liggett (Eds.), *Vitreoretinal surgery of the injured eye* (pp. 17–25). Philadelphia: Lippincott-Raven.

Landsbergis, P. A. (2003). The changing organization of work and the safety and health of working people: A commentary. *Journal of Occupational and Environmental Medicine, 45,* 61–72.

Landsbergis, P. A., Cahill, J., & Schnall, P. (1999). The impact of lean production and related new systems of work organization on worker health. *Journal of Occupational Health Psychology, 4*(2), 108–130.

Lawless, P. (1993, October). *Fear and Violence in the Workplace: A survey documenting the experience of American workers.* Minneapolis, MN: Northwestern National Life Insurance Co.

Leamon, T. B. (2001). The future of occupational safety and health. *International Journal of Occupational Safety and Ergonomics, 7,* 403–408.

Lemus-Ruiz, B. E. (1999). The local impact of globalization: Worker health and safety in Mexico's sugar industry. *International Journal of Occupational Medicine and Environmental Health, 5*(1), 56–60.

Levy, B. S., Wagner, G. R., Rest, K. M., & Weeks, J. L. (Eds.). (2005). *Preventing occupational disease and injury.* Washington, DC: American Public Health Association.

Liebler, D. (2006). The poisons within: Application of toxicity mechanisms in fundamental disease processes. *Chemical Research in Toxicology, 19,* 610–613.

Lipscomb, H. J., Epling, C. A., Pompeii, L. A., & Dement, J. M. (2007). Musculoskeletal symptoms among poultry processing workers and a community comparison group: Black women in low-wage jobs in the rural South. *American Journal of Industrial Medicine, 50,* 327–338.

Loewenson, R. (2001). Globalization and occupational health: A perspective from southern Africa. *Bulletin of the World Health Organization, 79,* 863–868.

Loomis, D., Bena, J. F., & Bailer, A. J. (2003). Diversity of trends in occupational injury mortality in the United States, 1980–96. *Injury Prevention, 9*(1), 9–14.

Loomis, D., & Richardson, D. (1998). Race and the risk of fatal injury at work. *American Journal of Public Health, 88,* 40–44.

Loomis, D., Richardson, D. B., Bena, J. F., & Bailer, A. J. (2004). Deindustrialisation and the long term decline in fatal occupational injuries. *Occupational and Environmental Medicine, 61,* 616–621.

Loomis, D., & Schulz, M. (2000). Mortality from six work-related cancers among African Americans and Latinos. *American Journal of Industrial Medicine, 38,* 565–575.

Lundberg, U. (1999). Stress responses in low-status jobs and their relationship to health risks: Musculoskeletal disorders. *Annals of the New York Academy of Sciences, 896,* 162–172.

Lussier, R. N., & Achua, C. F. (2004). *Leadership: Theory, application, skill development* (2nd ed.). Independence, KY: Thomson/South-Western.

Manning, G., & Curtis, K. (2007). *The art of leadership* (2nd ed.). Boston: McGraw-Hill Irwin.

Massey, D., & Denton, N. (1989). Hypersegregation in U.S. metropolitan areas: Black and Hispanic segregation along five dimensions. *Demography, 26.* 373–391.

McCauley, L. A. (2005). Immigrant workers in the United States: Recent trends, vulnerable populations, and challenges for occupational health. *AAOHN Journal, 53,* 313–319.

McCormick, E. J. (1976). *Human factors in engineering and design.* New York: McGraw-Hill.

McDade, J. E. (1999). Addressing the potential threat of bioterrorism—Value added to an improved public health infrastructure. *Emerging Infectious Diseases, 5,* 591–592.

McDiarmid, M., Oliver, M., Ruser, J., & Gucer, P. (2000). Male and female rate differences in carpal tunnel syndrome injuries: Personal attributes or job tasks? *Environmental Research, 83*(1), 23–32.

McGinnis, J., & Foege, W. (1993). Actual causes of death in the United States. *JAMA, 270,* 2207–2212.

McGwin, G., Jr., Enochs, R., & Roseman, J. M. (2000). Increased risk of agricultural injury among African-American farm workers from Alabama and Mississippi. *American Journal of Epidemiology, 152,* 640–650.

McKenzie, J. F., Pinger, R. R., & Kotecki, J. E. (2005). *An introduction to community health* (5th ed.). Sudbury, MA: Jones and Bartlett.

McLaughlin, C. P., & Kaluzny, A. D. (2007). *Continuous quality improvement in health care.* Sudbury, MA: Jones and Bartlett.

Medscape Today. (2004). *Trend of the month: Health insurance is most expensive employer paid benefit.* Retrieved April 25, 2009, from http://www.medscape.com/viewarticle/490517.

Merrill, R., & Timmreck, T. (2006). *Introduction to epidemiology.* Sudbury, MA: Jones and Bartlett.

Miniño, A. M., Anderson, R. N., Fingerhut, L. A., Boudreault, M. A., & Warner, M. (2006). Deaths: Injuries, 2002. *National Vital Statistics Reports, 54*(10).

Morewitz, S. J. (2006). *Chronic diseases and health care.* New York: Springer.

Mosisa, A. T. (2002). The role of foreign-born workers in the U.S. economy. *Monthly Labor Review, 125*(5), 3–14.

Mowday, R., Steers, R., & Porter, L. (1979). The measurement of organizational commitment. *Journal of Vocational Behavior, 14,* 224–247.

Murray, L. R. (2003). Sick and tired of being sick and tired: Scientific evidence, methods, and research implications for racial and ethnic disparities in occupational health. *American Journal of Public Health, 93,* 221–226.

Nahavandi, A. (2009). *The art and science of leadership* (5th ed.). Upper Saddle River, NJ: Pearson.

Naimi, T., Brewer, B., Mokdad, S., Denny, C., & Marks, J. (2003). Binge drinking among U.S. adults. *JAMA, 289,* 70–75.

Nakata, A., Ikeda, T., Takahashi, M., Haratani, T., Hojou, M., Fujioka, Y., et al. (2006). Impact of psychosocial job stress on non-fatal occupational injuries in small and medium-sized manufacturing enterprises. *American Journal of Industrial Medicine, 49,* 658–669.

Nas, T. (1996). *Cost-benefit analysis: Theory and application.* Thousand Oaks, CA: Sage.

National Center for Health Statistics. (2005). *Fastats A to Z: All injuries.* Retrieved April 4, 2006, from http://www.cdc.gov/nchs/fastats/injury.htm.

National Center for Health Statistics. (2006). *Health, United States, 2006.* Hyattsville, MD: Author.

National Highway Traffic Safety Administration. (2006). *Traffic safety facts (2005): Alcohol.* Retrieved September 15, 2006, from http://nrd.nhtsa.dot.gov.

National Institute for Occupational Safety and Health. (1996). *National occupational research agenda* (Publication No. 96-115). Cincinnati, OH: Author, 1996.

National Institute for Occupational Safety and Health. (2001). *Tracking occupational injuries, illnesses, and hazards: The NIOSH Surveillance Strategic Plan.* Retrieved April 2, 2009, from http://www.cdc.gov/niosh/docs/2001-118/pdfs/2001-118.pdf.

National Institute for Occupational Safety and Health. (2002). *Surveillance and prevention of occupational injuries in Alaska: A decade of progress, 1990–1999* (Introduction: Methods and approach to the problem). Retrieved May 12, 2008, from http://www.cdc.gov/niosh/docs/2002-115/pdfs/2002115c.pdf.

National Institute for Occupational Safety and Health. (2004). *Worker health chartbook, 2004* (Publication No. 2004-146). Cincinnati, OH: Author.

National Institute for Occupational Safety and Health. (2005). *A compendium of NIOSH economic research: 2002–2003.* Retrieved May 12, 2008, from http://www.cdc.gov/niosh/docs/2005-112/default.htm.

National Institute for Occupational Safety and Health. (2006). *NIOSH program portfolio.* Retrieved April 14, 2009, from http://www.cdc.gov/niosh/programs/surv/projects.html.

National Institute for Occupational Safety and Health. (2009). *Traumatic occupational injuries.* Retrieved April 10, 2009, from http://www.cdc.gov/niosh/injury.

National Institute for Occupational Safety and Health. (n.d.). *Quality of worklife questionnaire.* Retrieved April 10, 2009, from http://www.cdc.gov/niosh/topics/stress/qwlquest.html.

National Institute for Occupational Safety and Health. (n.d.). *Stress at work* (Publication No. 99-101). Retrieved June 11, 2009, from http://www.cdc.gov/niosh/docs/99-101.

National Institute on Alcohol Abuse and Alcoholism. (2006). *Early alcohol dependence linked to reduced treatment seeking and chronic disease.* Retrieved September 5, 2006, from http://www.niaaa.nih.gov.

National Institute on Deafness and Other Communication Disorders. (2007). *Noise-induced hearing loss.* Retrieved April 15, 2009, from http://www.nidcd.nih.gov/health/hearing/noise.asp.

National Institute on Drug Abuse. (2004). *The brain and addiction.* Retrieved September 22, 2006, from http://www.drugabuse.gov.

National Institute on Drug Abuse. (2005a). *Prescription drugs* (NIDA Community Drug Alert Bulletin). Retrieved September 22, 2006, from http://www.drugabuse.gov.

National Institute on Drug Abuse. (2005b). *Prescription drugs: Abuse and addiction.* Retrieved September 22, 2006, from http://www.drugabuse.gov.

National Institute on Drug Abuse. (2006a). *Treating prescription drug addiction.* Retrieved September 22, 2006, from http://www.drugabuse.gov.

National Institute on Drug Abuse. (2006b). *Understanding drug abuse and addiction* (NIDA Infofacts). Retrieved September 22, 2006, from http://www.drugabuse.gov.

National Safety Council. (2006). *Injury facts 2005–2006.* Itasca, IL: NSC Press.

National Safety Council. (2008). *Job safety analysis.* Retrieved March 25, 2009, from http://train.nsc.org/coc/course.aspx?aoid=7&cid=56.

Nicotine poisoning after ingestion of contaminated ground beef—Michigan, 2003. (2003). *Morbidity and Mortality Weekly Report, 52,* 1–6.

Nonfatal occupational injuries and illnesses among workers treated in hospital emergency departments—United States, 2003. (2006). *Morbidity and Mortality Weekly Report, 55,* 450–453.

Northouse, P. G. (2007). *Leadership: Theory and practice* (4th ed.). Thousand Oaks, CA: Sage.

Notifiable disease surveillance and notifiable disease statistics—United States, June 1946 and June 1996. (1996). *Morbidity and Mortality Weekly Report, 45,* 530–536.

Novick, L. F., Morrow, C. B., & Mays, G. P. (2008). *Public health administration principles for population-based medicine* (2nd ed.). Sudbury, MA: Jones and Bartlett.

Occupational exposure to formaldehyde in dialysis units. (1986). *Morbidity and Mortality Weekly Report, 35,* 399–401.

Occupational Safety and Health Administration. (1988). *Safety and health guide for the meatpacking industry.* Washington, DC: Author.

Occupational Safety and Health Administration. (1998). *OSHA's position on providing a drug-free workplace.* Retrieved September 15, 2006, from http://www.osha.gov.

Occupational Safety and Health Administration. (2004a). *Guidelines for retail grocery stores.* Washington, DC: Author.

Occupational Safety and Health Administration. (2004b). *Voluntary Protection Programs* (OSHA Fact Sheet). Retrieved April 15, 2009, from http://www.osha.gov/OshDoc/data_General_Facts/factsheet-vpp.pdf.

Occupational Safety and Health Administration. (2005, September 22). *OSHA fines BP Products North America more than $21 million following Texas City explosion* (News Release). Retrieved April 30, 2009, from http://www.osha.gov.

Occupational Safety and Health Administration. (2006). *OSHA's role.* Retrieved October 17, 2006, from http://www.osha.gov/oshinfo/mission.html.

Occupational Safety and Health Administration. (2007). *Guidance on preparing workplaces for an influenza pandemic.* Retrieved April 9, 2009, from http://www.osha.gov/Publications/OSHA3327pandemic.pdf.

Occupational Safety and Health Administration. (2008). *Safety and health topics: Eye and face protection: Standards.* Retrieved July 3, 2008, from http://www.osha.gov/SLTC/eyefaceprotection/standards.html.

Occupational Safety and Health Administration. (2009a). *Management leadership and employee involvement.* Retrieved April 23, 2009, from http://www.osha.gov/SLTC/etools/safetyhealth/comp1.html.

Occupational Safety and Health Administration. (2009b). *Overview of system components.* Retrieved April 23, 2009, from http://www.osha.gov/SLTC/etools/safetyhealth/components.html.

Occupational Safety and Health Administration. (2009c). *Safety & health culture.* Retrieved April 23, 2009, from http://www.osha.gov/SLTC/etools/safetyhealth/mod2_culture.html.

O'Driscoll, M. P., Brough, P., & Kalliath, T. J. (2004). Work/family conflict, psychological well-being, satisfaction and social support: A longitudinal study in New Zealand. *Equal Opportunities International 23*(1/2), 36–56.

Office of National Drug Control Policy. (2001). *Con to the question "Should marijuana be a medical option?"* Retrieved April 10, 2009, from http://medicalmarijuana.procon.org/viewsource.asp?ID=166.

Oh, J. H., & Shin, E. H. (2003). Inequalities in nonfatal work injury: The significance of race, human capital, and occupations. *Social Science & Medicine, 57*, 2173–2182.

Oppenheimer, G. M. (2005). Becoming the Framingham Study 1947–1950. *American Journal of Public Health, 95*, 602–610.

Padavic, I., & Reskin, B. (2002). *Women and men at work.* Thousand Oaks, CA: Pine Forge Press.

Partnership for Prevention. (2001). *Healthy workforce 2010.* Retrieved May 5, 2009, from http://www.prevent.org/images/stories/Files/publications/Healthy_Workforce_2010.pdf.

Plog, B. A., Niland, J., & Quinlan, P. J. (Eds.). (1996). *Fundamentals of industrial hygiene* (4th ed.). Itasca, IL: National Safety Council.

Ponder, R. D. (2005). *Leadership made easy.* Madison, WI: Entrepreneur Press.

Porter, L. W., Steers, R. M., Mowday, R. T., & Boulian, P. V. (1974). Organizational commitment, job satisfaction, and turnover among psychiatric technicians. *Journal of Applied Psychology, 59*, 603–609.

Preston, D. B., & Mansfield, P. K. (1984). An exploration of stressful life events, illness, and coping among the rural elderly. *Gerontologist, 24*, 490–495.

Prevent Blindness America. (2005). *Workplace eye safety.* Retrieved April 10, 2009, from http://www.preventblindness.org/safety/worksafe.html.

Prevention Institute. (2002). *Workplace policies to offer nutritious foods.* Retrieved June 2006 from http://www.preventioninstitute.org/pdf/CHI_Workplace_Policy.pdf.

PricewaterhouseCoopers. (2005). *Employers health care costs.* Retrieved April 5, 2006, from http://pwc.com/us/eng/about/ind/healthcare/rising.html.

Putz-Anderson, V. (Ed.). (1988). *Cumulative trauma disorders: A manual for musculoskeletal diseases of the upper limbs.* New York: Taylor & Francis.

Quick, J. C., Murphy, L. R., & Hurrell, J. J. (Eds.). (1992). *Stress and well-being at work: Assessments and interventions for occupational mental health.* Washington, DC: American Psychological Association.

Quick, J. C., Quick, J. D., Nelson, D., & Hurrell, J. J. (1997). *Preventive stress management in organizations.* Washington, DC: American Psychological Association.

Ready Business. (2009). *Emergency supplies.* Retrieved April 3, 2009, from http://www.ready.gov/business/plan/emersupply.html.

Respiratory illness associated with boot sealant products—2005–2006. (2006). *Morbidity and Mortality Weekly Report, 55*, 488–490.

Rice, C. (2007). Four priorities build bonds with stakeholders. *Leadership Excellence, 24*(3), 15.

Richardson, D., & Loomis, D. (1997). Trends in fatal occupational injuries and industrial restructuring in North Carolina in the 1980s. *American Journal of Public Health, 87*, 1041–1043.

Richardson, D., Loomis, D., Bena, J., & Bailer, A. (2004). Fatal occupational injury rates in southern and non-southern states, by race and Hispanic ethnicity. *American Journal of Public Health, 94*, 1756–1761.

Roberts, R. K., Swanson, N. G., & Murphy, L. R. (2004). Discrimination and occupational mental health. *Journal of Mental Health, 13*(2), 129–142.

Rosenman, K., Kalush, A., Reilly, M. J., Gardiner, J. C., Reeves, M., Luo, Z., et al. (2006, April). Federal monitoring system underestimates work-related injury and illness. *Journal of Occupational and Environmental Medicine,* pp. 357–365.

Rothman, K. J. (2002). *Epidemiology: An introduction.* New York: Oxford University Press.

Rothman, K. J., & Greenland, S. (2005). Causation and casual inference in epidemiology. *American Journal of Public Health, 95*(Suppl. 1), 144–150.

Rowitz, L. (2003). *Public health leadership: Putting principles into practice.* Sudbury, MA: Jones and Bartlett.

Rowitz, L. (2006). *Public health for the 21st century: The prepared leader.* Sudbury, MA: Jones and Bartlett.

Runyan, C. (2003). Introduction: Back to the future—Revisiting Haddon's conceptualization of injury epidemiology and prevention. *Epidemiology Reviews, 25,* 60–64.

Saha, A., Kulkarni, P. K., Chaudhuri, R., & Saiyed, H. (2005). Occupational injuries: Is job security a factor? *Indian Journal of Medical Sciences, 59,* 375–381.

Satcher, D. (1995). Emerging infections: Getting ahead of the curve. *Emerging Infectious Diseases, 1*(1), 1–8.

Satcher, D. (2006). The prevention challenge and opportunity. *Health Affairs. 25*(4), 1009–1011.

Sauter, S., Hurrell, J., Murphy, L., & Levi, L. (1997). Psychosocial and organizational factors. In J. Stellman (Ed.), *Encyclopaedia of occupational health and safety* (Vol. 1, pp. 34.1–34.77). Geneva: International Labour Office.

Schneider, M. J. (2006). *Introduction to public health* (2nd ed.). Sudbury, MA: Jones and Bartlett.

Schrijvers, C. T., van de Mheen, H. D., Stronks, K., & Mackenbach, J. P. (1998). Socioeconomic inequalities in health in the working population: The contribution of working conditions. *International Journal of Epidemiology, 27,* 1011–1018.

Schulte, P., Wagner, G. R., Ostry, A., Blanciforti, L. A., Cutlip, R. G., Krajnak, K., et al. (2007). Work, obesity, and occupational safety and health. *American Journal of Public Health, 97,* 428–436.

Seyle, H. (1975). Stress without distress. *Vie Médicale Au Canada Français, 4,* 964–968.

Shavers, V. L., Lawrence, D., Fagan, P., & Gibson, J. T. (2005). Racial/ethnic variation in cigarette smoking among the civilian US population by occupation and industry, TUS-CPS 1998–1999. *Preventive Medicine, 41,* 597–606.

Shi, L., & Singh, D. (2008). *Delivering health care in America: A systems approach* (4th ed.). Sudbury, MA: Jones and Bartlett.

Shopland, D. R., Anderson, C. M., Burns, D. M., & Gerlach, K. K. (2004). Disparities in smoke-free workplace policies among food service workers. *Journal of Occupational and Environmental Medicine, 46,* 347–356.

Simon, P., & Fielding, J. (2006). Public health and business: A partnership that makes cents. *Health Affairs, 25,* 1029–1039.

Simoni-Wastila, L., & Strickler, G. (2004). Risk factors associated with problem use of prescription drugs. *American Journal of Public Health, 94,* 266–268.

Simpson, C. L., & Severson, R. K. (2000). Risk of injury in African American hospital workers. *Journal of Occupational and Environmental Medicine, 42,* 1035–1040.

Smircich, L., & Morgan, G. (2006). *Leadership: The management of meaning.* Boston: McGraw-Hill Irwin.

Smith, G. S., Lincoln, A. E., Wong, T. Y., Bell, N. S., Vinger, P. F., Amoroso, P. J., et al. (2005). Does occupation explain gender and other differences in work-related eye injury hospitalization rates? *Journal of Occupational and Environmental Medicine, 47,* 640–648.

Smith, G. S., Wellman, H. M., Sorock, G. S., Warner, M., Courtney, T. K., Pransky, G. S., et al. (2005). Injuries at work in the US adult population: Contributions to the total injury burden. *American Journal of Public Health, 95,* 1213–1219.

Smith, P. M., & Mustard, C. A. (2004). Examining the associations between physical work demands and work injury rates between men and women in Ontario, 1990–2000. *Occupational and Environmental Medicine, 61,* 750–756.

Smith-Jackson, T. L., & Essuman-Johnson, A. (2002). Cultural ergonomics in Ghana, West Africa: A descriptive survey of industry and trade workers' interpretations of safety symbols. *International Journal of Occupational Safety and Ergonomics, 8*(1), 37–50.

Sorensen, G., Barbeau, E., Hunt, M. K., & Emmons, K. (2004). Reducing social disparities in tobacco use: A social-contextual model for reducing tobacco use among blue-collar workers. *American Journal of Public Health, 94,* 230–239.

Sorensen, G., Stoddard, A., Hammond, S. K., Hebert, J. R., Avrunin, J. S., & Ockene, J. K. (1996). Double jeopardy: Workplace hazards and behavioral risks for craftspersons and laborers. *American Journal of Health Promotion, 10,* 355–363.

Steinfeld, E., & Danford, G. S. (Eds.). (1999). *Enabling environments: Measuring the impact of environment on disability and rehabilitation.* New York: Kluwer Academic/Plenum.

Stellman, J. M. (2000). Perspectives on women's occupational health. *Journal of the American Medical Women's Association, 55*(2), 69–71, 95.

Stout, N. A., Jenkins, E. L., & Pizatella, T. J. (1996). Occupational injury mortality rates in the United States: Changes from 1980 to 1989. *American Journal of Public Health, 86,* 73–77.

Strong, L. L., & Zimmerman, F. J. (2005). Occupational injury and absence from work among African American, Hispanic, and non-Hispanic white workers in the national longitudinal survey of youth. *American Journal of Public Health, 95,* 1226–1232.

Subramanian, A., Desai, A., Prakash, L., Mital, A., & Mital, A. (2006). Changing trends in US injury profiles: Revisiting non-fatal occupational injury statistics. *Journal of Occupational Rehabilitation, 16,* 123–155.

Substance Abuse and Mental Health Services Administration. (2001). *Summary of findings from the 2000 National Household Survey on Drug Abuse.* (DHHS Publication No. SMA 01-3549). Rockville, MD: U.S. Department of Health and Human Services.

Substance Abuse and Mental Health Services Administration. (2002). *The NHSDA report: Substance use, dependence or abuse among full-time workers.* Retrieved September 15, 2006, from http://www.oas.samhsa.gov/2k2/workers/workers.cfm.

Substance Abuse and Mental Health Services Administration. (2006a). *Drug-free workplace programs.* Retrieved September 15, 2006, from http://www.samhsa.gov.

Substance Abuse and Mental Health Services Administration. (2006b). *Results from the 2005 National Survey on Drug Use and Health: National findings* (DHHS Publication No. SMA 06-4194). Rockville, MD: U.S. Department of Health and Human Services.

Substance Abuse and Mental Health Services Administration. (2006c). *Understanding drug abuse and addiction.* Retrieved September 15, 2006, from http://www.drugabuse.gov/pubs/teaching/Teaching3/Teaching.html.

Sull, D. N., & Spinosa, C. (2007, April). Promise-based management: The essence of execution. *Harvard Business Review*, pp. 79–86.

Sultz, H. A., & Young, K. M. (2009). *Health care USA: Understanding its organization and delivery.* Sudbury, MA: Jones and Bartlett.

Swanson, N. G. (2000). Working women and stress. *Journal of the American Medical Women's Association, 55*(2), 76–79.

Tanaka, S., Wild, D. K., Cameron, L. L., & Freund, E. (1997). Association of occupational and non-occupational risk factors with the prevalence of self-reported carpal tunnel syndrome in a national survey of the working population. *American Journal of Industrial Medicine, 32*, 550–556.

Task Force on Community Preventive Services (2005). *Guide to community preventive services/worksite health promotion.* Retrieved February 2, 2008, from http://www.thecommunityguide.org/worksite/index.html.

Taylor, P. (2002). *Public policy initiatives for older workers.* York, UK: Joseph Rowntree Foundation.

Ten great public health achievements—United States, 1900–1999. (1999). *Morbidity and Mortality Weekly Report, 48*, 241–243.

Testicular cancer in leather workers—Fulton County, New York. (1989). *Morbidity and Mortality Weekly Report, 38*, 111–114.

Texas American Safety Company. (2008). *Hearing protection.* Retrieved April 15, 2009, from http://www.tascosafety.com/earplugs/earplugs03.html#23006.

Tilson, H., & Berkowitz, B. (2006). The public health enterprise: Examining our twenty-first-century policy challenges. *Journal of Health Affairs, 25*, 900–910.

Tomiak, M., Gentleman, J. F., & Jette, M. (1997). Health and gender differences between middle and senior managers in the Canadian Public Service. *Social Science & Medicine, 45*, 1589–1596.

Török, T., Tauxe, R. V., Wise, R. P., Livengood, J. R., Sokolow, R., Mauvais, S., et al. (1997). A large community outbreak of salmonellosis caused by intentional contamination of restaurant salad. *JAMA, 278*, 389–395.

Trends in leisure-time physical inactivity by age, sex, and race/ethnicity—United States, 1994–2004. (2005). *Morbidity and Mortality Weekly Report, 54*, 991–993.

Trends in tuberculosis incidence—United States, 2006. (2007). *Morbidity and Mortality Weekly Report, 56*, 245–250.

Trust for America's Health. (2008). *Prevention for a healthier America: Investments in disease prevention yield significant savings, stronger communities.* Retrieved August 29, 2008, from http://www.healthyamericans.org.

Turnock, B. J. (2004). *Public health: What it is and how it works.* (3rd ed.). Sudbury, MA: Jones and Bartlett.

Turnock, B. J. (2007). *Essentials of public health*. Sudbury, MA: Jones and Bartlett.

Turnock, B. J. (2009). *Public health: What it is and how it works* (4th ed.). Sudbury, MA: Jones and Bartlett.

Uchitelle, L. (2005, October 23). For blacks, a dream in decline. *New York Times*.

U.S. Census Bureau. (2004). *U.S. interim projections by age, sex, race, and Hispanic origin*. Retrieved July 17, 2007, from http://www.census.gov/ipc/www/usinterimproj.

U.S. Chemical Safety and Hazard Investigation Board. (2006, June). *Case study: Polyethylene wax processing facility explosion and fire (No. 2005-02-I-TX)*. Retrieved April 30, 2009, from http://www.csb.gov/completed_investigations/docs/CSBMarcus OilCaseStudy.pdf.

U.S. Chemical Safety and Hazard Investigation Board. (2006, June 6). *Final report from U.S. Chemical Safety Board on 2004 explosion calls on Houston to enact stricter pressure vessel regulations (Press Release)*. Washington, DC: Author.

U.S. Department of Agriculture. (2009). *MyPyramid.gov*. Accessed March 31, 2009, from http://mypyramid.gov.

U.S. Department of Defense. (1999). *Department of Defense design criteria standard: Human engineering* (MIL-STD-1472F). Washington, DC: Author.

U.S. Department of Energy. (1991). Prevent eye injuries: Select and use appropriate eye protection. *Safety Note, 91–02*. Retrieved April 10, 2009, from http://www.hss.energy.gov/publications/safety_health_note/nsh9102.html.

U.S. Department of Health and Human Services. (2000, November). *Healthy people 2010* (2nd ed., 2 vols., with understanding and improving health and objectives for improving health). Washington, DC: U.S. Government Printing Office.

U.S. Department of Health and Human Services. (2006a). The health consequences of involuntary exposure to tobacco smoke. Retrieved April 3, 2009, from http://www.surgeongeneral.gov/library/secondhandsmoke/secondhandsmoke.pdf.

U.S. Department of Health and Human Services. (2006b). New surgeon general's report focuses on the effects of secondhand smoke (News Release). Retrieved April 2, 2009, from http://www.hhs.gov/news/press/2006pres/20060627.html.

U.S. Department of Health and Human Services, Office of the Assistant Secretary for Planning and Evaluation. (2005). *Overview of the uninsured in the United States: An analysis of the 2005 Current Population Survey*. Washington, DC: Author.

U.S. Department of Health and Human Services & U.S. Department of Agriculture. (2005). *Dietary guidelines for Americans*. Accessed June 2006, from http://www.health.gov/dietaryguidelines.

U.S. Department of Homeland Security. (2006). *Yearbook of immigration statistics: 2005*. Washington, DC: U.S. Department of Homeland Security, Office of Immigration Statistics.

U.S. Environmental Protection Agency. (2009). *Radiation protection: Health effects*. Retrieved April 9, 2009, from http://www.epa.gov/rpdweb00/understand/health_effects.html#radiationandhealth.

U.S. Eye Injury Registry. (2000). *Eye trauma epidemiology and prevention*. Retrieved April 15, 2009, from http://www.useironline.org/Prevention.htm.

U.S. Public Health Service, Office of the Surgeon General. (1986). *The health consequences of involuntary smoking: A report of the surgeon general* (DHHS Publication No. (CDC) 87-ni-8398). Rockville, MD: Public Health Service.

University of Minnesota, School of Public Health. (2003). *Guidelines for offering healthy foods at meetings, seminars and catered events.* Retrieved March 31, 2009, from http://www.sph.umn.edu/img/assets/9103/Nutrition_Guide.pdf.

University of Wisconsin Audiology Clinic. (2003). *Hearing protection for musicians and athletes.* Retrieved April 15, 2009, from http://www.surgery.wisc.edu/Oto/audiolo gyclinic/musiciansandathletes.shtml.

Vetter, N., & Matthews, I. (1999). *Epidemiology and public health medicine.* New York: Churchill Livingstone.

Washington State Department of Labor and Industries, SHARP Program. (2005). *Work-related musculoskeletal disorders of the neck, back and upper extremity in Washington State, 1994–2002* (Technical Report Number 40–8a-2004). Olympia, WA: Author.

Waters, T. R., Putz-Anderson, V., & Garg, A. (Eds.). (1994). *Applications manual for the revised NIOSH lifting equation.* Cincinnati, OH: National Institute for Occupational Safety and Health.

WebMD. (2007). *Hearing loss: Treatment overview.* Retrieved April 15, 2009, from http://www.webmd.com/a-to-z-guides/Hearing-Loss-Treatment-Overview.

Wegman, D. H., & McGee, J. P. (Eds.). (2004). *Health and safety needs of older workers.* Washington, DC: National Academies Press.

Weinrich, S. P., Greiner, E., Reis-Starr, C., Yoon, S., & Weinrich, M. (1998). Predictors of participation in prostate cancer screening at worksites. *Journal of Community Health Nursing, 15*(2), 113–129.

Welch, L. S., Goldenhar, L. M., & Hunting, K. L. (2000). Women in construction: Occupational health and working conditions. *Journal of the American Medical Women's Association, 55*(2), 89–92.

Wellness Council of America. (2008). *Worksite wellness.* Retrieved April 15, 2009, from http://www.preventdisease.com/worksite.wellness/worksite.wellness.html.

Wilkinson, R. G. (1999). Health, hierarchy, and social anxiety. *Annals of the New York Academy of Sciences, 896,* 48-63.

Williams, S., & Torrens, P. (2002). *Introduction to health services* (6th ed.). Albany, NY: Delmar Thomson Learning.

Willis, P. (1981). *Learning to labor.* New York: Columbia University Press.

Wilson, J. R., & Corlett, N. (Eds.). (2005). *Evaluation of human work* (3rd ed.). Boca Raton, FL: Taylor & Francis.

Wilson, M. G., Holman, P. B., & Hammock, A. (1996). A comprehensive review of the effects of worksite health promotion on health-related outcomes. *American Journal of Health Promotion, 10,* 429–435.

Winston, C. E. A. (1926). Public health at the crossroads. *American Journal of Public Health, 16,* 1075–1085.

Worker illness related to ground application of pesticide—Kern County, California, 2005. (2005). *Morbidity and Mortality Weekly Report, 55,* 486–487.

Workers' Memorial Day—April 28, 2009. (2009, April 24). *Morbidity and Mortality Weekly Report, 58*. Retrieved May 5, 2009, from http://www.cdc.gov/mmWR/preview/ mmwrhtml/mm5815a1.htm.

World Health Organization. (1999). *The world health report 1999: Making a difference.* Geneva: Author.

World Health Organization. (2005). *Preventing chronic disease: A vital investment.* Retrieved June 5, 2006, from http://www.who.int/chp/chronic-disease-report.

Worrall, L., & Cooper, C. L. (2001, Summer). Managing the work-life balance. *European Business Forum, 6*, 48–53.

Years of potential life lost before ages 65 and 85—United States, 1989–1990. (1992). *Morbidity and Mortality Weekly Report, 41*, 313–315.

Zeytinoglu, I. U., Seaton, M. B., Lillevik, W., & Moruz, J. (2005). Working in the margins: Women's experiences of stress and occupational health problems in part-time and casual retail jobs. *Women & Health, 41*(1), 87–107.

Zierold, K. M., & Anderson, H. A. (2006). Racial and ethnic disparities in work-related injuries among teenagers. *Journal of Adolescent Health, 39*, 422–426.

Zimmerman, F. J., Christakis, D. A., & Vander Stoep, A. (2004). Tinker, tailor, soldier, patient: Work attributes and depression disparities among young adults. *Social Science & Medicine, 58*, 1889–1901.

INDEX

operation plan by, 208; on influenza-related deaths, 208; on leading causes of mortality in the U.S., 38, 46; on lifetime costs of injuries in the U.S., 71; National Center for Injury Prevention and Control of, 136; NIOSH's research body headquartered in the, 44; on radiation exposure, 101; on rates and costs of chronic diseases, 47, 50; on secondhand smoke, 103; on similarity of prevention and treatment, 49; strategic workplace emergency response plan by, 168, 169, 176; surveillance as defined by, 31; on workplace emergency preparedness, 167

Census of Fatal Occupational Injuries (CFOI), 70

Certified ergonomics associate (CEA), 187

Certified human factors professional (CHFP), 187

Certified professional ergonomist (CPE), 187

Chain of infection, 28–29

Chicago Symphony, 228

Chronic diseases: American Cancer Society Workplace Solutions Pilot Study (2005–2006) on preventing, 19–24; CDC on rates and costs of, 47, 50; communicable diseases classified as, 200–201; employer best practices for preventing, 19–21; employer partnership with public health for preventing, 18; epidemiology of workplace, 38; high-risk personal behaviors leading to, 46, 51, 54; job stress impact on, 112–113; personal and population health costs related to, 49–50; pesticides associated with, 107–108; public health role in preventing, 52–54; WHO predictions on global epidemic of, 51; YPLL (years of potential life lost) due to, 50. *See also* Disease; Occupational injuries and illness

Cliff point, 188

CNS depressants, 136

Code of Federal Regulations (*CFR*): on

eye and face protection, 217–218; on noise exposures, 225

Cohort epidemiology study, 34

Comair Flight 5191 crash (2006), 182

Communicable diseases: control approach to, 201; definition of, 200; emerging infections, 209, 212–213; epidemiology of, 200–201; foodborne and waterborne, 202–203; hepatitis A, 205; hepatitis B, 72, 73, 205–206; hepatitis C, 72, 73, 206; incubation period of, 46, 49, 51, 54, 202; influenza (flu), 17, 208–212; *Morbidity and Mortality Weekly Report* (*MMWR*), 200; public health control of, 12; tuberculosis (TB), 203–204, 212. *See also* Disease; HIV/AIDS epidemic

Communication: Epi-X (Epidemic Information Exchange), 175; Turnock information model for emergency preparedness, 174, 175, 176. *See also* Surveillance systems

Complacency issue, 78

Component cause: definition of, 34; of workplace injuries, illnesses, chronic diseases, 35

Construction crane operation, 192–194

Contact lenses, 221

Contagious disease, 200

Control: applied to communicable disease programs, 201; public health and infectious diseases, 12; public health move to prevention from, 5, 6, 14–15; tuberculosis (TB), 204. *See also* Prevention

Coping: definition and ability of, 116; three stages of, 113

Core responsibilities of public health, 11

Coronary heart disease: as leading cause of death, 17; public health role in decline of, 12. *See also* Cardiovascular disease

Cost analysis (CA), 266, 269

Cost-benefit analysis (CBA), 268, 269

Cost-effectiveness analysis (CEA), 266–267, 269

CPSIA information can be obtained
at www.ICGtesting.com
Printed in the USA
BVOW11n2107240616
453372BV00001B/1/P